Issues in Clinical Child Psychology

Series Editor: Michael C. Roberts, University of Kansas, Lawrence, Kansas

For further volumes:
http://www.springer.com/series/6082

Anne McDonald Culp

Editor

Child and Family Advocacy

Bridging the Gaps Between
Research, Practice, and Policy

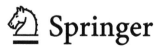 Springer

Editor
Anne McDonald Culp
Department of Child, Family, and Community Sciences
University of Central Florida
Orlando, FL, USA

ISSN 1574-0471
ISBN 978-1-4614-7455-5   ISBN 978-1-4614-7456-2 (eBook)
DOI 10.1007/978-1-4614-7456-2
Springer New York Heidelberg Dordrecht London

Library of Congress Control Number: 2013940912

Printed on acid-free paper

Springer is part of Springer Science+Business Media (www.springer.com)

Disclaimer

This volume is a product of the Society for Child and Family Policy and Practice (Division 37 of the American Psychological Association). Each chapter was reviewed by a minimum of two members of the book's Editorial Board with respect to scholarly significance of the material and the scientific and professional integrity of the process. *The findings and conclusions are those of the authors.* It has not been considered by the American Psychological Association Council of Representatives and does not necessarily reflect the official position of the organization as a whole.

Editorial Board

Preface

Act as if what you do makes a difference. It does.

William James

This book is intended to help people become passionate about initiating or renewing their advocacy skills for children and families in the United States. We as a society have too many children who live in families that are chronically or temporarily living below poverty level; we have too many children who are abused and neglected; we have too many children who are not receiving the education they need to reach their potential; in general, we have too many children being ignored in our country (Children's Defense Fund, 2012). As a student or professional in the human sciences and services, and a concerned citizen and fellow human, I believe you as a reader of this book feel a responsibility to do something, yet where do you start?

First and foremost, you must believe that you can improve the lives of children and families by creating a world where children are safe, that they can grow up healthy, and that they can be productive citizens as they age to adulthood. Yes, you want their parents to do the majority of the work of giving their children safe, healthy, and productive lives. Nonetheless, many parents confront obstacles that prevent them from providing resources necessary for their children's healthy development (Lieberman & Van Horn, 2009).

When situations are not conducive for parents to give their children safe, healthy, and productive lives, neighborhoods, communities, state government, federal government, and others step in to make sure that the constitutional rights of every child are secure. However, the systems and programs, which we as a society put in place, may not be working out as well as we had hoped. Funding, lack of training, lack of research, lack of public understanding and education all play a role in our systems weakening. When this happens, we must expand the arena of "helpers" and we find ourselves reaching out to citizens, especially those citizens being trained as professionals working with children, to step up and advocate for the decency of lives—the unalienable right of children to have safe, healthy, and productive lives in the United

States (and elsewhere in the world). The authors of the chapters of this book discuss the need to raise the standards for the quality of life for children in the United States.

Advocacy as an Ethical Responsibility

Many of us belong to professional organizations that have a code of ethical conduct. It is the moral compass for our professions. Within the ethical code document, there is usually a section which articulates standards and core values that reflect the highest of ethics. In almost all professions that work with children and families, there is a respect for the dignity and worth of each child and family member. We would all agree that we should not harm children. We shall not discriminate against children for being homeless, poor, or the many indicators of risk in which they themselves did not put themselves. We recognize that children, especially the very young, are at critical junctures in their lives in which certain interventions would be highly effective, and we recognize that not all children have the chance to function at their best.

We perform practices and teachings that promote healthy children and families, both in physical health and in mental health. These values provide a conceptual framework by which professionals define their work as clinicians, educators, and practitioners.

In the past few years it has become common for graduate curriculums to require a content knowledge base in public policy and advocacy (Kaslow et al., 2009). In fact, for professional psychology, the public policy curriculum is found within the construct of ethical and legal standards. The expected competencies in public policy and advocacy skills span across topics of assessment, diagnosis, intervention, research, supervision, and management. It permeates all curriculum constructs within doctoral work of clinical psychologists (Roldolfa et al., 2005). Each profession should identify the knowledge, the skill set, and the values that develop advocacy and public policy. However, there have been few resources to guide these efforts toward professional child and family advocacy. This book provides a research-based approach to address this need in many disciplinary fields.

Description of the Book

The book provides a functional model for integrating research and advocacy for children, youth, families, and communities to a large number of professions and practices. The work is a product of the ongoing professional agenda of the Society for Child and Family Policy and Practice, Division 37, of the American Psychological Association. The primary mission of the Society's work is to carry out research with children and families, advance education and training based on the research findings, and advocate for positive change in social and public policy. Based on this perspective, it is assumed that changes in social and public policy should be firmly grounded in scholarly research and that research development and funding should be influenced by social and public policy.

Many professionals lack training and experience in translating research into policy and utilizing research in advocacy efforts directed toward children, families, and communities. This volume provides a knowledge base for effective social and public policy as well as specific training for effective professional advocacy. One of the unique contributions of the book is that it serves as a model for psychological professional advocacy work in addition to specific guidelines applied to critical topics related to the well-being of children and families.

The book describes a range of advocacy skills: from grassroots efforts to testifying before legislative bodies, from efforts in neighborhoods and communities to efforts in state capitols and national efforts in Washington, DC. The authors translate research into action steps for changes in child and family policy. The authors describe how they use research to inform advocacy efforts at the community, state, and federal levels.

Definition of Child Advocacy

Advocacy involvement spans differing levels from service activities in school and communities, to grass root groups organizing for community social justice and change, to political lobbying, and to testifying before legislative bodies on behalf of quality of life issues for children's growth and development. This book spans each, but primarily focuses on how to make legislative policy changes on behalf of children and families. The advocacy work in the legislative arena is focused on public programs and social services, based on solid child development research, that assure safe and healthy (physical and mental) development for children and their families.

Organization of the Book

The organization of the book is based on a developmental ecological approach with four parts. The first part of the book provides two important chapters to provide the ground work for the remaining chapters: the state of the child in the United States; and an overview of the policy process which will provide an advocacy policy model for children and family issues.

The second part of the book presents substantive chapters providing a summary of research and advocacy related to key issues at the child and family levels of analysis. This part is reserved for chapters which concentrate on specific child issues. Each chapter defines the child issue, provides a research summary of the issue, and then specifies the advocacy goals. The authors underscore steps that have yielded success in policy change, whether it is local change in the community, or state or federal changes. Topics in this part include children's mental health, health disparities, homelessness, child abuse prevention, juvenile justice, media violence, working with Native American families, reform in child welfare, education, and early childhood and child care.

The third part of the book has four chapters in which authors share personal experience in the public policy domain. This part stands out as unique from Part II because the authors focus on the advocacy process within a child or family issue, rather than the child issue as the focus, as it is in Part II. For example, you will read first-hand accounts of testifying on Capitol Hill for IDEA, winning and losing policies for adolescent reproductive health, and how to engage families in your advocacy efforts.

The fourth part is an interesting chapter on the history of Division 37, whose primary function at the American Psychological Association is to promote child and family advocacy utilizing research-based evidence.

Each of the chapters' authors is committed to believing that you, the reader, can stand up and do what they have accomplished. They write their chapters in enough detail that you should be able to say, "I can do this!"

I would like to end with another quote relevant for advocates:

> Our greatest weakness lies in giving up. The most certain way to succeed is always to try just one more time.

> Thomas A. Edison

Orlando, FL, USA   Anne McDonald Culp

References

Kaslow, N. J., Grus, C. L., Campbell, L. F., Fouad, N. A., Hatcher, R. L., & Rodolfa, E. R. (2009). Competency assessment toolkit for professional psychology. *Training and Education in Professional Psychology*, *3*, 27–45.

Lieberman, A. F., & Van Horn, P. (2009). Child-parent psychotherapy: A developmental approach to mental health treatment in infancy and early childhood. In C. Zeanah (Ed.), *Handbook on infant mental health* (3rd ed., pp. 439–449). New York: Guilford Press.

Rodolfa, E., Bent, R., Eisman, E., Nelson, P., Rehm, L., & Ritchie, P. (2005). A cube model for competency development: Implications for psychology educators and regulators. *Professional Psychology: Research and Practice*, *36*, 347–354.

The Children's Defense Fund. (2012). *The State of America's Children Handbook*. Retrieved from http://www.childrensdefense.org/child-research-data-publications/

Acknowledgements

I am grateful to Judy Jones, Garth Haller and Rekha Udaiyar at Springer for the work and support they gave me. In addition, I would like to recognize an outstanding editorial board and an exceptional set of authors. The editorial board members contributed excellent reviews and provided passionate support throughout this endeavor. In particular, Dr. Carolyn Schroeder, Dr. Marion O'Brien, Dr. Cindy Miller-Perrin, Dr. Michael Roberts, and Dr. Jennifer Kaminski were always available to me when I needed meetings, phone conversations, and chapter reviews in need of immediate attention. I want to thank all of the authors for their extreme patience with the process. As they will tell you, I did not give up and would ask them to write additional specific steps of their successful advocacy work. The details in the chapters are evidence of their tenacity at rewriting the advocacy steps in words that the reader could visualize. Finally, I want to thank Rex Culp, my lifelong partner, who gave me countless "you can do it" cheers on days I needed it, and our daughter Kathanna Christine Culp, who always inspires my best work.

Contents

Contributors

Georgianna M. Achilles, Ph.D. Midstep Centers for Child Development, State College, PA, USA

Rene Anderson Department of Child and Family Studies, University of South Florida, Tampa, FL, USA

Mary I. Armstrong, Ph.D. Department of Child and Family Studies, University of South Florida, Tampa, FL, USA

Sandra Barrueco, Ph.D. The Catholic University of America, Washington, DC, USA

Ellen L. Bassuk, MD The National Center on Family Homelessness, Needham, MA, USA

Corey Anne Beach The National Center on Family Homelessness, Needham, MA, USA

Sandra J. Bishop-Josef, Ph.D. The Edward Zigler Center in Child Development & Social Policy, Yale University, New Haven, CT, USA

Bette L. Bottoms, Ph.D. University of Illinois, Chicago, IL, USA

Joseph J. Cocozza, Ph.D. National Center for Mental Health and Juvenile Justice, Policy Research Associates, Inc., Delmar, NY, USA

Natalie Coupe The National Center on Family Homelessness, Needham, MA, USA

Anne McDonald Culp, Ph.D. Department of Child, Family, and Community Sciences, University of Central Florida, Orlando, FL, USA

Daniel E. Dawes, JD National Working Group on Health Disparities and Health Reform, Washington, DC, USA

Debra K. DePrato, MD Institute for Public Health and Justice, Louisiana State University Health Sciences Center, New Orleans, LA, USA

Arielle R. Deutsch, Ph.D. Department of Psychological Sciences, University of Missouri, Columbia, MO, USA

Daniel Dodgen, Ph.D. Division for At-Risk Individuals, Behavioral Health and Community Resilience, U.S. Department of Health and Human Services, Washington, DC, USA

Kathleen Ferreira, Ph.D. Division of Training, Research, Education, and Demonstration, Department of Child and Family Studies, College of Behavioral and Community Sciences, Louis de la Parte Florida Mental Health Institute, University of South Florida, Tampa, FL, USA

Grace L. Francis, Ph.D. Beach Center on Disability, University of Kansas, Lawrence, KS, USA

Sharon Hodges, Ph.D., MBA Division of Training, Research, Education, and Demonstration, Department of Child and Family Studies, College of Behavioral and Community Sciences, Louis de la Parte Florida Mental Health Institute, University of South Florida, Tampa, FL, USA

Neil Jordan, Ph.D. Department of Psychiatry & Behavioral Sciences, Northwestern University Feinberg School of Medicine, Chicago, IL, USA

Karli J. Keator, M.P.H. National Center for Mental Health and Juvenile Justice, Policy Research Associates, Inc., Delmar, NY, USA

Lauren M. Littlefield, Ph.D. Department of Psychology, Washington College, Chestertown, MD, USA

Mary Ann McCabe, Ph.D. Department of Pediatrics, George Washington University School of Medicine, Washington, DC, USA

Cindy L. Miller-Perrin, Ph.D. Department of Psychology, Social Science Division, Pepperdine University, Malibu, CA, USA

Christina M. Murphy, MM The National Center on Family Homelessness, Needham, MA, USA

John P. Murray, Ph.D. Department of Psychology, Washington College, Chestertown, MD, USA

Center on Media and Child Health, Children's Hospital, Boston, MA, USA

Lap Nguyen, MS Department of Child, Family and Community Sciences, University of Central Florida, Orlando, FL, USA

Howard J. Osofsky, MD, Ph.D. Department of Psychiatry, Louisiana State University Health Sciences Center, New Orleans, LA, USA

Joy D. Osofsky, Ph.D. Departments of Pediatrics and Psychiatry, Louisiana State University Health Sciences Center, New Orleans, LA, USA

Stephen Phillippi Jr., Ph.D., LCSW School of Public Health, Louisiana State University Health Sciences Center, New Orleans, LA, USA

Sandie Plata-Potter, Ph.D. Department of Education, Mount Olive College, Mount Olive, NC, USA

Sharon G. Portwood, JD, Ph.D. Department of Public Health Sciences, University of North Carolina at Charlotte, Charlotte, NC, USA

Helen Raikes, Ph.D. Department of Child, Youth and Family Studies, University of Nebraska, Lincoln, NE, USA

Karen Saywitz, Ph.D. Department of Psychiatry and Biobehavioral Sciences, UCLA School of Medicine, Los Angeles, CA, USA

Cynthia Schellenbach, Ph.D. Department of Sociology, Anthropology, Social Work, and Criminal Justice, Oakland University, Rochester, MI, USA

Robert A. Siudzinski, Ph.D. Department of Education, Washington College, Chestertown, MD, USA

Elaine Slaton, MSA Slaton Associates, LLC, Tampa, FL, USA

Paul Spicer, Ph.D. Department of Anthropology, Center for Applied Social Research, University of Oklahoma, Norman, OK, USA

Lisa St. Clair, Ph.D. Department of Education and Child Development, Munroe-Meyer Institute, University of Nebraska Medical Center, Omaha, NE, USA

Rud Turnbull, LLM, LLB, JD Beach Center on Disability, University of Kansas, Lawrence, KS, USA

Donald Wertlieb, Ph.D. Department of Child Development, Tufts University, Boston, MA, USA

Brian L. Wilcox, Ph.D. Center on Children, Families and the Law, University of Nebraska, Lincoln, NE, USA

Diane J. Willis, Ph.D. Professor Emeritus, Department of Pediatrics, University of Oklahoma Health Sciences Center, Norman, OK, USA

Svetlana Yampolskaya, Ph.D. Department of Child and Family Studies, University of South Florida, Tampa, FL, USA

Part I
Introduction

Chapter 1
The Wellbeing of Children in the United States: Evidence for a Call for Action

Cynthia Schellenbach, Anne McDonald Culp, and Lap Nguyen

> *The gross national product does not allow for the health of our children, the quality of their education, or the joy of their play… it measures neither our wit nor our courage; neither our wisdom nor our learning; neither our compassion nor our devotion to our country; it measures everything, in short, except that which makes life worthwhile.*
>
> Robert F. Kennedy

When we examine the status of children and families in the United States today, it is clear that the state of the wellbeing of children and families in America does not meet the standards of our leaders a decade ago. Today, our children suffer from poverty in a country of great wealth; they may lack the educational skills that will allow them to be competitive in the future job market. Many of their parents experience chronic unemployment or transience, as well as periods of family instability. The lives of many children are scarred by abuse and neglect. Many children live in homes or neighborhoods which expose them to domestic or community violence. They are involved in an educational system that does not allow them to develop their full learning potential. Still others are homeless or confront food insecurity on a daily basis. As Marian Wright Edelman states

> Together we can and must build the powerful, proactive, united, courageous, and insistent voice required to enable all our children to get a healthy start; a quality early childhood

C. Schellenbach, Ph.D. (✉)
Department of Sociology, Anthropology, Social work, and Criminal
Justice, Oakland University, Rochester, MI, USA
e-mail: schellen@oakland.edu

A. McDonald Culp, Ph.D. • L. Nguyen, M.S.
Department of Child, Family, and Community Sciences, University of Central Florida,
Orlando, FL 32816-1250, USA

A. McDonald Culp (ed.), *Child and Family Advocacy: Bridging the Gaps Between Research, Practice, and Policy*, Issues in Clinical Child Psychology,
DOI 10.1007/978-1-4614-7456-2_1, © Springer Science+Business Media New York 2013

foundation; excellent and stimulating in and out of school experiences; and the comprehensive
continuum of support to make the successful transition to adulthood every child needs and
deserves (Children's Defense Fund, 2012, p.2).

The purpose of this book is to provide evidence-based models for social advocacy designed to improve the quality of life of children, youth, and families in our
communities today. When we examine the status of our nation and its citizens today,
we note that the United States has the highest gross national product of any country
in the world (Children's Defense Fund, 2012). In the face of this economic wealth,
glaring disparities exist among those living in poverty. Indeed, evidence indicates
that family economic wellbeing has significantly deteriorated in the decade since
2001 (Foundation for Child Development, 2012). Data suggest that families have
experienced a significant increase in poverty, a decrease in median family income, as
well as a decrease in family economic insecurity for middle-class and low-income
families (see also Aber, Morris, & Raver, 2012).

In addition to family economic instability, families have experienced profound
changes in family structure through the past 10 years. Demographic data derived
from the decade of the 2000s support the picture of a more diverse family life cycle,
including many different family structures such as married parents, gay and lesbian
parents, blended families, divorced, and single parent-headed households. These are
all examples of families, in which all family structures provide for the functions of
the private and public family (Cherlin, 2010).

There have been multiple significant changes in the family life cycle that have
affected children during the last 40 years in the United States. During the 1980s,
Glick (1988) presented the evidence for a linear family life cycle based on stage-
oriented transitions in the life course such as progressing from being single to
getting married to childbearing, launching adult children, the empty nest, and
finally widowhood. According to Cherlin (2010) this early empirical evidence did
underscore the importance of divorce, single parenthood, cohabitation, and remar-
riage. In 2000, a revised life cycle framework that emphasized the effects of race,
ethnicity, and social class on the family life course (Teachman, Tedrow, &
Crowder, 2000).

More recent analyses (Mclanahan, 2004) suggested that educational attainment
and income have prominent influences on the family life cycle. Specifically, the
family life cycle trajectories of those with higher educational attainment (e.g., a college degree) tended to have more positive outcomes in terms of less divorce and
more positive lifetime opportunities. Those with lower educational attainment
tended to have more negative outcomes (higher rates of divorce) and greater probability of negative lifetime opportunities. Cherlin (2010) emphasizes the divergent
life pathways and eventual outcomes based on educational attainment and income
apparent in the life courses of families in the future. Those children whose parents
have lower educational outcomes are likely to have more negative social and behavioral outcomes over the life course.

Risk Factors for Children, Youth, and Families in the United States

Although there are a multitude of risk factors that potentially affect the status of children in the United States, this review will focus on factors derived from two primary sources: the *State of America's Children Handbook* (Children's Defense Fund, 2012) and the *Child and Youth Well-Being Index* estimates of child wellbeing for 2001–2011 (Foundation for Child Development, 2012). These indices include poverty and economic wellbeing, physical health, educational attainment, emotional and behavioral wellbeing, housing and homelessness, juvenile justice, and other domains.

Poverty

The Foundation for Child Development (2012) reports that the economic wellbeing of children has declined in the last decade (2001–2011). In general, the evidence indicates that the probability of childhood poverty has increased from 15.6 % in 2001 to 21.4 % in 2011. In 2012, one in five children lived below the United States government poverty line. Sadly, our nation's youngest children under the age of five are the poorest age group in the country (25.9 %). Children of minority status are at highest risk for poverty. In fact, nearly two-thirds of African American children are in the lowest fifth of all income levels. It is important to note that one-third of the most significant increase in poverty among children was during the years 2001–2007, prior to the impact of the Great Recession. In fact, all increases in economic wellbeing for children since 1975 were lost during the last decade (Foundation for Child Development, 2012). There was no state in the nation that reported a decrease in poverty rates among children.

Many of these statistics utilize a measure of poverty based on the "poverty line" established by the US government. Researchers suggest that there are several other meaningful ways to define the meaning of poverty for children and families (Aber, Jones, & Raver, 2007). For example, subjective poverty defines poverty on the basis of individuals' perceptions and local economic conditions. Relative poverty is assessed by judging how far a family's income is from the national median for families. The family self-sufficiency standard assesses the needs of the family without benefit of outside assistance. The "poverty line" as defined by the US government is the lowest of all of these estimates of poverty. Based on these definitions, 15.5 million of poor American are children under the age of 18. In addition, 15.1 % of the population is considered "poor" and 21 % of all the children are considered "poor" by this lowest standard of the definition of poverty.

Based on demographic data, Cherlin (2010) notes significant differences in the life course trajectories of poor children in comparison to children of higher socioeconomic status. Families with parents with higher educational attainment tend to have more children with more positive life outcomes compared to children of parents with lower educational attainment. Only 4 % of low income children will experience an upward increase in social mobility over their life courses.

A decrease in parental secure employment has also contributed to the negative economic status of children. Evidence indicates that secure employment of parents has decreased over the past decade, with only 71 % of children having at least one parent with secure full-time employment in 2011. This rate is particularly high for children of single parent mother-headed households. The Foundation for Child Development (2012) reports that 6.5 million children were living with one unemployed parent in 2011.

Finally, there has been a 10 % decrease in median family income as well. All of these factors contribute to the decline in economic wellbeing of children in the United States. Children suffer not only from poverty and parental unemployment but they also confront hunger as well. In a report for the United States Department of Agriculture, Nord, Coleman-Jensen, and Andrews (2010, 2012) state that 20 % of all children experience food insecurity. More than one of five children do not know when or where they will have their next meal. About 85 % of households with food insecure children had a working adult, including 70 % with a full-time worker. Fewer than half of these households with a food insecure child included an adult educated past high school. Thus, job opportunities and wage rates for workers with lower educational attainment are identified as important factors affecting the food security of children (Nord et al, 2010, 2012).

Researchers from a decade of work underscore that poverty predicts long-term problems in physical–biological outcomes, cognitive–academic outcomes, and social–emotional outcomes (Duncan & Brooks-Gunn, 1997; Aber, Morris, & Raver, 2012). There are several pathways through which poverty affects child outcomes including biological, ecological or contextual, and academic pathways.

The majority of the chapters in Part II of this volume discuss poverty as a contributing factor to the child and family issue highlighted in the chapter. For example, children's mental health services are not as readily available, many times absent, in communities dominated by poverty (McCabe, Wertlieb, & Saywitz, this volume). Health reform is aimed at making sure those with less advantage and accesses have decent health insurance coverage (Dawes, this volume). Homelessness among children and families is directly associated with family unemployment and poverty (Murphy, Bassuk, Coupe, & Beach, this volume). Access to affordable child care is limited if a family has very little income (Raikes, St. Clair, Kutuka, & Potter, this volume); and certain populations, such as Native American families are disproportionately affected by high poverty rates (Willis & Spicer, this volume).

In a recent SRCD social policy report, Aber, Morris, and Raber (2012) discuss policy implications associated with poverty. They recommend merging the research studies on prevention with studies in developmental science to help make decisions for program curriculum. The many factors associated with poverty have high levels of significance for our nation's budget in health and educational outcomes.

Physical Health

According to data derived from the Children's Defense Fund (2012), one in ten children or almost eight million children are uninsured. Again, minority children are more likely to be uninsured in comparison to other groups. For example, Hispanic children (14 %) were twice as likely as non-Hispanic Caucasian children to be uninsured for health care (Dawes, this volume).

Twelve percent of children in families with incomes less than $35,000 had no health insurance compared to 2 % of children in families with incomes of $100,000 or more. Although the Medicaid and CHIP programs provided coverage to more than 60 % of low income children, many remain uninsured (Bloom, Cohen, & Freeman, 2011). The adolescent pregnancy rate has been decreasing since the 1990s. Although the United States has the highest teen birth rate among industrialized nations, the birth rate is actually the lowest rate recorded at 34.3 births for every 1,000 teens aged 15–19. In 2010, 40.8 % of all births were to single parent mothers.

Researchers suggest that the daily experience of poverty causes children and their parents to react to repeated or chronic exposure to stressors that lead to long-term physiological costs such as negative changes to the cardiovascular system, the immune system, and the neuroendocrine and cortical systems (Shonkoff et al., 2012). Indeed, parents suffer the consequences of exposure to the chronic stressors of life in poverty, experiencing higher rates immune diseases and cardiovascular problems in adulthood in comparison to higher income comparison groups.

In Part II of this volume, researchers define and delineate issues and recommend advocacy steps to take to maximize health coverage for all children and families.

Social and Emotional Health

The experience of living in poverty includes ecological factors that lead to negative social and psychological adjustment (Aber et al., 2012). The structural and physical characteristics of inferior housing exert a negative influence on child development. Low-income housing is also likely to have a toxic influence from exposure to unsanitary conditions, pollutants, and overcrowding. Murphy, Bassuk, Coup, and Beach (this volume) describe strategies for ending homelessness among children and families.

Moreover, studies demonstrate that children living in unsafe neighborhoods are likely to have a higher incidence of stress and anxiety in comparison to those who live in safe neighborhoods. Exposure to community violence in high-risk neighborhoods can negatively affect children's social, emotional, and cognitive development (Leventhal & Brooks-Gunn, 2000). Exposure to natural disasters has disturbing consequences to children's social and emotional health if we do not react quickly and help first responders in these communities devastated by hurricanes, tsunamis, and other natural disasters (Osofsky & Osofsky, this volume). Murray (this volume) summarizes the history of research on the exposure to media violence and how it relates to children's social and emotional behavior.

The peer environment for low-income children and families may also be directly related to higher rates of negative peer behaviors and delinquency (Cocozza, DePrato, Phillippi, & Keator, this volume). The neighborhood environment may also exert a negative influence on the development of negative social behaviors among children and adolescents. In all chapters of Parts II and III of this volume, the authors highlight further research findings and recommendations for advocacy steps and outcomes so that our nation can move forward in supporting programs and treatments in social and emotional health to better the lives of our children and their families.

Educational Achievement

According to evidence from the Organization for Economic Cooperation and Development, graduation trends in 34 member countries was at 82 % compared to 76 % graduation rate in the United States (OECD, 2011). At present, three million individuals eligible by age have not earned a high school diploma. Based on standardized testing from 2000 through 2009, students in the United States showed a decline in reading scores, as well as "below average" rating in math literacy.

Moreover, evidence from the High Scope Perry Preschool Project (Schweinhart et al., 2005), utilizing a sample of 123 children born in poverty between the years of 1962 and 1967 (aged 3–4 years) were tracked by the researchers for over 40 years. Remarkably, 97 % of the original sample was retained throughout the 40 years. At age 40, the participants in the High Scope Perry Preschool Project were more likely to have graduated from high school, to be gainfully employed, and to have higher IQ scores over time. Thus, the impact of an effective early intervention or prevention program is likely to have a lasting positive impact on high-risk children and families for many years to come (Raikes et al., this volume).

Chapters in Part II of this volume underscore a research and advocacy plan to promote education reform in the twenty-first century and address the urgent educational needs of our nation's children and adolescents as they prepare for productive lives in the future (Littlefield & Siudzinski, this volume).

Child Abuse and Neglect

Based on data derived from the statistics from the Department of Health and Human Services, there were approximately three million reported cases of child maltreatment including physical abuse, sexual abuse, neglect, and psychological maltreatment in 2010 (U.S Department of Health and Human Services, 2011). Of these reports, 436,000 were substantiated following investigation by Child Protective Services. In 2010, 1,560 children died as a direct result of child abuse and neglect. Researchers suggest that these estimates are lower than the actual rates of abuse and neglect. This occurs because of variation in definitions and differences in reporting sources. Based on these data, child abuse and neglect are serious risks that endanger the physical and social wellbeing of our nation's children.

Chapters in Part II of this volume provide research and advocacy agenda that address child abuse prevention and the urgent need for prevention and intervention for these vulnerable children. Specifically, the chapters on child maltreatment prevention (Miller-Perrin & Portwood, this volume) and child welfare reform (Armstrong, Yampolskaya, Jordon, & Anderson, this volume) summarize the research and advocacy needs on this topic.

One prominent advocacy outcome, implementing home visitation services for families with newborns, is in the Patient Protection and Affordable Care Act (P.L. 111-148). President Obama is establishing the Maternal, Infant, and Early Childhood Home Visiting Program. Obviously, we as child advocates need to follow this bill closely and promote the bill in obtaining the funding it needed for prevention of child abuse and neglect.

Conclusions and a "Call to Action"

We have ample evidence that children and families in our country are in need of a new beginning. We present evidence in Part II of this volume of the best environments for children to thrive in their development and make positive contributions to society. We are in a national crisis with the need to change our social and public policies to benefit children. We need advocates to make those changes, so that all children are educated equally and are taught to reach their potential and that all children and families get services and attention as early as the prenatal period of life. We have ample evidence now that the earlier we support children and families, the more likely they are to succeed in our society, and the less likely they are to represent a cost to our society. Rather than waiting for families to fall apart, let us take a stand and get support, both financial and programmatic, to the children as early as possible and as soon as possible.

> We are now faced with the fact that tomorrow is today. We are confronted with the fierce urgency of now. In this unfolding, conundrum of life and history there is such a thing as being too late ... we must move past indecisiveness to action. Dr. Martin Luther King, Jr.

References

Aber, J. L., Jones, S. M., & Raver, C. C. (2007). Poverty and child development: New perspectives on a defining issue. In J. L. Aber, S. J. Bishop-Josef, S. M. Jones, K. T. McLearn, & D. A. Phillips (Eds.), *Child development and social policy: Knowledge for action* (pp. 149–166). Washington, DC: American Psychological Association.

Aber, J. L., Morris, P., & Raver, C. (2012). Children, families and poverty: Definitions, trends, emerging science and implications for poverty. *Social Policy Report, 26*(3). Washington, DC: Society for Research in Child Development.

Bloom, B., Cohen, R. A., & Freeman, G. (2011). Summary health statistics for U.S. children: National health interview survey, 2010. *U. S. Dept. of Health, Education and Welfare, Public Health Service, Health Resources, 12*(250), 1–80.

Cherlin, A. J. (2010). *Public and private families: A reader.* New York, NY: McGraw-Hill.

Children's Defense Fund. (2012). *The state of America's children handbook.* Washington, DC: Children's Defense Fund.

Duncan, G. J., & Brooks-Gunn, J. (1997). *Consequences of growing up poor.* New York, NY: Russell Sage Foundation for Child Development.

Foundation for Child Development (2012). *The child well-being index.* New York, NY: Foundation for child development.

Glick, P. C. (1988). Fifty years of family demography: A record of social change. *Journal of Marriage and Family, 50*(4), 861–873.

Leventhal, T., & Brooks-Gunn, J. (2000). The neighborhoods they live in: The effects of neighborhood residence on child and adolescent outcomes. *Psychological Bulletin, 126*(2), 309–337.

Mclanahan, S. (2004). Diverging destinies: How children are faring under the second demographic transition. *Demography, 41*(4), 607–627.

Nord, M., Coleman-Jensen, A., Andrews, M., & Carlson, S. (2010). Household food security in the United States, 2009. *United States Department of Agriculture, 108.*

Nord, M., Coleman-Jensen, A., Andrews, M., & Carlson, S. (2012). Household food security in the United States, 2011. *United States Department of Agriculture, 108.*

Organization for Economic Cooperation and Development (OECD). (2011). *Education at a glance 2011: OECD Indicators.* OECD: Author. http://dx.doi.org/10.1787/eag-2011-en

Patient Protection and Affordable Care Act (Pub.L. 111-148).

Schweinhart, L. J., Montie, J., Xiang, Z., Barnett, W. S., Belfield, C. R., Nores, M. (2005). Lifetime effects: The high scope perry preschool study through age 40. *Monographs of the High Scope Educational Research Foundation.* Ypsilanti, MI: High Scope Press.

Shonkoff, J. P., Garner, A. S., The Committee on Psychosocial Aspect of Child and Family Health, Committee on Early Childhood, Adoption, and Dependent Care, and Section on Developmental and Behavioral Pediatrics, Siegel, B. S., Dobbins, M. I., Earls, M. F., Garner, A. S., et al. (2012). The lifelong effects of early childhood adversity and toxic stress. *Pediatrics, 129*(1), 232–246.

Teachman, J., Tedrow, L., & Crowder, K. (2000). The changing demography of America's families. *Journal of Marriage and the Family, 62*(4), 1234–1246.

U.S Department of Health and Human Services (USDHHS). (2011). *Child maltreatment 2011.* U.S. Department of Health and Human Services Administration of Children and Families Administration on Children, Youth and Families Children's Bureau.

Chapter 2
Advocating for Children, Youth, and Families in the Policymaking Process

Sandra J. Bishop-Josef and Daniel Dodgen

Policymaking happens in a context that is dynamic and complex, but not unknowable. Policymakers are influenced by many factors. These include budget, constituents, science, experts, anecdotes, recent news, and the campaign/election cycle, among others. The weight of each of these factors will vary depending on the issue and on how much the various factors are in alignment or conflict. Advocating on behalf of children and youth can be particularly challenging because most people feel they already know a lot about children. Furthermore, children and youth, particularly those from disadvantaged backgrounds, typically do not have a voice of their own in policy decisions that affect them. Thus, it is incumbent upon those who have knowledge about and care for children to advocate on their behalf.

Effective advocacy must take into consideration the factors that influence policy. Critical steps to creating a strong voice for children include: defining the problem; reviewing research relevant to solving the problem; setting a specific advocacy goal(s); and bringing research to bear on the policymaking process, to reach the advocacy goal(s). This chapter will address each of these steps, providing guidance and resources to prepare advocates to engage in the policymaking process.

S.J. Bishop-Josef, Ph.D. (✉)
The Edward Zigler Center in Child Development & Social Policy, Yale University, New Haven, CT, USA
e-mail: sandra.bishopjosef@gmail.com

D. Dodgen, Ph.D.
Division for At-Risk Individuals, Behavioral Health and Community Resilience, U.S. Department of Health and Human Services, Washington, DC, USA

A. McDonald Culp (ed.), *Child and Family Advocacy: Bridging the Gaps Between Research, Practice, and Policy*, Issues in Clinical Child Psychology, DOI 10.1007/978-1-4614-7456-2_2, © Springer Science+Business Media New York 2013

Defining the Problem

Given the competing sources of information described above, effective advocates must frame the problem for their audience, using as many of these sources as possible. To address a problem, policymakers need facts, including data on incidence and prevalence of the problem, gathered from reliable sources. While national data can be of interest, policymakers are particularly interested in data that are specific to their constituencies: what are the facts related to the problem in their state, district, or local area? Advocates can access many sources of data, including federal, state, or local government web sites (e.g., http://www.childstats.gov/) and publications and reports from various advocacy organizations (e.g., http://www.aecf.org/MajorInitiatives/KIDSCOUNT.aspx). In addition to statistics, policymakers appreciate anecdotes that provide real life examples of the problem, as experienced by their constituents. Advocates, through their work and connections in the community, can be a rich source of stories that put a human face on social problems and pique policymakers' interest. Items from local media also help frame the issue and bolster the relevance of the issue for policymakers.

Garnering Research Relevant to Solving the Problem

For many pressing social problems, there is research relevant to how they might be ameliorated or even solved. This can include both research on the factors contributing to the problem at hand and research focusing on approaches to the problem (programs, policies) that have proven effective in other settings, including program evaluations. Policymakers deal with a vast range of issues on a daily basis, from health to transportation to business to education and beyond. They must rely on experts in each of these areas to provide the research background they need. Advocates, with their professional expertise and knowledge of specific areas of research, can play this important role in the policymaking process (Zigler & Gilliam, 2009).

Setting Advocacy Goals

Once the problem has been defined and the relevant research gathered, advocates must set specific advocacy goals. This process involves advocates going beyond their area of expertise and looking at factors in the policy arena: What issues are other advocates addressing at this time? What are the related funding opportunities currently available? What issues are politically popular or pressing now? The most important concern in this step is setting realistic goal(s), given the current circumstances. There are often windows of opportunity for particular efforts and advocates must take advantage of them (Golden, 2007). Various professional organizations publish regular newsletters and blogs that advocates can use to keep abreast of the national (and sometimes state) policy scene (e.g., The Society for Research on Child Development's [SRCD] *Policy Watch*, http://www.srcd.org/index. php?option=com_content&task=view&id=266&Itemid=652; Zero to Three's *Baby Monitor*, http://www.zerotothree.org/public-policy/newsletters/; Child Welfare League of America's Children's Monitor blog, http://childrensmonitor.wordpress. com/). Relationships with other advocates at the state and local level, as well as with state-level child advocacy organizations (e.g., Connecticut Voices for Children, ctvoices.org), can provide advocates with information on more local, recent policy concerns. Armed with information on current circumstances, advocates can then discern what advocacy goals seem realistic at this time. The recent school shooting tragedy in Newtown Connecticut illustrates how a major news event can create an opportunity to discuss an issue—in this case gun control—that had previously been very challenging to raise.

Bringing Research to Bear on Policymaking

Finally, to work toward their advocacy goal(s), advocates must deliver the relevant research to policymakers (Maton & Bishop-Josef, 2006). To function effectively in the policy arena, advocates must have an understanding of how the policymaking process works. This includes knowledge about how a bill becomes a law, the role of committees and legislative staff, the role of executive branch agencies and their regulatory functions, etc. Some professional organizations have published excellent, yet brief, guides to the federal policymaking process (e.g., American Psychological Association [APA], 2010). Policymaking on the state or local level is likely to vary by locale, but advocates working at these levels can partner with state or local advocacy organizations to learn more about how the process works in their particular locale (e.g., Connecticut Voices for Children; http://www.ctvoices.org/advocacy/advocacy-toolkit). Some professional societies also focus on the state level (e.g., Zero to Three, http://www.zerotothree.org/public-policy/action-center/state-advocacy-tools.html). Hodges and Ferreira in this volume discuss the role of communities in local policy formation.

Advocates must also understand the culture of the policy world, which can be very different from that of research and practice settings (Shonkoff, 2000). It is a very fast-paced environment and policymakers often need information extremely quickly, sometimes within a day or even less. Policymakers are not likely to be interested in nuances of the research findings, preferring instead that advocates provide them with the "bottom line." Communication has to be very brief: research should be summarized in short (1–5 pages maximum) policy briefs. Policymakers typically focus on action; however interesting the information advocates offer might be, if the policymaker cannot do something with the information, it is not likely to be useful to him/her.

Mindful of the process and culture of policymaking, there are several ways advocates can bring research to bear on it. Again, professional societies and advocacy groups assist in these efforts, by maintaining web pages focused on advocacy (e.g., APA, http://www.apa.org/about/gr/advocacy/network.aspx; Zero to Three, http://www.zerotothree.org/public-policy/action-center/). Contacting professional societies or advocacy groups and contributing to their efforts can be an effective way of beginning one's own advocacy work. As described by Hodges et al. in this volume, family-run organizations can also be effective advocates and advocacy partners.

Possible activities to bring research to bear on policy include:

Join a policy alert listserv. Several professional societies and advocacy groups have email listservs to alert their members when a policy proposal is being considered (e.g., APA's Public Policy Action Network [PPAN], http://www.capwiz.com/apa-policy/home/; Children's Defense Fund's Email Alerts, http://www.childrensdefense.org/take-action/online.html). Listserv members receive email notices and respond by calling or emailing their legislators to provide support for or voices against the given proposal.

Write an op-ed or letter to the editor for the local newspaper. The media can be a very effective tool for impacting policy, despite the fact that working with the media can be difficult (Thompson & Nelson, 2001; Zigler & Gilliam, 2009). Legislative staffers monitor local newspapers to get a sense of how their constituents think on various issues. Writing an op-ed or a letter to the editor can therefore be an effective means of gaining legislators' attention. Instructions for how to write op-eds and letters to the editor are available (e.g., http://www.childrensdefense.org/take-action/advocacy-that-works/write-an-oped.html).Wilcox and Deutsch in this volume provide a compelling example of successful advocacy using the media.

Write/email legislators or legislative staff. Advocates can send letters or policy briefs to legislators or their staff. The most important rule here is: *be brief and clear.* Legislators and staff have extremely busy schedules and are unlikely to read more than a page or two. Bullet points can be an effective way of communicating information concisely. Make sure the information is presented clearly, with no professional jargon. Ask a friend who knows nothing about the topic to determine if it is clear what the problem is, what the data show, and what the relevant research suggests with regard to possible solutions. Be sure to tell the legislator or staff what you want him/her to do in response to the information you are providing and how it fits with what they are already concerned about or working on. If you can, provide some local data or add an anecdote about a local example. Examples of policy briefs can be found on the Internet (e.g., Future of Children, http://futureofchildren.org/future-ofchildren/publications/docs/21_01_PolicyBrief.pdf; SRCD's *Social Policy Reports Briefs*, http://www.srcd.org/index.php?option=com_content&task=view&id=229&Itemid=524; Zero to Three, http://www.zerotothree.org/public-policy/policy-toolkit/5x12-card-trifold-final-12-1-10.pdf). Sample letters are included in APA's advocacy guide: http://www.apa.org/about/gr/advocacy/pi-guide.pdf

Meet with legislators or their staff. Members of Congress return to their home states/districts regularly throughout the year, so advocates can meet with them in their home state. Or advocates can request a meeting if they are visiting Washington, DC. The points for writing to legislators also apply here, particularly brevity, as you may only be granted a short meeting. Be sure to have a written document (as described in the previous section) to leave with them.

Testify before the legislature. Through repeated contact with policymakers, over time, some advocates develop strong relationships with them. Given the time pressure in the policymaking process, legislative staff often rely on advocates they already know when they need assistance. In some cases, advocates will be asked to testify before a Congressional committee or the state legislature, during a hearing. Advocates can also contact state legislators or their staff and volunteer to testify. The parameters for testimony are typically defined and narrow, with regard to both length and content. Advocates often have to submit the testimony in advance of the hearing. The chapter by Francis and Turnbull in this volume discusses testifying in more detail, using the Individuals with Disabilities Education Act (IDEA) as an example (cf. McCartney & Phillips, 1993).

Comment on proposed regulations. On the federal level, once a bill has been passed by Congress and signed into law by the President, executive branch agencies (e.g., Department of Health and Human Services, Department of Education, etc.) develop regulations on exactly how the law will be implemented. Often, there is a call for public comment on proposed regulations published in the *Federal Register* (www.federalregister.gov). Advocacy groups and professional societies sometimes publicize these calls, as well. Advocates can easily submit comments on these proposed regulations, thereby potentially having impact on how laws in their area of concern affect children and families.

At the federal, state, and local levels, policymakers and elected officials create programs and initiate change. However, the implementation of these changes is usually left to career civil servants and political appointees. These individuals often have greater subject matter expertise and may be more receptive to the information social scientists can provide that will help them implement legislative action.

Pursue training. There are opportunities to pursue training in advocacy, both through workshops and in formal education programs. Professional societies offer workshops on advocacy (e.g., APA). For those interested in pursuing degrees in areas related to child and family policy, these are offered by several schools, including those in the University-Based Child and Family Policy Consortium (http://www.childpolicyuniversityconsortium.com/members.html).

Apply for a policy fellowship or internship. Several professional societies offer fellowships or internships in policy settings. Professionals or students spend a period of time (several months to a year or more) working in government settings (Congress, executive branch agency) or the society's government relations office, funded by the society. These opportunities allow for an in-depth exposure to the policy arena. APA (http://www.apa.org/about/gr/fellows/index.aspx) and SRCD (http://www.srcd.org/policy-media/policy-fellowships) offer fellowships and internships related to child and family policy.

In many of these activities designed to bring research to bear on the policymaking process, the issue of relationships is important. Policymakers often rely on a relatively small set of advisors or other sources of information when looking for research relevant to their current policy concerns (cf. Meyer, Alteras, & Adams, 2006; Tseng, 2012).

In sum, there are many opportunities and ways for concerned advocates, armed with their professional expertise, to attempt to impact the policymaking process. While it is true that there are many voices and factors competing for the attention of policymakers and attempting to influence them, it is also true that the policymaking process can and does lead to positive changes. Becoming involved in this process requires considerable effort, including often going outside one's comfort zone; the potential benefits to children, youth and families justify these efforts.

References

American Psychological Association. (2010). *A psychologist's guide to federal advocacy: Advancing psychology in the public interest.* Washington, DC: American Psychological Association, Public Interest Government Relations Office. Retrieved from http://www.apa.org/about/gr/advocacy/pi-guide.pdf

Golden, O. (2007). Policy looking to research. In J. L. Aber, S. J. Bishop-Josef, S. M. Jones, K. T. McLearn, & D. A. Phillips (Eds.), *Child development and social policy knowledge for action.* Washington, DC: American Psychological Association.

Maton, K. I., & Bishop-Josef, S. J. (2006). Psychological research, practice and social policy: Potential pathways of influence. *Professional Psychology: Research and Practice, 37,* 140–145.

McCartney, K., & Phillips, D. (1993). *An insider's guide to providing expert testimony before congress.* Washington, DC: Society for Research in Child Development.

Meyer, J. A., Alteras, T. T., & Adams, K. B. (2006). *Toward more effective use of research in state policymaking.* Washington, DC: The Commonwealth Fund.

Shonkoff, J. (2000). Science, policy and practice: Three cultures in search of a shared mission. *Child Development, 71,* 181–187.

Thompson, R. A., & Nelson, C. A. (2001). Developmental science and the media. Early brain development. *American Psychologist, 56,* 5–15.

Tseng, V. (2012). The uses of research in policy and practice. *Social Policy Reports, 26*(2), 3–16.

Zigler, E. F., & Gilliam, W. S. (2009). Science and policy: Connecting what we know to what we do. *Zero to Three, 30*(2), 40–46.

Part II
Selected Child Issues in Need
of Advocacy Effort

Chapter 3
Promoting Children's Mental Health: The Importance of Collaboration and Public Understanding

Mary Ann McCabe, Donald Wertlieb, and Karen Saywitz

In the present chapter we strive to help readers understand the opportunities and impediments for child mental health advocacy. We emphasize the critical importance of enhancing public understanding of the science regarding children's mental health for public investment in this area. We also build a case for the value of collaboration across stakeholders for effective advocacy and discuss one initiative in depth that is built on this premise—a Summit of child mental health scholars and experts partnering with communication scientists. The collaboration embodied by the Summit illustrates one promising approach to advocacy supported by the scholarship regarding bridging research, practice, and policy.

What We Know About Child Mental Health

Children's mental health is a fundamental aspect of their healthy development. Although many children in contemporary society are thriving, too many others are not provided with the conditions necessary to build a strong foundation for healthy productive lives (National Scientific Council on the Developing Child, 2007a, 2007b). In order to capture this wide spectrum, it is helpful to conceptualize advocacy regarding children's mental health in terms of a continuum of promotion, prevention, and treatment. According to the Office of the US Surgeon General,

M.A. McCabe, Ph.D. (✉)
Department of Pediatrics, George Washington University School of Medicine, Washington, DC 20052, USA
e-mail: mamccabe@cox.net

D. Wertlieb, Ph.D.
Department of Child Development, Tufts University, Boston, MA, USA

K. Saywitz, Ph.D.
Department of Psychiatry and Biobehavioral Sciences, UCLA School of Medicine, 760 Westwood Plaza, Los Angeles, CA 90095, USA

A. McDonald Culp (ed.), *Child and Family Advocacy: Bridging the Gaps Between Research, Practice, and Policy*, Issues in Clinical Child Psychology, DOI 10.1007/978-1-4614-7456-2_3, © Springer Science+Business Media New York 2013

"growing numbers of children and families are suffering needlessly because their emotional, behavioral, and developmental needs are not being met by the very institutions that were explicitly created to take care of them. It is time that we as a Nation took seriously the task of preventing mental health problems and treating mental illness in youth" (U.S. Public Health Service, 2000, p. 1).

Indeed, mental health problems in children and adolescents have grown to alarmingly high prevalence rates in the United States. Approximately two in ten or 20 % of children have a diagnosable mental, emotional, or behavioral disorder. (For annual sources of information, see the Anne E. Casey Foundation (http://datacenter. kidscount.org/) and the Federal Information Interagency Forum on Child and Family Statistics (http://www.childsats.gov/).) Further, most mental disorders in adults can be traced to an onset during childhood (Kessler & Wang, 2008; National Research Council and Institute of Medicine, 2009). Yet, only 20 % of those children in need receive mental health services (U.S. Public Health Service, 2000). This has been referred to as the "20/20 problem:" 20 % of children in the United States have a mental health problem and only 20 % of those children receive mental health services.

This has been attributed to a lack of both funding and providers (Cooper et al., 2008; Knitzer & Cooper, 2006). Many of those who access care do not receive state of the art treatment; often it is not available until late in the process when problems have become entrenched and more resistant to treatment (Cooper et al., 2008). Moreover, there are grave disparities in access to quality care for children with special needs and children from ethnic minorities (U.S. Public Health Service, 1999). (For additional information on mental health disparities, see the Office of Minority Health and Health Disparities, Centers for Disease Control (http://www.cdc.gov/ omhd/) and the National Institute on Minority Health and Health Disparities, National Institutes of Health (http://www.nimhd.nih.gov)). The mental health system itself is poorly funded and fragmented, with too many children and families falling through the cracks, and there is a workforce shortage of professionals trained specifically to work with children and diverse cultures (Annapolis Coalition, 2007).

The economic costs to society of ignoring child mental health are great. According to the Agency for Healthcare Research and Quality (2009), childhood mental disorders account for the largest category of spending of health dollars for children from birth to 17 years of age. A recent estimate for the annual cost of mental disorders in children and youth is $247 billion (National Research Council and Institute of Medicine, 2009). Additional costs are incurred outside the health care system in special education, child welfare, and juvenile justice.

Defining Child Mental Health

Advancing public policy in children's mental health has been hampered by the absence of a clear and unifying definition. This has discouraged the cross-fertilization of knowledge across the range of scientific disciplines concerned with child development, education, and health. Further, the field of mental health has historically focused on mental illness rather than mental health; only recently have we witnessed a greater appreciation for resilience, health promotion, and prevention. This illness or deficit paradigm has further discouraged the integration of scientific knowledge and policies about children's mental health along the full continuum, from healthy child development through evidence-based prevention and treatment of mental disorders.

Effective advocacy requires a broad definition of child mental health as being a critical part of healthy development, incorporating mental, social, emotional, and behavioral health and including the growing scholarship in developmental science, mental health science, neuroscience, education, pediatrics, mental health services, and interventions. This broad definition is consistent with the recent National Research Council and Institute of Medicine report, *Preventing Mental, Emotional, and Behavioral Disorders Among Young People: Progress and Possibilities* (National Research Council and Institute of Medicine, 2009). It is also consistent with the *Report of the Surgeon General's Conference on Children's Mental Health* (U.S. Public Health Service, 2000) which emphasized, "mental health is a critical component of children's learning and general health. Fostering social and emotional health in children as part of healthy child development must therefore be a national priority" (U.S. Public Health Service, 2000, p. 3).

Addressing the Impediments to Effective Advocacy

Fortunately, we are in the midst of a remarkable expansion in new knowledge. Discoveries in genetics, neurobiology, child development, mental health treatment, and economics offer an unprecedented opportunity to catalyze cost-effective, science-based policies and practices to promote the health and wellbeing of our children (National Scientific Council on the Developing Child, 2008; National Research Council and Institute of Medicine, 2009). We now know that childhood experiences have lifelong effects; the interactions of genes and early experiences shape the very architecture of the brain and provide individuals with a strong or weak foundation for future health, behavior, and learning (National Scientific Council on the Developing Child, 2004a, 2004b, 2005). Creating the right conditions for healthy emotional, social, and behavioral development early are likely to be more effective and less costly than addressing problems at a later stage. As the last 2 decades of research suggest, many child mental health problems are both preventable (National Research Council and Institute of Medicine, 2009) and treatable (Sturmey & Herson, 2012). A continuum of evidence-based interventions, as well as increased public interest and government investment, will be needed to promote healthy emotional, social, and behavioral development, to prevent problems in high-risk populations, and to effectively treat disorders when they arise.

Perhaps the greatest opportunity for cost savings and effective advocacy can be found in *early childhood*—through promoting children's mental health, preventing conditions in children at risk, and providing evidence-based early intervention. However, McLearn, Knitzer, and Carter (2007) proposed four reasons for relative neglect of mental health in early childhood policy and programs: (1) the focus on early childhood learning originally overshadowed the importance of social and emotional development for school preparedness; (2) a myth that young children do not experience mental health conditions; (3) the stigma for parents and families, particularly in some cultures; and (4) the political complexity of the health system for young children. Regarding the latter, these authors further emphasized the "blurry" line between promoting children's mental health and treating mental health conditions, the difficulty of identifying problems within the child vs. within the parent–child relationship, and the relative dearth of developmentally appropriate diagnostic categories within the DSM-IV (American Psychiatric Association, 2000). With the nation undergoing complex transformation of the health care system, as well as the emergence of new diagnostic schemes by the American Psychiatric Association (Diagnostic and Statistical Manual (DSM)) and World Health Organization (International Classification of Diseases (ICD)), it is likely that some of these controversies and confusions may continue.

It is particularly difficult for young children and their families to receive outcomes-based treatment (Cooper et al., 2008; McLearn et al., 2007), despite the fact that investing early in children's mental health can lead to future savings in special education, juvenile justice, and child welfare, as well as increased work productivity and better physical health. Similarly, we are well aware of the critical benefits of nurturing environments for promoting health and wellbeing, and in countering the deleterious effects of poverty on children's mental, emotional, and behavioral health (Biglan, Flay, Embry, & Sandler, 2012; National Scientific Council on the Developing Child, 2004b; Yoshikawa, Aber, & Beardslee, 2012), yet there has been little public investment for widespread evidence-based prevention in troubled environments.

There has been significant growth in basic developmental science regarding the trajectories of (and contexts for) social, emotional, and behavioral development, yet much of this knowledge resides within the "silos" in which it was created. In particular, it is not readily incorporated by those designing and studying programs and interventions (National Research Council and Institute of Medicine, 2000). Similarly, there have been impressive gains in developing evidence-based practices for preventing and treating mental health conditions in children, yet there are critical gaps in dissemination and implementation of these services in the community. We are becoming increasingly aware of the need for a more strategic approach in this regard (Chambers, 2007; Fixsen, Naoom, Blasé, Friedman, & Wallace, 2005; Shoenwald & Hoagwood, 2001; APA Task Force on Evidence-Based Practice with Children and Adolescents, 2008; Wallace, Blasé, Fixen, & Naoom, 2008; Wandersman et al., 2008).

A final but critical reason for slow progress in policies that effectively promote children's mental health is the public's (and policymakers') lack of understanding of the growing body of science. Indeed, promoting public recognition of the importance of young children's mental health has been a key element of several influential national reports (e.g., *From Neurons to Neighborhoods,* National Research Council and Institute of Medicine, 2000; *Surgeon General's Action Agenda for Children's*

Mental Health, U.S. Public Health Service, 2000; *Achieving the Promise: Transforming Mental Health Care in America*, The President's New Freedom Commission on Mental Health, 2003; *Preventing mental, emotional, and behavioral disorders among young people: Progress and possibilities,* National Research Council and Institute of Medicine, 2009). Yet the process of knowledge transfer and translation about children's mental health continues to be fragmented according to diverse networks of practitioners, researchers, advocates, families, funders, and policymakers. Effective public policies in child mental health require public understanding of the science in the silos.

The Importance of Collaboration: The Example Within Psychology

Psychology can serve as one example of a professional discipline that pursues advocacy for child mental health. The evolution of advocacy efforts in psychology illustrates the increasing recognition of the critical role of collaboration—first within psychology and ultimately across fields concerned with child mental health. (See Appendix for the range of advocacy efforts in child mental health.) Following the release of the *Report of the Surgeon General's Conference on Children's Mental Health: A national action agenda* (U.S. Public Health Service, 2000), the APA Board of Directors established a Working Group on Children's Mental Health which crossed the areas (directorates within the organization) of science, practice, education, and public interest. This working group produced a report, *Developing Psychology's National Agenda for Children's Mental Health: APA's Response to the Surgeon General's Action Agenda for Children's Mental Health* (APA Working Group on Children's Mental Health, 2001). The report identified five central strategies to guide APA in developing and implementing activities that would promote and further the eight goals as stated in the Surgeon General's report. In turn, the APA Board of Directors established the Task Force on Psychology's Agenda for Child and Adolescent Mental Health which further defined implementation plans to advance child mental health (APA Task Force on Psychology's Agenda for Child and Adolescent Mental Health, 2004). Finally, this report became the transitional work plan for forming a more lasting Interdivisional Task Force on Child and Adolescent Mental Health (ITDF) within APA in 2005. The IDTF enabled more lasting collaboration across the many specialties within psychology research and practice that are concerned with child and family mental health.[1]

---

[1]The current members of the IDTF include the following divisions within APA: Developmental Psychology; Society of Clinical Psychology; Educational Psychology; School Psychology; Society for Community Research and Action: Division of Community Psychology; Intellectual and Developmental Disabilities; Society for Child and Family Policy and Practice; Psychoanalysis; The American Psychology-Law Society; Family Psychology; Society of Clinical Child and Adolescent Psychology; Society of Pediatric Psychology.

The Goal: Expanding Collaboration and Convening a Summit

We present here one activity within the ongoing advocacy of the IDTF; namely, an interdisciplinary Summit held in 2009. While collaboration across psychology through the IDTF has advanced progress in advocacy, we[2] believed that it was necessary to expand this collaboration to include colleagues from other disciplines who share an investment in promoting children's mental health. It seemed critical to search for consensus among otherwise seemingly competing or contradictory advocacy goals.

In order to inform public attitudes and public policy about children's mental health, we felt that it would be imperative to work in a *coalition* across the disciplines and stakeholders in children's mental health. Indeed, the collaborative process begun at the Summit reflects what Cohn (2006) describes as the work of an "advocacy coalition." He argues that individuals and organizations can be more effective in informing public policy by working collaboratively in advocacy coalitions over an extended period. Specifically, coalitions can identify scholarly ideas and evidence that reconcile the views of diverse stakeholders who otherwise may not achieve common ground. By working in tandem, coalitions can enhance their political influence and affect the perspective of policymakers. In addition, the Summit was designed to identify not the work of individual scholars but a body of research, or what Cohn (2006) referred to as "schools of thought," which he argued carry more influence for policymakers. He suggests that when policymakers are made aware of widely held academic schools of thought on an issue such as children's mental health, they can incorporate this body of research into their own understanding of the issue and narrow the range of potential solutions.

Key Considerations for the Summit

We felt that the timing was ripe for a national Summit to call attention to children's mental health. Cohn (2006) refers to this issue of timing as "policy windows" or the changing political and socioeconomic forces for decision makers that make them more attentive to an issue, to evidence related to it, and to opportunities for more effective advocacy. The timing of the Summit drew upon emerging changes in mental health parity, in the broader landscape of health care, and in emphasis on reducing health disparities. Indeed, we recognized that our society and multiple intersecting policy contexts were at a "tipping point" (Gladwell, 2000), poised for significant progress in addressing the needs of children.

---

[2]The summit planning group included: Barry Anton, Mary Campbell, Mary Ann McCabe (Chair), Karen Saywitz, Stephen Shirk, Patrick Tolan, and Donald Wertlieb.

The Summit also capitalized on another "policy window" by focusing in early childhood. As noted earlier, it is strategic to focus advocacy efforts in early childhood (birth to eight) because it is the best time to promote healthy development, and because early intervention provides the best opportunity to prevent mental health problems and health disparities. However, there are additional advantages to focusing our efforts on young children: (1) The science of early childhood development has already demonstrated the importance of child mental health for healthy development (e.g., National Research Council and Institute of Medicine, 2000; National Scientific Council on the Developing Child, 2004a, 2004b, 2005, 2007a, 2007b, 2008); (2) There have already been important successes in improving public understanding that early child development is critical, thereby informing more effective public policy. (See the information on early childhood development at the National Conference of State Legislatures (http://www.ncsl.org/), the National Governor's Association, Center for Best Practices (http://www.nga.org/cms/center), and the National Summit on America's Children in the U.S. House of Representatives (http://www.house.gov/)); and (3) Economic science has shown clear benefits to investing in early childhood (Heckman, 2007, 2008).

In order to improve public (and policymakers') understanding of child mental health, we recognized that it would be critical to collaborate with communication scientists. Just as there are differing theoretical approaches and skills in mental health interventions, so, too, are there different theoretical and empirical approaches to communication with the public (McCabe & Browning, 2010; Welch-Ross & Fasig, 2007). Benjamin (2007) describes the key difference between two such approaches within communication science–social marketing and strategic frame analysis™. Social marketing is most often used as a means to educate the public and encourage healthier individual decisions (e.g., stop smoking, exercise). In contrast, he argues that strategic frame analysis™ serves to better educate the public on more lasting social and public policy issues where science and cultural beliefs do not coincide.

The communication scientists at FrameWorks Institute who conduct strategic frame analysis™ were ready partners for our Summit. FrameWorks Institute (http://frameworksinstitute.org/ecd.html) had already formed a strong collaboration with the Harvard Center on the Developing Child in related efforts (http://developing-child.harvard.edu/), and this prior research provided framing of early childhood that served as a foundation for framing children's mental health (National Scientific Council on the Developing Child, 2004a, 2004b, 2005, 2007a, 2007b, 2008). Their preliminary research on child mental health was beginning to suggest that the following would be key considerations for effective framing: shifting the public focus away from mental illness; anchoring mental health as a critical part of healthy development; emphasizing the importance of families and environments; connecting the antecedents of mental health to long-term outcomes; relating child and adult mental health; clarifying notions about the long-term effects of intervention and early intervention; and providing a clear message that treatment can be effective (FrameWorks Institute, 2009a, 2009b).

Action Steps: Designing the Summit

Partnering with the interdisciplinary Society for Research in Child Development (SRCD) and the University of Denver, the Summit was convened in Denver in 2009, entitled, *Healthy Development: A Summit on Young Children's Mental Health* (SRCD, 2009).[3] The Summit size and format was based on the "convening model" of the Johnson Foundation at Wingspread (http://www.johnsonfdn.org/). Researchers and practitioners from the following disciplines were represented at the Summit: anthropology, economics, education, nursing, pediatrics, psychiatry, psychology, social work, and sociology. In addition, parents, policymakers, advocates, federal agency staff, and communication science experts also participated. See this volume, Chap. 15 on Family Engagement, for a detailed model of engaging parents in the children's mental health arena.

We designed the Summit to bring together representatives from *diverse stakeholder groups*, with communication scientists, to cross silos, encourage collaboration, and begin to build consensus regarding what the science tells us about children's mental health. It was intended to generate the difficult dialog inherent in diverse perspectives but necessary for progress. While there are a range of sources of knowledge, the Summit emphasized science as the most trusted source of knowledge and the arbiter across diverse stakeholder perspectives. The Summit was dedicated to Dr. Jane Knitzer, whose career was devoted to advancing scientifically based mental health policy (Cooper & Ardoin, 2009).

The Summit agenda focused on three main questions: What does the science say about young children's mental health? What promotes it and what derails it? What science constitutes useful information for communication science to improve public understanding? To catalyze the discussions of both the small breakout groups as well as the larger group of Summit participants, a few invited experts presented information from two perspectives: mental health (and developmental) science and communication science. Mental health science experts focused on what the public needs to know so that it grasps the importance of children's mental health for healthy development. Communication science experts articulated their process for developing scientifically informed and empirically tested frames to promote the public's understanding of child mental health, which fit well with the framework of science as the source of knowledge.

---

[3] Summit funders included: SRCD, American Orthopsychiatric Association, APA, Society of Clinical Child and Adolescent Psychology, Society of Pediatric Psychology, Anne E. Casey Foundation, APA Division of School Psychology, National Association of School Psychologists, National Association of Social Workers, Society for Child and Family Policy and Practice, Society of Clinical Psychology, Society for Developmental and Behavioral Pediatrics, Society for Prevention Research, APA Division of Family Psychology. APA Division of Intellectual and Developmental Disabilities, APA Division of Psychoanalysis and the section on Childhood and Adolescence, the Child, Adolescent and Family Caucus of APA, Society for Community Research and Action, and the IDTF. Institutional Sponsors included the University of Denver and Nemours Health and Prevention Services.

The Summit discussions were organized according to four different areas of children's mental health, outlined by Tolan and Dodge (2005): healthy development, promotion, prevention, and interventions. The real work of the meeting happened in these four small groups:

- *Group* 1: Importance of mental health for normal child development
- *Group* 2: Everyday challenges for parents and child mental health
- *Group* 3: Prevention opportunities in child mental health
- *Group* 4: Child mental disorders: treatment works

Activities at the Summit

Each of the small groups was charged with building consensus for the following question, "Among those findings that are empirically supported, what are the most critical and useful ideas to improve public understanding of child mental health?" The points of consensus that emerged from the Summit can be found in the full report (SRCD, 2009).

Examples of these points of consensus within each of the small groups can be found here.

The Importance of Mental Health for Normal Child Development

- Providing support for children's optimal social and emotional development results in positive outcomes for individuals and society, including healthier behavior, greater school success, improved relationships, and economic savings.
- These caregivers need to receive support. Families, parents, caregivers, teachers, and others who care for and work with children need to be better informed about milestones of normal, healthy child development to both reassure caregivers when development proceeds within typical limits and to identify early warning signs that indicate when assistance is necessary.
- Children and families can be prepared for stress points and transitions. They can learn the skills to be resilient in periods of stress and challenge, thus protecting and promoting mental health.

Everyday Challenges for Parents

- Families can be strengthened and parents can increase their skills through interventions designed to promote children's mental health.
- Decreasing poverty will increase resources to promote children's mental health.
- One-stop facilities that provide integrated health care and human services enable parents to meet their children's needs, which include safety, education, health, and happiness.

Prevention Opportunities in Child Mental Health

- Healthy prenatal choices, e.g., refraining from smoking, alcohol, or drug use, and avoiding unintentional toxic exposure, protect the developing brain and are critical for child mental health.
- Organized community-wide assessment, planning, and action using evidence-based approaches can reduce the prevalence of childhood mental, emotional, and behavioral disorders.
- Promoting social and emotional learning in school programs leads to success in school and life and prevents mental health problems.

Effective Treatment for Childhood Mental Health Problems

- Similar to the obstacles they encounter in the health care system, children and families face many barriers to receiving evidence-based treatments for children's mental disorders. These barriers include a lack of trained providers, lack of public financing, limited private insurance coverage, and stigma.
- More research is needed to develop effective, developmentally appropriate, and culturally responsive treatments and to bring them from the development stage to actual delivery. Research can guide the tailoring of interventions to the particular needs of children and families.

A number of converging themes also emerged across the small and large group discussions at the Summit, including: the importance of a broad and clear definition of child mental health; the central importance of families, parents, and caregivers; the importance of resilience for mitigating the impact of stress and transitions; the view of prevention from a developmental framework, to include individuals, families, neighborhoods, and communities; the challenges for ensuring widespread access to evidence-based treatments for children and families, including the need to identify common effectiveness factors and address workforce issues; and the overarching premise that mental health should be addressed where children live, play, work, and grow.

Outcomes of the Summit

The Summit report was mailed to over 400 key stakeholders in policy and practice. In addition, planners and participants of the Summit again partnered with SRCD in 2010 to present the report of the Summit at a briefing for Congressional staff and the wider policy audience. Highlights of the briefing and speaker slides can be found online (SRCD, 2010). Illustrating the importance of translation for the policy audience,

Examples of Messages for the Policy Audience Stemming from the Summit

- It is a *critical time* for policymakers to focus on young children's mental health—across the diverse areas of: child care, early education, welfare reform, child welfare, disasters, health disparities, health care reform, health care delivery systems, mental health parity, school bullying, and teacher preparation
- Children's mental health is not confined to a single area of policy, but is linked to policies related to health, education, and safety
- Investing in *young* children's mental health can result in *savings* for both individuals and society and can result in enhanced educational attainment, work productivity, and health into adulthood

Examples of Specific Policy Recommendations Stemming from the Summit

Promotion

- Make mental health supports available in early care and education settings
- Teacher preparation programs should include training in social and emotional learning

Prevention

- Consider the impact of the built environment (e.g., safe playgrounds) and housing
- Use evidence-based prevention programs in schools and other child settings

Treatment

- Promote interdisciplinary training and collaboration (e.g., integrated health care, developmental consultation in schools)

we have provided some examples of key messages and specific policy recommendations stemming from the Summit here.

Summit participants were asked to complete a 15-question evaluation form following the meeting. A complete description of their feedback is included in the Summit report (SRCD, 2009). Of note, the majority of respondents felt that the Summit was an important step in achieving cross-discipline dialogue and that it would influence their future work in teaching, research, advocacy, and communication. Participants recommended that the objectives and central themes of the Summit be carried forward to a wider group of stakeholders to raise funds, build coalitions, and cultivate leadership.

By the close of the Summit, participants identified the need for even wider collaboration in future work, including: federal, state, and local legislators; professional organizations; leaders in business; associations representing families and other caregivers; nonprofit organizations; advocates for racial, ethnic, cultural, and language minority groups; insurers; and federal, state, and local systems in child welfare, health care, education, law enforcement, and justice. Indeed, as noted in the close of the summit report, "Diverse domains have legitimate claim to both the problems and solutions, and those bridges that can be built are likely to enhance the effectiveness of efforts in the field" (SRCD, 2009, p. 21).

Next Steps and Looking Forward

Following 3 years of empirical research, including both the expert perspectives on what scientific evidence is important for the public to understand and the conflicting realities of what the public currently believes, in 2010 researchers from FrameWorks Institute released their findings on the strategic framing™ that has been shown to enhance public support for investment in children's mental health (FrameWorks Institute, 2010). This new frame builds on previous ones (National Scientific Council on the Developing Child, 2004a, 2004b, 2005, 2007, 2008) for early child development (e.g., brain architecture, toxic stress) and centers on the concept of stability or "levelness" (including the metaphor of a table that was employed by one subject). This frame incorporates aspects of the individual child's biology, environment, experience, and the importance of early intervention when levelness falters (FrameWorks Institute, 2010). (See the FrameWorks website (http://www.frameworksinstitute.org/cmh) for more of these results on framing and the underlying research process.)

A critical next step has become educating other messengers for the policy audience about these empirically tested frames. FrameWorks researchers presented these results at the 2011 APA Convention [4] (Erard, 2011; Kendall-Taylor, 2011) and were invited to present again as an invited session for the Society for Child and Family Policy and Practice at the 2012 APA Convention (Erard, 2012; Kendall-Taylor, 2012). The FrameWorks scientists also presented their framing results to the members of the National Consortium of Child and Adolescent Mental Health Services in 2012 (Kendall-Taylor & Lindland, 2012)—these are the messengers from the various professional associations and stakeholder groups who conduct federal advocacy work regarding issues in child mental health.

The Summit and its follow-up activities have been crucial steps in the long-term collaborative advocacy work that will be necessary to inform more effective public policies in children's mental health. Indeed, both advocacy work and the policy-making process are incremental in this way. The planners of the Summit (psychologists), along with some key participants in pediatrics, psychiatry, and social work,

---

[4]Note that the 2011 session is available as a Continuing Education module with APA (http://apa.bizvision.com/).

are currently working toward a second Summit to further expand collaboration. We envision that this next meeting will focus not on what we *know* but on what we *do*, changing our frames and changing our usual partners in order to more effectively promote children's mental health.

Telling this story of the Summit is yet another way in which we pursue our commitment to bridging the gaps across research, practice, and policy. Our hope is that as you consider how you might use your skills to participate and lead advocacy initiatives, novice readers will be better informed of the fundamental need to reframe public discourse on child mental health—from an individual problem of treating illness caused by genes set in stone to a shared responsibility for societal changes that promote healthy emotional, social, and behavioral development of all children in order to improve lifelong outcomes that benefit society as a whole. For experienced readers, we hope the Summit demonstrates the added value of partnering with communication scientists and working to cross silos, find common ground, and leverage impact by translating scientific discoveries into ideas that the public, the media, civic leaders, and policy makers can understand. In turn, these new understandings can be used to create innovative policies and programs that promote children's mental health.

The Range of Advocacy Efforts for Child Mental Health

Advocacy for children's mental health takes many forms with diverse targets and goals. The following are some important examples to acquaint the reader with the range of efforts—within which the Child Mental Health Summit is situated: The Children's Defense Fund (CDF) (http://www.childrensdefense.org) sustains a focus on mental health in a context of priorities for health care, education, and eradication of poverty. Prevent Child Abuse America (http://www.preventchildabuse.org) has its eponymous mission, but the essential links to child mental health permeate its policies and practices. Mental Health America (MHA) (http://www.mental-healthamerica.net) aims for broad systems change and concerns itself with all ages, yet the agenda specific to children's mental health is robust. The National Alliance on Mental Illness (NAMI) (http://www.nami.org) organizes grassroots on particular issues, but maintains a focus on children's needs in those contexts.

Increasingly we see focused collaboration among stakeholders with specific commitment to children's mental health. For example, Children's Mental Health Matters (http://www.childrensmentalhealthmatters.org) networks partners in its home state of Maryland, the Child Mind Institute (http://www.childmind.org) catalyzes national stakeholders from multiple sectors, the federal agency Substance Abuse and Mental Health Services Administration (http://www.samhsa.gov/children) operates sophisticated advocacy for children, and on a global level, groups such as the World Health Organization (http://www.who.int/) allocate resources for child mental health advocacy.

References

Agency for Healthcare Research and Quality. (2009). *The five most costly children's conditions, 2006: Estimates for the U.S. civilian noninstitutionalized children, ages 0–17.* Retrieved from http://www.meps.ahrq.gov/mepsweb/data_files/publications/st242/stat242.shtml

American Psychiatric Association. (2000). *Diagnostic and statistical manual of mental disorders* (4th ed.). Washington, DC: Author.

American Psychological Association, Task Force on Evidence-Based Practice with Children and Adolescents. (2008). *Disseminating evidence-based practice for children and adolescents: A Systems approach to enhancing care.* Retrieved from http://www.apa.org/practice/resources/evidence/children-report.pdf

American Psychological Association, Task Force on Psychology's Agenda for Child and Adolescent Mental Health. (2004). *Report of the task force on psychology's agenda for child and adolescent mental health.* Retrieved from http://www.apa.org/pi/cyf/child_adoles_mental-health_report.pdf

American Psychological Association, Working Group on Children's Mental Health. (2001). *Developing psychology's national agenda for children's mental health: APA's response to the Surgeon General's Action Agenda for Children's Mental Health.* Retrieved from http://www.apa.org/pi/cyf/dpnacmh.pdf

Annapolis Coalition. (2007). *An action plan for behavioral health workforce development: A framework for discussion.* Retrieved from http://www.annapoliscoalition.org/resources/1/Action%20Plan%20-%20Full%20Report.pdf

Benjamin, D. (2007). *Differences between strategic frame analysis and social marketing.* Retrieved from http://www.frameworksinstitute.org/assets/files/framebytes/framebyte_social_marketing.pdf

Biglan, A., Flay, B. R., Embry, D. D., & Sandler, I. N. (2012). The critical role of nurturing environments for promoting human well-being. *American Psychologist, 67,* 257–271.

Chambers, D. (2007). Disseminating and implementing evidence-based practices for mental health. In M. Welch-Ross & L. Fasig (Eds.), *Handbook on communicating and disseminating behavioral science* (pp. 365–389). Thousand Oaks, CA: Sage.

Cohn, D. (2006). Jumping into the political fray: Academics and policy-making. *IRPP Policy Matters, 7,* 8–36.

Cooper, J. L., Aratani, Y., Knitzer, J., Douglas-Hall, A., Masi, R., Banghart, P., et al. (2008). *Unclaimed children revisited: The status of children's mental health policy in the United States.* New York: National Center for Children in Poverty. Retrieved from http://nccp.org/publications/pdf/text_853.pdf

Cooper, J. L., & Ardoin, M. (2009). Obituary: Jane Knitzer (1941–2009). *The American Journal of Orthopsychiatry, 79,* 439–440.

Erard, M. (2011, August). Metaphors as cognitive tools: The case of child mental health. In M. A. McCabe (Chair), *Public policy and the science of child mental health: How communication science bridges the divide.* Symposium conducted at annual meeting of the American Psychological Association, Washington DC.

Erard, M. (2012, August). Metaphors as cognitive tools: The case of child mental health. In M. A. McCabe (Chair), *Public policy and the science of child mental health: How communication science bridges the divide.* Invited symposium conducted at annual meeting of the American Psychological Association, Orlando, FL.

Fixsen, D., Naoom, S. F., Blasé, K. A., Friedman, R. M., & Wallace, F. (2005). *Implementation research: A synthesis of the literature.* Tampa, FL: University of South Florida.

FrameWorks Institute. (2009a). *Child mental health: A review of the scientific discourse: A FrameWorks research report.* Retrieved from http://frameworksinstitute.org/assets/files/PDF_childmentalhealth/childmentalhealthsummaryexcerpt.pdf

FrameWorks Institute. (2009b). *Conflicting models of mind in mind: Mapping the gaps between the expert and the public understandings of child mental health as part of strategic frame analysis*™. Retrieved from http://frameworksinstitute.org/assets/files/PDF_childmentalhealth/childmentalhealthculturalmodels.pdf

FrameWorks Institute. (2010). *How to talk about children's mental health: A FrameWorks message memo.* Retrieved from http://www.frameworksinstitute.org/assets/files/CMH_MM.pdf

Gladwell, M. (2000). *The tipping point: How little things can make a big difference.* Boston, MA: Little Brown.

Heckman, J. (2007). The economics, technology, and neuroscience of human capability formation. *Proceedings of the National Academy of Sciences of the United States of America, 104,* 13250–13255.

Heckman, J. (2008). *Schools, skills, synapses.* Retrieved from http://www.heckmanequation.org/content/resource/schools-skills-synapses

Kendall-Taylor, N. (2011, August). Rethinking child mental health: Seeing perceptual barriers to policy in media and mind. In M. A. McCabe (Chair), *Public policy and the science of child mental health: How communication science bridges the divide.* Symposium conducted at annual meeting of the American Psychological Association, Washington, DC.

Kendall-Taylor, N. (2012, August). Rethinking child mental health: Seeing perceptual barriers to policy in media and mind. In M. A. McCabe (Chair), *Public policy and the science of child mental health: How communication science bridges the divide.* Invited symposium conducted at annual meeting of the American Psychological Association, Orlando, FL.

Kendall-Taylor, N. & Lindland, E. (2012, January). *Strategic framing of child mental health.* Paper presented at the quarterly meeting of the National Consortium of Child and Adolescent Mental Health Services, Washington, DC.

Kessler, R. C. & Wang, P. S. (2008). The descriptive epidemiology of commonly occurring mental disorders in the United States. *Annual Review of Public Health, 29,* 115–129. Retrieved from 10.1146/annurev.pubhealth.29.020907.090847

Knitzer, J., & Cooper, J. (2006). Beyond integration: Challenges for children's mental health. *Health Affairs, 25,* 670–679. doi:10.1377/hlthaff.25.3.670 no. 3 670–679.

McCabe, M. A., & Browning, A. (2010). Disseminating and communicating your applied research findings to the public. In V. Maholmes & C. Lomonaco (Eds.), *Applied research in child and adolescent development: A practical approach* (pp. 247–266). New York, NY: Taylor & Francis.

McLearn, K., Knitzer, J., & Carter, A. (2007). Mental health: A neglected partner in the healthy development of young children. In J. L. Aber, S. J. Bishop-Josef, S. M. Jones, K. T. McLearn, & D. A. Philips (Eds.), *Child development and social policy* (pp. 233–248). Washington, DC: American Psychological Association.

National Research Council and Institute of Medicine. (2000). *From neurons to neighborhoods: The science of early childhood development.* Washington, DC: National Academies Press.

National Research Council and Institute of Medicine. (2009). *Preventing mental, emotional, and behavioral disorders among young people: Progress and possibilities.* Washington, DC: National Academies Press.

National Scientific Council on the Developing Child. (2004a). *Children's emotional development is built into the architecture of their brains*: Working paper #2. Retrieved from http://developingchild.harvard.edu/library/reports_and_working_papers/wp2/

National Scientific Council on the Developing Child. (2004b). *Young children develop in an environment of relationships*: Working paper #1. Retrieved from http://developingchild.harvard.edu/library/reports_and_working_papers/wp1/

National Scientific Council on the Developing Child. (2005). *Excessive stress disrupts the architecture of the developing brain:* Working paper #3. Retrieved from http://developingchild.harvard.edu/library/reports_and_working_papers/wp3/

National Scientific Council on the Developing Child. (2007). *The science of early childhood development: Closing the gap between what we know and what we do.* Retrieved from http://developingchild.harvard.edu/index.php/resources/reports_and_working_papers/science_of_early_childhood_development/

National Scientific Council on the Developing Child. (2007). *The timing and quality of early experiences combine to shape brain architecture:* Working paper #5. Retrieved from http://developingchild.harvard.edu/resources/reports_and_working_papers/

National Scientific Council on the Developing Child. (2008). *Mental health problems in early childhood can impair learning and behavior for life:* Working paper #6. Retrieved from http://developingchild.harvard.edu/library/reports_and_working_papers/wp6/

Schoenwald, S. K., & Hoagwood, K. (2001). Effectiveness, transportability, and dissemination of interventions: What matters when? *Psychiatric Services, 52,* 1190–1197.

Society for Research in Child Development. (2009). Report of *healthy development: A summit on young children's mental health.* Partnering with Communication Scientists, Collaborating across Disciplines and Leveraging Impact to Promote Children's Mental Health. Washington, DC: Author. Retrieved from http://www.apa.org/pi/families/Summit-report.aspx

Society for Research in Child Development SRCD. (2010, May 3). *Briefing on the report: Healthy development: The summit on young children's mental health* [Congressional Briefing]. Retrieved from http://www.srcd.org/index.php?option=com_content&task=view&id=415&Itemid=1

Sturmey, P., & Hersen, M. (Eds.). (2012). *Handbook of evidence-based practice in clinical psychology* (Child and adolescent disorders, Vol. I). Ney York, NY: Wiley.

The President's New Freedom Commission on Mental Health. (2003). *Achieving the promise: Transforming mental health care in America.* Final report. (DHHS Publication No. SMA-03-3832). Washington, DC: U.S. Government Printing Office.

Tolan, P. H., & Dodge, K. A. (2005). Children's mental health as a primary care and concern: A system for comprehensive support and service. *American Psychologist, 60,* 601–614.

U.S. Public Health Service. (1999). *Mental health: A report of the Surgeon General.* Rockville, MD: Department of Health and Human Services. Retrieved from http://www.surgeongeneral.gov/library/mentalhealth/home.html

U.S. Public Health Service. (2000). *Report of the Surgeon General's Conference on Children's Mental Health: A national action agenda.* Rockville, MD: Department of Health and Human Services. Retrieved from http://www.ncbi.nlm.nih.gov/books/NBK44233/

Wallace F., Blase, K., Fixsen, D., & Naoom, S. (2008). *What we know about: Implementing the findings of research: Bridging the gap between knowledge and practice.* Educational Research Service.

Wandersman, A., Duffy, J., Flaspohler, P., Noonon, R., Lubell, K., Stillman, L., et al. (2008). Bridging the gap between prevention research and practice: The interactive systems framework for dissemination and implementation. *American Journal of Community Psychology, 41,* 171–181. doi:10.1007/s10464-008-9174-z.

Welch-Ross, M., & Fasig, L. (Eds.). (2007). *Handbook on communicating and disseminating behavioral science.* Thousand Oaks, CA: Sage.

Yoshikawa, H., Aber, J. L., & Beardslee, W. R. (2012). The effects of poverty on the mental, emotional, and behavioral health of children and youth: Implications for prevention. *American Psychologist, 67,* 272–284.

Chapter 4
Health Reform: A Bridge to Health Equity

Daniel E. Dawes

Disparities in Health Status and Health Care Among Vulnerable Populations

Racial and ethnic minorities and other vulnerable populations have long experienced severe and pervasive disparities in health status and outcomes, and faced barriers to obtaining quality health care and public health services. This is especially evident in behavioral health. According to several ground-breaking reports, African Americans, Hispanics, American Indians/Alaska Natives, Asian/Pacific Islander Americans, and lesbian, gay, bisexual, and transgender (LGBT) individuals are particularly at risk for mental illness, substance use, and other chronic conditions (Institute of Medicine, 2002, 2011; U.S. Department of Health and Human Services, 2001).

Racial and ethnic minorities and lower socioeconomic status children experience a greater burden from mental illness than the general population (U.S. Department of Health and Human Services, 2001), report more severe symptoms and experience more persistent disorders than other groups (Breslau et al., 2006; U.S. Department of Health and Human Services, 2001; Williams et al., 2007). Consider for example:

- Lower socioeconomic status children are more likely to receive a diagnosis of attention deficit hyperactivity disorder (Agency for Healthcare Research and Quality, 2012).
- The suicide rate among American Indians and Alaska Natives is 50 % higher than the national average (U.S. Department of Health and Human Services, 2001).

D.E. Dawes, J.D. (✉)
National Working Group on Health Disparities and Health Reform, Washington, DC, USA
e-mail: daniel.dawes@gmail.com

A. McDonald Culp (ed.), *Child and Family Advocacy: Bridging the Gaps Between Research, Practice, and Policy*, Issues in Clinical Child Psychology,
DOI 10.1007/978-1-4614-7456-2_4, © Springer Science+Business Media New York 2013

- African Americans are 30 % more likely to report having serious psychological distress than Caucasians (Center for Disease Control, 2007).
- Latino/Hispanic youth experience disproportionately more anxiety-related and delinquency problem behaviors, depression, and substance use than Caucasian youth (U.S. Department of Health and Human Services, 1999).
- Asian women have the highest suicide rate of all women over age 65 (U.S. Department of Health and Human Services, 2001).
- Racial and ethnic minorities and other lower socioeconomic status children and adolescents experience significantly higher rates of obesity among U.S. children and adolescents (Center for Disease Control, 2012a, 2012b), which has been shown to lead to bullying and behavioral health problems (Janssen, Craig, Boyce, & Pickett, 2004).

Lesbian, gay, and bisexual individuals also experience significant behavioral health disparities. They are approximately two and a half times more likely than heterosexuals to have a mental health disorder in their lifetime (Cochran, Sullivan, & Mays, 2003). Moreover, according to the Institute of Medicine's report, *The Health of Lesbian, Gay, Bisexual, and Transgender People* (2011), LGBT youth may exhibit higher rates of depression, substance use, and attempted suicide than heterosexual youth (Institute of Medicine, 2011).

In addition to experiencing behavioral health disparities, vulnerable populations have also endured critical health care disparities. Since 2003, the Agency for Healthcare Research and Quality has published annual reports tracking the disparities in health care and the quality of health services across the United States. These reports have consistently documented and confirmed that although there has been significant improvement in health care quality over the years, there has not been similar success in reducing disparities in health care (Agency for Healthcare Research and Quality, 2011a, 2011b). This assessment is bolstered by the fact that behavioral health services meet the needs of only 13 % of racial and ethnic minority children and youth (Stagman & Cooper, 2010). Despite the fact that minorities are less likely to receive mental health services, when they do access services, those services tend to be ineffective and of low quality (Cooper et al., 2008; U.S. Department of Health and Human Services, 2003). Another example of health care disparities include people with severe mental illness experiencing higher mortality rates—dying 25 years earlier than the general population, oftentimes due to treatable medical conditions (National Alliance on Mental Illness, 2008; National Association of State Mental Health Program Directors, 2008).

These statistics provide only a sketch of a problem that is complex and arcane, especially when the social[1] and physical determinants of health are considered.

---

[1]Social determinants of health are conditions, in which people are born, live, learn, work, play, worship, and age that impact health status and quality of life such as safe housing, fresh and healthy foods, quality education, transportation, and exposure to crime. Physical determinants of health include the natural environment such as green space, built environment such as buildings, sidewalks, and bike lanes, and exposure to toxic substances. (Center for Disease Control—Healthy People 2020).

Indeed, the health disparities confronting other vulnerable populations are many and varied. Nevertheless, vulnerable populations may experience symptoms that are undiagnosed, under-diagnosed, or misdiagnosed for cultural, linguistic, or historical reasons. For racial and ethnic minorities alone, this equates to approximately 83,000 racial and ethnic minorities dying (U.S. Department of Health and Human Services, 2009) and over $60 billion in direct healthcare expenditures in the United States each year (LaVeist, Gaskin, & Richard, 2009). Overall, the economic burden of racial and ethnic health disparities in the United States equates to $300 billion in direct and indirect costs annually (LaVeist et al., 2009).

Solutions to Health Care Disparities

Elevating Health Equity Across Government Agencies

Eliminating disparities in behavioral health status and health care is essential to improving health outcomes and services to underserved children, youth, and families. The lack of attention to the behavioral health needs of racial and ethnic minorities, LGBT individuals, people with disabilities, and other vulnerable populations in federal and state policies, as well as the inadequate provision of culturally competent behavioral health care in these communities, demonstrates a clear need for encouraging collaboration and finding ways to close the gap in health status and health care. Therefore, one solution is to promote and elevate minority health and health equity across federal agencies responsible for developing and implementing health policies.

Instituting a More Robust Data Collection and Reporting System

There is inconsistency in the collection, documentation, examination, and utilization of demographic data throughout the healthcare and public health systems, which means there is no comprehensive or interoperable system in place to accurately track disparities in health status and health care as well as gauge the level of health care and preventive services vulnerable populations are receiving (Institute of Medicine, 2009). If there is no accurate and granular demographic data, then it is difficult to identify and track the health conditions and inequities that vulnerable populations experience disproportionately, and it is difficult to develop culturally and linguistically effective interventions and solutions for tackling these disparities (Institute of Medicine, 2009). In addition, failure to collect accurate data on vulnerable individuals means that it is more difficult to ensure access to preventive services, quality health services, and appropriate treatments (American Psychological

Association, 2009). Therefore, another solution to reducing and eliminating health disparities is to improve standards for the collection of data as well as improve and expand data collection and reporting efforts.

Enhancing Behavioral Health Disparities Research

The rates of mental health, behavioral health, and substance use disorders are not adequately studied in many racial and ethnic minority groups, most notably American Indians, Alaska Natives, Asian Americans, Native Hawaiians, and Pacific Islanders, resulting in a scarcity of quality research (U.S. Department of Health and Human Services, 2001, 2012). Epidemiological studies often fail to include data on vulnerable, high-risk subgroups such as persons who are exposed to violence, or who are homeless, incarcerated, institutionalized, or in foster care (Williams et al., 2007). Moreover, studies examining issues impacting LGBT individuals have failed to adequately include adolescents as well as bisexual and transgender individuals (Institute of Medicine, 2011). This means diagnostic criteria developed with one particular group may not be directly applicable to other groups, such that instruments of assessment and diagnosis may be less appropriately applied in different groups (Low & Hardy, 2007). Therefore, in order to understand the complex issues and challenges to reducing health disparities, more comprehensive research studies that target health disparities have to be conducted.

Prevention, Early Intervention, and Promotion of Wellness to Address Health Disparities

Individuals who are homeless, incarcerated, or institutionalized experience higher rates of mental health, behavioral health, and substance use disorders (Breakey et al., 1989; Koegel, Burnam, & Farr, 1988; Teplin, 1990; Vernez, Burnam, McGlynn, Trude, & Mittman, 1988). African Americans and Hispanics are over-represented in these high-risk populations (U.S. Department of Health and Human Services, 2001). For instance, although Hispanic girls ages 12–17 are at higher risk for suicide than other youths, only 32 % of Hispanic girls at risk for suicide received mental health treatment (Substance Abuse and Mental Health Services Administration, 2003). Recognizing the critical need to invest in prevention, early intervention, and public health programs to decrease the escalating rates of chronic diseases and health disparities, as well as the costs associated with these conditions, federal, state, and local policies are needed to support behavioral health and public health activities, including immunizations, screenings, testing, and various public health programs targeting disparities.

Integrated Care and Quality Improvement to Reduce Health Disparities

Disparities are observed in most aspects of health care, including care for chronic conditions such as mental health disorders and substance use, HIV/AIDS, cancer, diabetes, heart disease, respiratory diseases, and end-stage renal disease (Agency for Healthcare Research and Quality, 2006). Several barriers deter people from receiving preventative services and treatment, including cost, fragmentation of services, lack of availability of services, and societal stigma toward mental illness. Additional barriers deterring vulnerable populations, include mistrust/fear of treatment, racism and discrimination, differences in communication (U.S. Department of Health and Human Services, 2001), and lack of culturally and linguistically appropriate services (Swartz et al., 1998).

Many racial and ethnic individuals are more likely to experience poor communication and more difficulties interacting with their health care providers, as well as difficulty accessing health care information (Agency for Healthcare Research and Quality, 2004). There is also a greater unmet need for alcoholism and substance use treatment as well as mental health care among African Americans and Latinos relative to Caucasians (Wells, Klap, Koike, & Sherbourne, 2001). Consequently, policies are needed that recognize the importance of improving the coordination and integration of primary and behavioral health services for vulnerable populations and instituting programs that address the quality and underlying disparities of these services.

Increasing the Cultural and Linguistic Competence[2] of Health Professionals

As a result of the diversity in their symptoms, racial and ethnic minorities and other vulnerable populations may have mental health conditions that do not correspond directly to general categories of illness and mental disorders, which require knowledgeable and culturally competent mental and behavioral health professionals (American Psychological Association, 2009). When services take culture into account and address the culture of the community being served, there is an increase in service utilization and a decrease in early termination of treatment (American Psychological Association, 2009). Therefore, another solution to the

---

[2]Cultural competence "refers to awareness of unique, and defining characteristics of the populations for which health professionals provide care…. [and] entails understanding the importance of social and cultural influence on patients' health beliefs and behaviors." Some scholars have used cultural responsiveness, cultural sensitivity, or cultural humility, but "cultural competence moves beyond sensitivity or awareness to action" (Harvard Catalyst, 2010, Cultural competence in research, Boston, MA www.mfdp.med.harvard.edu.

comprehensive strategy of reducing health disparities among vulnerable populations is to develop model curricula, guidelines, and other programs aimed at increasing the cultural and linguistic competence of health professionals as well as promoting interdisciplinary collaboration among the health professions.

Goals of the Advocacy Effort

During 2008 when it became apparent that discussions were taking place around health reform, health equity advocates took action to inform policymakers about the impact of health disparities in the United States. In February of 2009, when serious negotiations over several health reform proposals were taking place in key committees[3] of the House and Senate, advocates realized that this was a rare opportunity to advance a health equity agenda and address health disparities once and for all in a more comprehensive manner. However, health equity advocacy coalitions and organizations were not well-coordinated or consistent in their legislative requests. Some health equity advocates were only focused on health care quality improvement issues, some focused primarily on data collection and reporting issues, and others were focused primarily on health workforce development issues, prevention and wellness issues, or language access issues. This caused much consternation on Capitol Hill because the drafters of the health reform legislative proposals were not sure who to seek counsel from and whose priorities to include.

The disorganization found among health equity advocates attenuated the argument for including robust health equity-related provisions in health reform legislation. Drafters of the health reform bills wanted assurance that any language submitted by health equity advocates had been properly vetted and agreed upon by the majority of advocates. Consequently, the need to unite and mobilize, as well as streamline efforts, and create a one-stop shop for information sharing and collaboration, became increasingly important if health equity advocates wanted to be effective in realizing their goals.

In March 2009, when it was clear that health disparities was not being addressed at all during health reform negotiations, a group of 35 organizations, associations, and coalitions banded together. The result of this mobilization and grassroots effort was the formation of the *National Working Group on Health Disparities and Health Reform* convened by the American Psychological Association, with the overarching goal of advancing a health equity agenda and ensuring that health reform legislation in the House and Senate included provisions to address health disparities. Related targeted goals included: (1) developing a robust advocacy strategy, (2) drafting model legislative language and incorporating that in health reform proposals, (3) monitoring and analyzing any legislative proposals to ensure that they included

---

[3] Senate Health, Education, Labor, and Pensions Committee, Senate Finance Committee, House Energy and Commerce Committee, House Ways and Means Committee, and House Education and Labor Committee.

health equity-related provisions, and (4) monitoring the implementation of provisions aimed at addressing disparities in health status and health care through prevention and wellness programs, integrated care, quality measure development, and other programs and initiatives.

Members of the *National Working Group on Health Disparities and Health Reform* worked closely with the Congressional Black Caucus Health Braintrust (CBCHB) under the leadership of Congresswoman Donna M. Christensen, as well as with the Congressional Hispanic Caucus (CHC), and the Congressional Asian Pacific American Caucus (CAPAC), which collectively make up the TriCaucus. The group also worked closely with the Congressional Native American Caucus, The White House, and key committees in Congress to negotiate these provisions. By the beginning of April 2009, the group grew to more than 250 organizations, associations, and coalitions across the country representing diverse stakeholders, including consumers, racial and ethnic minorities, people with disabilities, children, women, LGBT individuals, community health centers, hospitals and other healthcare entities, health professionals, insurers, and businesses.

Disparities in health status and health care are a critical matter, but have been terribly underrated—treated as a secondary issue in health policy. This was evident during health reform despite the group's efforts to educate policymakers about the number of individuals who die each year as a result of racial and ethnic disparities and the tremendous impact the costs of these disparities have on the United States. Nevertheless, the group, finding strength in numbers and harnessing the power of collaboration, pushed forward arguing that it was imperative for policymakers to acknowledge the severity of the problem and enact health reforms to curb them.

As months went by and opponents of health reform started to increase their advocacy efforts against the bill, the health equity advocates frequently and consistently argued that the goal of eliminating health disparities should be a key component of health reform since it will improve health status, save lives, and increase longevity and quality of life for the nation's most vulnerable populations. The group's tag line became: *Health Reform should be reform for all, not reform for some*! The group ardently voiced support for the notion that cost-savings would be realized not only by improving the health of populations and communities that experience health disparities and barriers to health care and public health services, but by reducing the costs resulting from the disproportionate burden of disease faced by these populations.

Health equity advocates urged lawmakers and the Obama administration to ensure that any final comprehensive health reform legislation included provisions to address health inequities and to reduce and eliminate health care disparities. The group advocated for, at a minimum, the inclusion of several health equity-related priorities, including:

1. *High quality, affordable health care coverage must be available to everyone, particularly populations and communities that have traditionally suffered health disparities and barriers to coverage.* Coverage must include prevention, wellness, chronic disease management, behavioral health, and support services, such as social work and language services.

2. Health insurance coverage alone does not ensure access to health services. *A full range of culturally and linguistically appropriate health care and public health services must be available in every community and accessible to all.* A greater investment is necessary to expand grants and demonstration projects to support community-based programs designed to reduce health disparities and barriers to health services through education and outreach, health promotion and disease prevention activities, and health literacy education and services. In addition, reimbursement for Medicaid, the Children's Health Insurance Program (CHIP) or any other subsidized public insurance plans must be adequate to ensure a sufficient pool of providers willing to treat beneficiaries.

3. *Every community must have the health workforce and infrastructure necessary to provide a full range of health care and public health services.* A greater investment must be made in programs under Title VII and VIII of the Public Health Service Act, the National Health Service Corps, AIDS Education and Training Centers, Minority Fellowship Program, and Graduate Medical Education programs to strengthen the recruitment, retention, training, and continuing education of primary care, behavioral health, public health, and other health professionals, and increase their diversity, distribution, cultural competence, and knowledge of treating the unique needs of different populations. Support must also be provided to sustain and expand institutions that have traditionally served health disparity populations, such as community health centers and public hospitals.

4. *All efforts to reduce health disparities and barriers to quality health services require better data.* Federal, state, and local governments and health care and public health providers must be required to support the collection and accurate reporting of standardized demographic data on patients and the community, and be provided the resources to do so. Data and findings should be disseminated to inform policy decisions and assist in efforts to eliminate health disparities.

5. *Recognition of diversity is critical to improving health care quality.* Quality improvement and pay-for-performance policies must take into account the needs and challenges of populations and communities that have traditionally suffered health disparities and barriers to health services, and reward efforts that reduce disparities and barriers. Resources should be provided to design and implement evidence-based quality improvement strategies, such as the medical/health home model, to eliminate disparities and barriers to health care delivery. Studies must be done to ensure that efforts to improve quality of care for the general population do not inadvertently exacerbate health disparities.

Advocacy Action Steps

Once health equity advocates formed a working group on health disparities and health reform, which ultimately included over 300 national organizations, associations, and coalitions, they immediately went to work developing and implementing a flexible advocacy strategy around communications and media, grassroots, and outreach to Congress and the Obama Administration, including TriCaucus members. This flexible approach allowed group members to sequentially and simultaneously develop and implement certain components of the advocacy strategy depending on various existing and emerging factors. Overall, the convening of this group resulted in enhanced cooperation, efficient and more targeted use of resources to overcome challenges and leverage opportunities, and the creation and execution of a more effective strategy to inform members of Congress and the Obama Administration about health disparities and their impact on the health status and care of vulnerable populations as well as the cost burden to the United States.

The first step in organizing the group and ensuring better facilitation of information dissemination among group members internally was to create a master list of all organizations, associations, and coalitions committed to the inclusion of health equity provisions in health reform. Each organization was urged to specify their areas of expertise around health disparities in regard to quality improvement, behavioral health, prevention and public health, research, and workforce development so that congressional members and staff could more easily identify experts when needed to give briefings or share information on specific health equity issues.

The second action step was to identify and recruit external champions of health equity in Congress and the Administration as well as with organizations who had not joined the group yet, including health care, behavioral health, and public health experts in Washington, DC and around the country who could help advance this cause. The intent of this action step was to get health equity included in the larger health reform discussions that were taking place around prevention and wellness, quality improvement, workforce development, insurance expansion, and comparative effectiveness research. For many health equity advocates, addressing health disparities elimination as a singular issue was worrisome because of the belief that it would not receive enough attention to get included in a larger health reform proposal or even if it was included in a larger health reform proposal, opponents of health equity would be able to more easily strike the health equity-related provisions.

The third action step of the strategy was to collect and share stories about different populations that were experiencing inequities in health care and public health. One story included the fate of a 49-year-old African American woman, Esmin Green. Ms. Green had a serious mental illness (SMI) and experienced disparate treatment in a hospital emergency room while waiting there for 24 h for mental health care. Paramedics had brought her to the hospital emergency room on the morning of June 18, 2008. Hospital records stated that she was exhibiting agitation and psychosis and was involuntarily admitted after refusing health care. During the first week of July, major news media aired a video showing Ms. Green sitting in a waiting room at a hospital in New York for nearly 24 h when she collapsed from her chair. Once she collapsed, neither fellow patients nor the hospital's staff moved to help her, even as she moved her legs on the floor trying to get up. Two security guards and a member of the hospital's medical staff can be seen on the video, briefly stopping to look at Ms. Green before walking away. She stopped moving about

30 min after falling and was dead when a nurse finally examined her another 30 min after that. Advocates used this story to serve as a wake-up call and show that mental health and mental health care disparities are real, as well as to highlight the lack of compassion toward individuals with mental health problems and the need for more culturally competent health professionals.

After collecting stories from across the country, health equity advocates then developed targeted messaging to respective congressional members and committees. In the fourth action step of the strategy, advocates initiated a postcard campaign and drafted letters to congressional leadership explaining the importance of addressing health disparities and urging them to support the inclusion of health equity-related provisions in health reform legislation. These postcards and sign-on letters were intended for each organization, association, or coalition to lend their name as a signatory and increase attention to the issue of health disparities. In so doing, advocates hoped this would help to ensure legislative responsiveness to this issue. One goal for these postcards and letters was to demonstrate the tremendous support for a health equity agenda that advocates had created and sustained so that they could not be ignored. A second goal was to provide leverage to congressional members and staff to move forward with a health equity agenda in health reform. Each letter had 250–300-plus national, regional, and local organizations, associations, and coalitions signed on, and thousands of postcards delivered to health champions in Congress.

After the foundation had been laid in terms of identifying and recruiting internal and external health equity champions, collecting compelling health equity stories to share with policymakers, and writing to Congress about the importance of including a health equity agenda in health reform, health equity advocates then executed their fifth action step, which involved developing health equity principles, talking points, legislative outlines, and legislative language to share with the key congressional committees charged with drafting the health reform bill. Once these items were vetted by members of the group, health equity advocates then proceeded to tirelessly advocate for their inclusion in congressional white papers and legislative proposals. The group also developed a simple website to house and categorize, by specific health disparity population, all materials that were created to facilitate use of stakeholder recommendations and to serve as an additional resource for congressional staff when crafting health reform legislation.[4]

The sixth action step by the group involved holding congressional meetings and briefings to educate members of Congress about this critical issue and to serve as a reminder that health equity advocates were persistent and adamant about the inclusion of robust provisions in health reform to address health disparities. These meetings focused on reaching out to members of key committees in Congress, which had jurisdiction over the health reform bills. As these Hill visits were being organized, members of the group found it helpful to establish a listserv to communicate

---

[4] Several of the materials have been archived on the National Health Law Program's website www.healthlaw.org and may be accessed by clicking on the tab "Issues" and then clicking on the tab "Health Disparities."

meetings that were secured, in case individual organizations were interested in meeting with a particular member of Congress or had members of their own organizations who were constituents of the representative or senator. The group also sought the placement of health disparities experts on panels during congressional hearings and during meetings on health reform to ensure that this issue would continue to receive maximum attention.

During health reform negotiations, the *National Working Group on Health Disparities and Health Reform* underscored the fact that it had been almost 10 years since President Bill Clinton signed into law the *Minority Health and Health Disparities Research and Education Act of* 2000 (Pub.L. 106-525, 114 Stat. 2495), a critical, but limited law on health disparities research, and that the United States could not afford to wait another 10 years to get more comprehensive legislation around health equity passed.

The health equity provisions that advocates secured in health reform endured multiple attacks from those opposed to health equity or just simply ignorant about these issues. For several months, the group made the argument that including health equity provisions in health reform would result in greatly improved health and thousands of lives saved. Advocates thought this moral argument would be sufficient to ensure the inclusion of health disparities provisions—and it seemed to resonate with many members of Congress and their staff, but then the focus shifted to costs and cost-savings. Obviously, it was important for the group to react and slightly reframe their message to accommodate this focus and demonstrate the cost burden that health and health care disparities have on our country. That was easier said than done. Up to this point, group members had tried their best to engage in proactive advocacy, but the shift in focus by policymakers forced members of the working group to employ a more reactive advocacy strategy to accommodate this new shift and ensure their continued relevance in the larger debate on health reform.

When congressional staff requested information on the costs of health disparities and the cost-savings that would be realized by reducing these disparities, the group was only able to share two very small studies focusing on Colorado and California. Fortunately, the Joint Center for Political and Economic Studies released a groundbreaking report[5] on the costs of health disparities in our country, which clearly put things into perspective (LaVeist et al., 2009). The numbers were more frightening than many thought. But at least now, health equity advocates were able to convince congressional staff that they needed to address health disparities in health reform.

Unfortunately, demonstrating the cost-savings that would accrue to the United States if it reduced and eliminated health disparities was not enough to convince policymakers for long because the focus for health reform shifted once again. This time, policymakers moved away from calling health reform "comprehensive health reform" to "health insurance reform."

---

[5]From 2003 to 2006 the combined cost of health disparities totaled $1.24 trillion in our country. This report also found that in the same time period, eliminating certain health disparities would have reduced direct health care expenditures by $229.4 billion.

At first, many members of the group thought this was a smart shift—vilifying the insurance companies, but then advocates became very concerned when many government officials started taking a very narrow approach to health reform—primarily discussing health insurance coverage provisions and barely mentioning the other provisions around quality, prevention, and workforce. As a result, health equity advocates argued that health insurance coverage is very important, but addressing it alone would not necessarily equate to access and access would not necessarily equate to quality services, treatment, and better outcomes. The group further argued that they envisioned health reform legislation that ensured equity and accountability, provided individuals with the ability to access comprehensive and culturally and linguistically appropriate health care and public health services, and achieve health outcomes consistent with the rest of the population.

After fighting to make sure that other health equity provisions remained a priority during this shift to "health insurance reform," advocates endured additional battles and had to make sure that they remained diligent in their advocacy in order to keep the health equity provisions of the bill intact.

Outcome and Next Steps

In March 2010, Congress passed and President Barack Obama signed into law, two pieces of legislation, which collectively make up the health reform law—the *Patient Protection and Affordable Care Act* (Pub.L. 111-148) and the *Health Care and Education Reconciliation Act of* 2010 (Pub.L. 111-152). This law incorporates numerous health equity-related provisions that will serve as a bridge to effectively and efficiently address health disparities and achieve health equity. In general, the efforts of this working group on health disparities and health reform were hugely successful. It is a testament to the power of collaboration and determination to address, in a more comprehensive manner, pervasive health disparities among vulnerable populations.

Although there are laws in place that address discrimination in healthcare access, disparate treatment between protected classes in health services, and parity between mental/substance use benefits and medical/surgical benefits, no other law prioritizes health equity and the reduction of health disparities like the health reform law. Indeed, this landmark law contains substantive provisions, which address a critical issue in health status and health care—eliminating the root causes of disparities among vulnerable, underserved, and often marginalized populations, including mental and behavioral health disparities.

Collectively, the health equity-related provisions found in the quality improvement, prevention and wellness, data collection, comparative effectiveness research, workforce development, and health insurance sections are intended to address inequities in a comprehensive manner. However, there is still much work to be done to ensure that the needs of vulnerable populations remain a priority, especially as these provisions are implemented. Federal budget constraints will continue to pressure health care cost reduction, opponents of health equity will try to continue chipping away at the health equity provisions of the law, and there will be additional hurdles to overcome both politically, legally, and administratively. This is especially evident with the United States Supreme Court decision[6] on June 28, 2012 upholding the constitutionality of the health reform law and its provisions aimed at addressing health disparities, but weakening a key aspect of the statute's efforts to expand health insurance coverage to vulnerable populations—the Medicaid expansion provision. The Supreme Court decision prohibits the federal government from conditioning receipt of existing Medicaid funding by states on their expansion of the Medicaid program to include individuals under 133 % of the federal poverty level. This ruling essentially left Medicaid expansion under the health reform law optional for states, which may lead to fewer uninsured or underinsured individuals having access to affordable health insurance coverage.

Consequently, health equity advocates—whether students, faculty members, community leaders, or practicing health professionals—will have to continue to diligently and tirelessly advocate for adequate funding from Congress and the Administration for the many health equity provisions that fall under discretionary funding or to protect programs that received mandatory appropriations under the law. Health equity advocates will have to continue providing sound information and feedback to regulators who are and will be drafting the regulations to implement the law so that health equity and the reduction of disparities remain a priority in health reform. Health equity advocates will have to also make sure they are aware of key advisory groups, commissions, and task forces that were established by the law to ensure proper representation of the issues impacting vulnerable populations. They will have to make sure that they are participating in the development of national strategies relative to health disparities reduction so that their voices are heard. Lastly, advocates will have to keep a watchful eye on political and legal efforts to amend health reform to make sure that these efforts do not weaken the protections secured under the law for the most vulnerable individuals.

As health equity advocates know too well, the improvements and changes to health care and public health systems will not occur overnight, but will take several years to materialize. As Dr. Martin Luther King, Jr. once reminded advocates, "Change does not roll in on the wheels of inevitability, but comes through continuous struggle." The health equity provisions that were secured in the health reform law are only a fraction of the public policies needed to completely eliminate disparities in health status and health care in the United States. There is still much work to be done in developing, strengthening, and implementing public policies that aim to achieve health equity for vulnerable populations.

---

[6]*National Federation of Independent Business v. Sebelius* (11-393).

References

Agency for Healthcare Research and Quality. (2004). *National healthcare disparities report: Summary*. Rockville, MD: Agency for Healthcare Research and Quality. Retrieved August 22, 2011, from http://www.archive.ahrq.gov/qual/nhdr04/nhdr2004.pdf

Agency for Healthcare Research and Quality. (2006). *National healthcare disparities report*. Rockville, MD: Agency for Healthcare Research and Quality. Retrieved August 22, 2011, from http://www.ahrq.gov/qual/nhdr06/nhdr06.htm

Agency for Healthcare Research and Quality. (2011a). *National healthcare disparities report*. Rockville, MD: Agency for Healthcare Research and Quality. Retrieved August 22, 2012, from http://www.ahrq.gov/qual/qrdr11.htm

Agency for Healthcare Research and Quality. (2011b). *National healthcare quality report*. Rockville, MD: Agency for Healthcare Research and Quality. Retrieved August 22, 2012, from http://www.ahrq.gov/qual/qrdr11.htm

Agency for Healthcare Research and Quality. (2012). *Clinician summary: Attention deficit hyperactivity disorder in children and adolescents*. Rockville, MD: Agency for Healthcare Research and Quality. Retrieved September 10, 2012, from http://effectivehealthcare.ahrq.gov/ehc/products/191/1149/adhd_clin_fin_to_post.pdf

American Psychological Association. (2009). *Psychological and behavioral perspectives on health disparities*. Communique. Washington, DC: American Psychological Association.

Breakey, W. R., Fischer, P. J., Kramer, M., Nestadt, G., Romanoski, A. J., Ross, A., et al. (1989). Health and mental health problems of homeless men and women in Baltimore. *Journal of the American Medical Association, 262*, 1352–1357.

Breslau, J., Aguilar-Gaxiola, S., Kendler, K., Maxwell, S., Williams, D., & Kessler, R. (2006). Specifying race-ethnic differences in risk for psychiatric disorder in a USA national sample. *Psychological Medicine, 36*(1), 57–68.

Center for Disease Control (CDC). (2007). Table 61. *Health, United States, 2007 with chartbook on trends in the health of Americans*. Hyattsville, MD: CDC.

Center for Disease Control (CDC). (2012a). National Center for Health Statistics. *Health, United States, 2011: With special feature on socioeconomic status and health*. Hyattsville, MD: CDC. Retrieved May 29, 2012, from http://www.cdc.gov/nchs/data/hus/hus11.pdf#listfigures

Center for Disease Control (CDC). (2012b). *Childhood obesity facts*. Hyattsville, MD: CDC. Retrieved May 29, 2012, from http://www.cdc.gov/obesity/data/childhood.html

Cochran, S., Sullivan, J., & Mays, V. (2003). Prevalence of mental disorders, psychological distress, and mental health services use among lesbian, gay, and bisexual adults in the United States. *Journal of Consulting and Clinical Psychology, 71*, 53–61.

Cooper, J., Aratani, Y., Knitzer, J., Douglas-Hall, A., Masi, R., Banghart, P., et al. (2008). *Unclaimed children revisited: The status of children's mental health policy in the United States*. New York, NY: National Center for Children in Poverty.

Health Care and Education Reconciliation Act of 2010 (Pub.L. 111-152).

Institute of Medicine. (2002). *Unequal treatment: Confronting racial and ethnic disparities in healthcare*. Washington, DC: The National Academies Press.

Institute of Medicine. (2009). *Race, ethnicity, and language data: Standardization for health care quality improvement*. Washington, DC: The National Academies Press.

Institute of Medicine. (2011). *The health of lesbian, gay, bisexual and transgender people: Building a foundation to better health*. Washington, DC: The National Academies Press.

Janssen, I., Craig, W., Boyce, W., & Pickett, W. (2004). Associations between overweight and obesity with bullying behaviors in school-aged children. *Pediatrics, 113*, 1187–1194.

Koegel, P. M., Burnam, A., & Farr, R. K. (1988). The prevalence of specific psychiatric disorders among homeless individual in the inner city of Los Angeles. *Archives of General Psychiatry, 45*, 1085–1093.

LaVeist, T., Gaskin, D., & Richard, P. (2009). *The economic burden of health inequalities in the United States*. Joint center for political and economic studies report, Sept 2009.

Low, N., & Hardy, J. (2007). Psychiatric disorder criteria and their application to research in different racial groups. *BMC Psychiatry, 7*, 1. doi:10.1186/1471-244X-7-1.

Minority Health and Health Disparities Research and Education Act of 2000 (Pub.L. 106-525, 114 Stat. 2495).

National Alliance on Mental Illness. (2008). *Mental illness: Facts and numbers.* Arlington, VA: National Alliance on Mental Illness. Retrieved September 7, 2012, from http://www.nami.org/ Template.cfm?Section=About_Mental_Illness&Template=/ContentManagement/ ContentDisplay.cfm&ContentID=53155

National Association of State Mental Health Program Directors. (2008). *Measurement of health status for people with serious mental illnesses.* Alexandria, VA: National Association of State Mental Health Program Directors. Retrieved September 7, 2012, from http://www.nasmhpd. org/docs/publications/MDCdocs/NASMHPD%20Medical%20Directors%20Health%20 Indicators%20Report%2011-19-08.pdf

National Federation of Independent Business v. Sebelius (11-393)

Patient Protection and Affordable Care Act (Pub.L. 111-148).

Stagman, S., & Cooper, J. (2010). *Children's mental health: What every policymaker should know.* New York, NY: National Center for Children in Poverty.

Substance Abuse and Mental Health Services Administration (SAMHSA). (2003). *Risk of suicide among Hispanic females aged 12 to 17.* National household survey on drug abuse report. Rockville, MD: Substance Abuse and Mental Health Services Administration. Retrieved September 1, 2011, from http://www.oas.samhsa.gov/2k3/LatinaSuicide/LatinaSuicide.htm

Swartz, M., Wagner, R., Swanson, J., Burns, B., George, L., & Padgett, D. (1998). Administrative update: Utilization of services. *Community Mental Health Journal, 34*(2), 133–144.

Teplin, L. A. (1990). The prevalence of severe mental disorder among male urban jail detainees: Comparison with the epidemiologic catchment area program. *American Journal of Public Health, 80*, 663–669.

U.S. Department of Health and Human Services (HHS), Public Health Service, & Office of the Surgeon General. (1999). *Mental health: A report of the surgeon general.* Rockville, MD: Department of Health and Human Services, U.S. Public Health Service.

U.S. Department of Health and Human Services (HHS), Public Health Service, & Office of the Surgeon General. (2001). *Mental health: Culture, race and ethnicity—A supplement to mental health: A report of the surgeon general.* Rockville, MD: U.S. Department of Health and Human Services, Substance Abuse and Mental Health Services Administration, Center for Mental Health Services.

U.S. Department of Health and Human Services (HHS), & New Freedom Commission on Mental Health. (2003). *Achieving the promise: Transforming mental health care in America—Final report.* Rockville, MD: New Freedom Commission on Mental Health.

U.S. Department of Health and Human Services (HHS), Advisory Committee on Minority Health, Office of Minority Health. (2009). *Ensuring that health care reform will meet the health care needs of minority communities and eliminate health disparities: A statement of principles and recommendations.* Rockville, MD: Office of Minority Health. Retrieved September 10, 2011, from http://minorityhealth.hhs.gov/Assets/pdf/Checked/1/ACMH_HealthCareAccessReport.pdf

U.S. Department of Health and Human Services (HHS), Office of Minority Health. (2012). *Native Hawaiian/other Pacific Islander profile.* Rockville, MD: U.S. Department of Health and Human Services. Retrieved May 29, 2012, from http://minorityhealth.hhs.gov/templates/content.aspx?lvl=3&lvlID=4&ID=8593

Vernez, G. M., Burnam, M. A., McGlynn, E. A., Trude, S., & Mittman, B. (1988). *Review of California's program for the homeless mentally ill disabled* (Report no. R3631-CDMH). Santa Monica, CA: RAND.

Wells, K., Klap, R., Koike, A., & Sherbourne, C. (2001). Ethnic disparities in unmet need for alcoholism, drug abuse, and mental health care. *The American Journal of Psychiatry, 158*, 2027–2032.

Williams, D., Gonzalez, H., Neighbors, H., Nesse, R., Abelson, J., Sweetman, J., et al. (2007). Prevalence and distribution of major depressive disorder in African Americans, Caribbean Blacks, and Non-Hispanic Whites: Results from the National Survey of American Life. *Archives of General Psychiatry, 64*, 305–315.

Chapter 5
Child Maltreatment Prevention

Cindy L. Miller-Perrin and Sharon G. Portwood

Child maltreatment is a pervasive problem that affects families and communities in the United States and throughout the world. Most credit the "discovery" of child maltreatment to Henry Kempe, a physician from Colorado, who in 1962 published an article in the *Journal of the American Medical Association* on the "battered child syndrome" (Kempe, Silverman, Steele, Droegemueller, & Silver, 1962). Since the publication of Kempe's seminal article, progress in the field has been rapid, mobilized by the efforts of many, including grassroots organizations, mental health professionals, university researchers, lawmakers, medical personnel, social service professionals, and criminal justice workers. These efforts have contributed significantly to furthering our understanding of child maltreatment and to the myriad ways that families and professionals can work together to prevent abuse and neglect. This chapter provides a brief overview of the problem of child maltreatment and describes successful research-based prevention strategies. The chapter also describes specific advocacy efforts and action steps and outcomes that should provide a critical component to alleviating the problem of child maltreatment.

C.L. Miller-Perrin, Ph.D. (✉)
Department of Psychology, Social Science Division, Pepperdine University,
Malibu, CA, USA
e-mail: Cindy.Perrin@pepperdine.edu

S.G. Portwood, J.D., Ph.D.
Department of Public Health Sciences, University of North Carolina at Charlotte,
Charlotte, NC, USA

A. McDonald Culp (ed.), *Child and Family Advocacy: Bridging the Gaps Between Research, Practice, and Policy*, Issues in Clinical Child Psychology,
DOI 10.1007/978-1-4614-7456-2_5, © Springer Science+Business Media New York 2013

Nature and Scope of the Problem

Definitions of Child Maltreatment

The 1974 Child Abuse Prevention and Treatment Act (CAPTA) defined child mal-treatment as "Any recent act or failure to act on the part of a parent or caretaker which results in death, serious physical or emotional harm, sexual abuse or exploita-tion; or an act or failure to act which presents an imminent risk of serious harm" (U.S. DHHS, 2011, p. vii). CAPTA was most recently reauthorized in 2010, retain-ing this definition which serves as a foundation for each US State to determine its own definitions of child abuse and neglect (U.S. DHHS, 2010).

The lack of standard definitions of child maltreatment across the United States contributes to significant difficulties in tracking, reporting, and responding to the problem of child maltreatment. In its 2008 document, *Child Maltreatment Surveillance: Uniform Definitions for Public Health and Recommended Data Elements*, the Centers for Disease Control and Prevention (CDC), created uniform definitions for each of the four major types of child maltreatment in an effort to decrease this definitional ambi-guity (Leeb, Paulozzi, Melanson, Simon, & Arias, 2008). The CDC defines three acts of commission (physical abuse, sexual abuse, psychological abuse) and one act of omission (neglect) as follows (Leeb et al., 2008, p. 11):

- Physical Abuse: The intentional use of physical force against a child that results in, or has the potential to result in, physical injury.
- Sexual Abuse: Any completed or attempted (non-completed) sexual act, sexual contact with, or exploitation (i.e., noncontact sexual interaction) of a child by a caregiver.
- Psychological Abuse: Intentional caregiver behavior (i.e., act of commission) that conveys to a child that he/she is worthless, flawed, unloved, unwanted, endangered, or valued only in meeting another's needs. Psychologically abusive behaviors may include blaming, belittling, degrading, intimidating, terrorizing, isolating, restraining, confining, corrupting, exploiting, spurning, or otherwise behaving in a manner that is harmful, potentially harmful, or insensitive to the child's developmental needs, or can potentially damage the child psychologi-cally or emotionally.
- Neglect: Failure by a caregiver to meet a child's basic physical, emotional, medi-cal/dental, or educational needs—or combination thereof.

Although delineating the four major types of child maltreatment reduces defini-tional ambiguity, it is important to note that there is considerable overlap among the various forms of child maltreatment (Finkelhor, 2008; Stevens, Ruggiero, Kilpatrick, Resnick, & Saunders, 2005). Findings from the National Survey of Adolescents, for example, indicated that approximately 17 % of the 831 adolescents sampled were multiply victimized, experiencing both sexual and physical assault (Stevens et al., 2005). Although largely unrecognized until relatively recently, child maltreatment experts are increasingly focusing on the importance of examining the interrelation-ships among different forms of child maltreatment (e.g., Finkelhor, 2008).

Incidence and Prevalence of Child Maltreatment

There are two primary sources of information about the extent of child maltreatment: *incidence studies* which examine official estimates of the number of new cases of child maltreatment occurring within a specific time period, and *prevalence studies* which examine the proportion of a population that reports a history of childhood maltreatment. The most often cited official statistics on child maltreatment come from the National Child Abuse and Neglect Data System (NCANDS) and the National Incidence Study (NIS).

NCANDS is a federally sponsored data collection system that disseminates information annually about child abuse and neglect reports received across the United States. Now in its 21st edition, *Child Maltreatment 2010* includes state-level data on the number of child abuse and neglect reports received by state Child Protective Services (CPS) agencies (U.S. DHHS, 2011). According to the most recent report, CPS agencies across the United States received approximately three million reports of child maltreatment (including physical and sexual abuse, neglect, and psychological maltreatment) in 2010. Of these reports, approximately 436,000 were substantiated (i.e., a case in which CPS has investigated a report and concluded that a "preponderance of evidence" indicates that abuse occurred), which converts to a rate of approximately 9 out of every 1,000 children. Approximately 18 % of these cases were specific instances of physical abuse, 78 % were instances of neglect, 9 % were instances of sexual abuse, and 8 % were instances of psychological maltreatment. Data from the same survey also indicate that in 2010, approximately 1,560 children died as a result of child abuse and neglect with approximately 23 % of those deaths a result of physical abuse exclusively, 37 % the result of neglect exclusively, and 41 % the result of some combination of maltreatment types (U.S. DHHS, 2011).

Although incidence data from these sources are invaluable in estimating the extent of child maltreatment in the United States, these data are not without their limitations. Official statistics such as those provided by NCANDS, for example, reflect only those cases of child maltreatment reported to CPS. In addition, the definitions of child maltreatment, investigative procedures, and data collection procedures are determined at the state level, which all vary from agency to agency (U.S. DHHS, 2010). The NIS data improves upon the limitations of the NCANDS data by employing uniform definitions of abuse and including a relatively broad definition of abuse designed to measure not only reports to CPS agencies but also the number of cases of child maltreatment reported to police and sheriff's departments, schools and day care centers, hospitals, and other mental health and social service agencies. Table 5.1 shows the trends in incidence rates across NIS studies over the past several years.

The second NIS (NIS-2) found that nearly one million children were reported for child maltreatment in 1986, for a rate of 14.8 per 1,000 children in the United States (Sedlak, 1990). NIS-3, which was published in 1996, found that the number of reported cases of child maltreatment increased significantly between 1986 and 1993, with over 1.5 million children reported for child maltreatment in 1993 (a rate of 23.1 per 1,000 children) (Sedlak & Broadhurst, 1996). The most recent National

Table 5.1 Rate per 1,000 children meeting harm standard for child maltreatment in NIS studies

Type of maltreatment	NIS-2 (1986)	NIS-3 (1993)	NIS-4 (2005/2006)
All forms of maltreatment	14.8	23.1	17.1
Physical abuse	4.3	5.7	4.4
Sexual abuse	1.9	3.2	1.8
Emotional/psychological abuse	2.5	3.0	2.0
Child neglect	7.5	13.1	10.5

Incidence Study, NIS-4, was published in 2010 and shows an overall decrease in the general incidence of child maltreatment with approximately 1.3 million children reported for maltreatment for a rate of 17.1 per 1,000 children (Sedlak et al., 2010). These figures indicate a 29 % decline since NIS-2 which includes reductions in rates of physical abuse, sexual abuse, and emotional abuse in recent years, but not in child neglect. Similar patterns of decline have been observed in cases of physical and sexual abuse reported to CPS (U.S. DHHS, 2010).

The prevalence of child maltreatment has also been examined through the use of self-report surveys which ask respondents about their experiences as victims of child maltreatment. Self-report surveys include the obvious advantage that they provide access to information about maltreatment that is not reported to official agencies. One such survey is the Juvenile Victimization Questionnaire, recently developed by Finkelhor et al. (Finkelhor, Ormrod, Turner, & Hamby, 2005a, 2005b; Finkelhor, Turner, Ormrod, & Hamby, 2009). The survey is administered via telephone to obtain information on a variety of forms of childhood victimization either directly from youth (ages 10–17) or indirectly from a parent or other adult caretaker for younger children (ages 0–9). The most recent survey was administered in 2008 to a large nationally representative sample of 4,549 American children and findings indicated that approximately 10 % of the youth and parents surveyed reported some experience of child maltreatment (i.e., physical, psychological/emotional, neglect, or sexual) in the previous year and nearly 19 % at some point during their lifetime (Finkelhor et al., 2009).

The Financial Costs of Child Maltreatment

The costs of child maltreatment in terms of its negative effects on the psychological functioning of victims, the detrimental impact on families, and the serious repercussions for the child welfare system have long been recognized. Only recently, however, has the financial burden associated with child maltreatment been estimated. The financial costs of child maltreatment include expenses associated with mental and physical health care, special education, loss in productivity, and the resources of law enforcement, child welfare, and the criminal justice system (Fanga, Brown, Florence, & Mercy, 2012).

The first estimates of the financial burden associated with child maltreatment in the United States were provided by Prevent Child Abuse America in 2003 which estimated the annual cost at $94 billion (as cited in Wang & Holton, 2007). More recently, Fanga et al. (2012) estimated the cost of child maltreatment using the best available secondary data to develop cost per case estimates. These researchers concluded that the estimated average lifetime cost per child maltreatment death is approximately $1.3 million, most of which is attributable to productivity losses, or the earnings the child would have made over his or her lifetime. For victims of non-fatal child maltreatment, the estimated average lifetime cost per victim was over $200,000 and included expenses associated with short-term childhood health care costs, adult medical expenses, productivity losses, as well as child welfare, criminal justice, and special education costs. Furthermore, when considering all cases of child maltreatment reported during the year of analysis, the researchers estimated a total lifetime economic burden of $124 billion in financial costs.

Solutions to the Problem of Child Maltreatment

Based on its global magnitude, financial costs, as well as its association with a range of short- and long-term negative physical and mental health outcomes, child maltreatment has been identified by the World Health Organization as a public health concern requiring an emphasis on prevention and the root causes of the problem (Butchart, Harvey, Mian, Furniss, & Kahane, 2006). The solutions presented in this section will therefore focus on primary prevention interventions, supported by research, aimed at preventing child maltreatment before it occurs. A number of approaches have appeared and include strategies ranging from those that focus on micro-level systems (e.g., individual children and parents) to those that focus on macro-level systems (e.g., communities) (for reviews, see Child Welfare Information Gateway, 2011; MacMillan et al., 2009; and chapter 12 on child welfare reform of this volume). Because the nature of child sexual abuse differs significantly from other forms of child maltreatment, this review will limit its scope to the major approaches directed at the other forms of maltreatment (for a review of child sexual abuse prevention approaches, see Wurtele & Miller-Perrin, 2012). These approaches vary not only in terms of the ecological level targeted but also in terms of the quality and quantity of evidence to support each particular approach.

Public Awareness Campaigns

One approach to the prevention of child maltreatment that primarily targets the individual ecological level, albeit broadly, is public education through mass media campaigns. Such campaigns employ a variety of media advertisements including public service announcements on radio, television, and billboards as well as various print sources (e.g., in newspapers, magazines, and brochures). The goal of such campaigns is to increase individuals' knowledge and awareness about child maltreatment, with the assumption that such efforts will result in lower levels of abuse. The Adults and Children Together (ACT) Against Violence Campaign is an example of a media campaign designed to help adults teach young children nonviolent ways to resolve conflicts and deal with frustration and anger. The primary message of the campaign is to "teach carefully" suggesting that adult behavior, especially the verbal and physical expression of anger and aggression, serves as a model for children that can affect their future behavior (ACT Against Violence, n.d.). A similar program in Canada, the "Violence: You Can Make a Difference" campaign, uses the media to raise awareness about both child maltreatment and marital violence, provides tips on anger management, and provides information for abuse victims (Godenzi & De Puy, 2001).

Although limited, there is some research evidence indicating the effectiveness of public education campaigns. Just prior to the dramatic increase in reporting of child maltreatment during the 1980s in the United States, for example, several media campaigns were aimed at increasing local as well as national public awareness about maltreatment (Daro & Gelles, 1992). A more systematic link between public education and increased reporting was demonstrated in studies examining a multi-media campaign conducted in the Netherlands from 1991 to 1992 (Hoefnagels & Baartman, 1997; Hoefnagels & Mudde, 2000). This campaign employed a variety of media and educational efforts, including a televised documentary, public service announcements, a radio program, teacher training, and various print materials (e.g., posters, newspaper articles). Hoefnagels and Baartman (1997) evaluated the program and found that it was effective in increasing awareness of abuse, as shown by a dramatic increase in the number of calls received by a national child abuse hotline in the period after the campaign. Other evaluations of media campaigns have demonstrated effectiveness in enhancing knowledge and awareness about child maltreatment, increasing abuse disclosures, and changing adults' beliefs about their responsibility to prevent child maltreatment (see Lalor & McElvaney, 2010; Schober, Fawcett, & Bernier, in press).

Parent Education and Support Programs

Parent education and support programs are prevention approaches which focus on both individual and dyadic ecological levels to enhance parent–child interactions and build specific skills and knowledge. In addition to educating parents about child development and improving parenting skills, such programs also attempt to modify attitudes associated with harsh parenting, reduce negative emotions such as anger and stress, and provide settings where parents can share their concerns and work on problem solving with one another (Child Welfare Information Gateway, 2011; Lundahl, Nimer, & Parsons, 2006). Most of these programs focus on education and support of parents, but some programs also include structured parent–child interactions as well as specific interventions for children (e.g., Chaffin et al., 2004; Webster-Stratton & Reid, 2003). Although many of these programs target high-risk populations such as low income, pregnant women, some experts argue that all parents or prospective parents might benefit from such programs (Krug, Dahlberg, Mercy, Zwi, & Lozano, 2002).

In general, parent education and support programs have gained increased empirical support in recent years with several studies demonstrating their effectiveness in improving parental psychological adjustment, increasing parenting skills, improving parents' beliefs about child development and age-appropriate interventions, reducing parent–child conflict, improving child behavior, increasing parents' use of social supports, and enhancing parents' sense of efficacy, control, and confidence (e.g., Long, Edwards, & Bellando, 2009; Peterson, Tremblay, Ewigman, & Saldana, 2003). Unfortunately, very few studies have examined the efficacy of such programs in reducing the risk of child maltreatment or its risk factors in particular, and those that have frequently did not incorporate strong methodology using randomized control trials (Lundahl et al., 2006).

One exception is the American Psychological Association's Adults and Children Together (ACT) Against Violence Parents Raising Safe Kids program, a cost-effective program based on behavioral and social learning theories available to all parents of young children regardless of risk (ACT; Silva, 2007). The program trains caregivers in a variety of areas that have been empirically linked to child maltreatment, including nonviolent discipline, child development, anger management, social problem-solving skills, the effects of media on children, and methods to protect children from exposure to violence. A recent evaluation of the program found that, compared to controls, participating parents engaged in less physically aggressive discipline (e.g., spanking and hitting with an object). Participants also demonstrated improved knowledge, behaviors, and beliefs regarding violence prevention and parenting (Knox, Burkhart, & Hunter, 2011). Using an experimental design with random assignment to groups, Portwood, Lambert, Abrams, and Nelson (2011) also found that ACT achieved positive results in areas related to effective parenting, including reductions in the use of harsh discipline and an increase in nurturing behavior, and that participation increased social support for those parents with the greatest need.

Another successful parent education program that evaluated actual reductions in abuse reports is a study conducted by Chaffin et al. (2004) which examined the efficacy of parent–child interaction therapy (PCIT) using a randomized trial with physically abusive parents. PCIT is a behavioral parent training program designed to provide training through didactic instruction, modeling, role-playing, and coaching (Long et al., 2009). In this study, parents were randomly assigned to one of the three intervention conditions: (a) PCIT, (b) PCIT plus individualized enhanced services, or (c) a standard community-based parenting group. At approximately 2.5 year follow-up, 19 % of PCIT parents had a re-report for physical abuse compared to 49 % of parents who received the standard community-based parenting group.

Other success stories of the power of parent education are those addressing shaken baby syndrome (SBS). Dias et al. (2005) examined the effectiveness of a hospital-based prevention program designed to educate all parents of newborn infants about the dangers of violent infant shaking. Prior to their infant's discharge, both mothers and fathers viewed an 11-minute video and received a 1-page leaflet about the potential damage of violent infant shaking and ways to handle persistent infant crying. Both parents were also asked to sign a commitment statement indicating that they had received and understood the educational materials. The program resulted in a 47 % reduction in the incidence of abusive head injuries during the 5.5-year study period. Although 93 % of parents indicated that they were aware of the dangers associated with violent infant shaking prior to receiving the educational materials, a simple program with a powerful message, if delivered at the most opportune time, has the potential to effectively prevent child maltreatment (Miller-Perrin & Perrin, 2013). Other studies have also demonstrated the effectiveness of video interventions for increasing awareness about caregiving practices connected to SBS (Russell, Trudeau, & Britner, 2008).

Although few studies have addressed the specific program components that lead to the efficacy of parent education and support programs, researchers are beginning to identify specific program components that seem to be particularly effective in enhancing parenting skills, reducing risk of abuse, changing attitudes and emotions, and reducing children's problem behaviors. In a recent meta-analysis conducted by the Centers for Disease Control and Prevention (2009), for example, effective components included teaching parents various skills in emotional communication and positive parent–child interactions and providing parents with the opportunity to demonstrate and practice these skills. Others have identified uniquely effective components such as offering a mixture of office and home visits, as well as a combination of both behavioral and nonbehavioral management practices (Lundahl et al., 2006).

Home Visiting Programs

Home visiting programs are designed to facilitate positive and secure attachments between parents and their children by connecting at-risk parents with mentors who visit their homes to provide various forms of support. Although the specifics of such programs vary, the Child Welfare Information Gateway (2011, p. 7) recently identified several primary issues addressed during home visits including: (a) the mother's personal health and life choices; (b) child health and development; (c) environmental concerns such as income, housing, and community violence; (d) family functioning, including adult and child relationships; and (e) access to services. Such programs therefore target multiple ecological levels including individual, dyadic, familial, and community. Both theory and research evidence suggest that prevention programs that focus on multiple levels of the ecological model tend to be more effective than programs which focus on a single ecological level (Nation et al., 2003; Weis, Sandler, Durlak, & Anton, 2005).

Home visiting programs and their evaluation as a potential tool to combat child maltreatment began to flourish in the United States in the 1990s. Currently, more than half of the nation's states have parent support initiatives underway (Daro, 2006). These early intervention programs have received considerable state and federal support. In 2010, for example, federal legislation provided over $88 million in grants to support and expand the implementation of evidence-based home visiting programs (Child Welfare Information Gateway, 2011).

One of the most well-established home visiting programs is the Hawaii Healthy Start Program which is part of a series of programs known as Healthy Families America (HFA), a joint effort of the National Committee to Prevent Child Abuse and the Ronald McDonald House Charities (Daro, 1998). Although the program was originally created by the Hawaii Family Stress Center in Honolulu in 1985, it expanded across that state and currently exists in several states across the United States (e.g., Culp & Schellenbach, 2007; Daro, McCurdy, & Harding, 1998; Duggan et al., 2007). The program offers a variety of voluntary services to high-risk parents, defined by demographic and socioeconomic factors such as marital status, education, family support, limited prenatal care, and history of substance abuse. In general, these programs begin before at-risk mothers give birth, are intensive (visits occur at least once a week), and provide social support as well as instruction on parenting and child development (Daro et al., 1998; Healthy Families America, 1994).

In a carefully controlled evaluation of the Hawaii Healthy Start Program, Daro et al. (1998) randomly assigned families into one of two groups: (1) those families who qualified for the program and whose children had been born on even-numbered days were offered Healthy Start services; and (2) those families who qualified for the program and whose children had been born on odd-numbered days were not offered services. Follow-up 12 months after birth indicated that, relative to controls, Healthy Start mothers were more involved with their children, more sensitive to their needs, and the children were more responsive to their mothers and at less risk of physical abuse. More recent research has provided further evidence of the effectiveness of HFA programs including increased parenting attitudes and child health, and decreased reports of serious abuse, physical aggression and harsh parenting, and serious abuse and neglect (Dumont, Mitchell-Herzfeld, Greene, Lee, Lowenfels, Rodriguez, & Dorabawila, 2008; Harding, Galano, Martin, Huntington, & Schellenbach, 2007).

Another well-known home visiting program was established by Olds and colleagues and is recognized as an important success story in child maltreatment prevention (Wekerle & Wolfe, 1998). Originally called the Prenatal/Early Infancy Project, the program began in the 1970s and pairs young single mothers with public health nurses (Olds, Henderson, Chamberlin, & Tatelbaum, 1986). The project is currently referred to as the Nurse-Family Partnership (NFP) and provides prenatal and early childhood services to young mothers to help them understand child health and development and to strengthen their confidence in themselves and in their capacity for change. More specifically, the program is designed to accomplish the following goals: (a) enhance the health of the infant: (b) improve parental caregiving; and (c) provide life course development support (e.g., educational, occupational, and pregnancy planning) (Olds, 1997). The first implementation of the project was conducted in Elmira, New York where a nurse visited each mother an average of 9 times during her pregnancy and 23 times during the first 2 years of the child's life (Olds, 1997).

The NFP program has undergone a number of carefully controlled evaluations and demonstrated its effectiveness in preventing child maltreatment. The first evaluation examined the records of children involved in the Elmira study during their second year after birth and found that children who were nurse-visited showed a 56 % reduction in emergency room visits for injuries and ingestions compared to control children (Olds et al., 1986). In addition, there was an 80 % reduction in substantiated incidents of child maltreatment in a group of single, low-income, teen mothers, considered at high risk for abuse. Furthermore, at 15-year follow-up child abuse and neglect were identified less often in the families who received home visitation compared to those who had not (Olds et al., 1997, 1998). A review of the 27-year program of research on NFP concluded that the program has been successful in achieving two of its most important goals including the improvement of parental care (i.e., fewer injuries associated with child abuse and neglect) and improved maternal life course (i.e., greater employment) (Olds, 2006).

Recently, a review of the home visiting literature was conducted by Mathematical Policy Research under the guidance of a Department of Health and Human Services (DHHS) interagency working group as part of the Home Visiting Evidence of Effectiveness (HomVEE) initiative (Paulsell, Avellar, Sama Martin, & Del Grosso, 2011). The review summarized various home visiting models in terms of their evidence of effectiveness and found that out of 22 models, nine programs met DHHS criteria for evidence of effectiveness. Furthermore, the review found that the two models with the most favorable impacts in terms of DHHS criteria were the HFA and NFP programs, providing further evidence of the effectiveness and promise of these approaches in the prevention of child maltreatment.

Although studies of other home visiting programs have also found positive results, such as enhanced parenting knowledge and skills, more appropriate developmental expectations, safer home environments, fewer child injuries, and less use of corporal punishment among program participants compared to controls (Culp et al., 2004; Culp, Culp, Anderson, & Carter, 2007; Daro, 2011; Daro & McCurdy, 1994; Wekerle & Wolfe, 1993), many reviews of evaluation studies assessing the effectiveness of home visiting programs have been mixed (Chaffin, 2004; Daro, 2011; MacMillan et al., 2009). Some experts, for example, have seriously questioned the effectiveness of home visiting programs and concluded that despite rigorous randomized control trial studies, programs have produced mostly disappointing outcomes (Chaffin, 2004; Chaffin & Friedrich, 2004; MacMillan et al., 2009). Duggan and colleagues, for example, examined the effectiveness of the Healthy Start program by conducting a large, well-designed randomized trial and found little evidence that the program was effective in preventing either self-reported or officially reported child maltreatment (Duggan, Fuddy, et al., 2004; Duggan, McFarlane, et al., 2004). In addition, a recent review of home visiting programs by MacMillan et al. (2009) concluded that "home-visiting programs are not uniformly effective in reducing child physical abuse, neglect, and outcomes such as injuries" (p. 250).

Although many professionals recognize the limitations of current programs and research, many also recognize the potential of home visiting programs for preventing child maltreatment. Daro and Connelly (2002) suggest several limitations associated with home visiting programs that may impact their effectiveness in preventing child maltreatment. First, a significant number of families drop out of treatment before service goals are fully met. In addition, it is not clear whether home visiting programs empower families to access community resources, thereby fulfilling their broader goal of integrating families into their communities. It may also be the case that specific factors, such as various characteristics of participants (e.g., maternal age, child age, etc.), may explain the differential effectiveness of home visiting programs observed across studies (Dumont et al., 2008). Daro (2011) has argued that since such programs have demonstrated general effectiveness in improving child and family functioning, they are valuable regardless of whether they show evidence of directly preventing child maltreatment. It may be that only with further refinement will the effectiveness of such programs be demonstrable through rigorous research designs (Hahn, Mercy, Bilukha, & Briss, 2005).

Community Prevention Strategies

In recent years, primary prevention efforts have begun to focus on strategies and programs that emphasize change at the community level (Daro & Dodge, 2009). These prevention strategies are typically designed to improve the larger community environment of children through wide-scale dissemination of information, expansion of service and support for parents, and provision of efficient delivery of services (Miller-Perrin & Perrin, 2013). The goal of such interventions is to address the complex and interactive nature of child maltreatment by targeting multiple systems and integrating complementary services—all with an ecological emphasis that aims to change and improve not only the family's social environment but the social institutional structures as well (Corcoran, 2000; Daro & Dodge, 2009).

One of the most widely researched community-level prevention strategies is the Triple P—Positive Parenting Program, a multilevel parenting and family support program originally developed by a group of researchers at the University of Queensland in Australia. According to Turner and Sanders (2006), the primary goal of the Triple P program is to "promote family harmony and reduce parent–child conflict by helping parents develop a safe, nurturing environment and promote positive, caring relationships with their children, and to develop effective, non-violent management strategies for dealing with a variety of childhood behavioral problems and common developmental issues" (p. 184). The program includes a series of integrated intervention levels that increase in intensity in order to meet the varying levels of need among families. For example, interventions, which focus on positive parenting, range from less intense broad public or universal forms of dissemination of parenting information (e.g., newspaper articles, radio spots, website) to brief parenting sessions offered in various primary care facilities to more intensive behavioral family interventions for multiple-risk families (Prinz, Sanders, Shapiro, Whitaker, & Lutzer, 2009; Turner & Sanders, 2006).

A series of controlled outcome studies assessing the quality of parenting has demonstrated the effectiveness of the various levels of intervention among a variety of populations and problem areas (Prinz et al., 2009; Sanders, 2008). In addition, controlled evaluation studies have demonstrated the program's effectiveness in terms of community-wide outcomes. In one study, for example, Prinz et al. (2009) randomly assigned 18 counties in South Carolina to either the Triple P program or a control group who received "services-as-usual." Results suggested a relative lack of growth in child maltreatment in the counties receiving the Triple P program compared to the control counties which showed considerable growth in substantiated maltreatment. Related indicators such as out-of-home placements and hospital admissions for child injuries also showed significant decreases in the intervention counties compared to the control counties. Prevention programs such as Triple P are promising because they have the potential to mobilize various community constituents to not only prevent child maltreatment but to positively impact other community outcomes such as economic development and health care (Child Welfare Information Gateway, 2011).

Goals of the Advocacy Effort

With the emergence of a growing body of research evidencing that a number of program models hold great promise for preventing child maltreatment, significant advocacy efforts have focused on securing funding for the implementation, maintenance, and/or expansion of prevention programming, as well as the further evaluation, refinement, and modification of existing programs to ensure that they meet a range of diverse family needs. As indicated, parent education and support programs, including public education and awareness efforts, services directed to at-risk parents, and home visiting programs, are among the most common approaches to preventing child maltreatment (Daro & Connelly, 2002). Accordingly, the remainder of this chapter will highlight efforts aimed at supporting home visitation to illustrate how individuals can engage in advocacy for child abuse prevention.

The first step in advancing prevention programming is, of course, to ensure that decision makers are aware of the problem, as well as its costs and consequences. As discussed in the preceding sections, a great deal of relevant, high quality research is available; it is the role of advocates to ensure that this information reaches those audiences that can play a role in affecting policy change, including not only legislators and other public officials, but also human service professionals, first responders, the faith community, and the general public. Individuals who are uncomfortable with the thought of working as an advocate, or who are just beginning to gain experience with advocacy, may already be very comfortable in the role of teacher or trainer. While those working in the field of child maltreatment are very familiar with the scope of the issue, other groups, including policymakers, often lack basic knowledge about child maltreatment and its impact. Paradoxically, increased public awareness of the occurrence of child maltreatment can lead to a diffusion of responsibility, with individuals assuming that *someone* is already taking the formal steps necessary to address what is widely recognized as a serious social problem (Abrams & Portwood, 2010). Accordingly, education remains an important advocacy goal.

In addition, providing relevant information to policymakers and their staff is one means of working toward another essential goal of advocates—establishing a good working relationship with those individuals who have the power to make actual policy changes. Given that they are responsible for responding to so many issues, legislators and their staff members seek to identify individuals who display a high level of professionalism and upon whom they can rely to obtain timely, accurate, and useful information. Establishing a regular channel for communication between policymakers and content experts is the ideal way to ensure that policy reflects the best science available (Dodgen, 2000; Portwood & Dodgen, 2005).

A critical goal in advocating for prevention programs, including home visiting programs, is to obtain appropriate levels of funding. Obviously, unless the necessary resources are available, prevention programs will not be offered, or will be offered to only a few of those who could benefit from these services. Unfortunately, child abuse prevention has been severely underfunded, with expressed concerns for the safety and well-being of children rarely translating directly into policy (Portwood & Dodgen, 2005). In fact, the CAPTA, originally enacted in 1974, remains the sole federal policy aimed specifically at child abuse prevention (Portwood, 2006), and it must be reauthorized at regular intervals in order to remain law, requiring advocates to expend considerable resources simply to maintain the status quo. In fact, in almost four decades since its passage, CAPTA has never been fully funded—even in those years when the economy was booming. While, as discussed below, there have been some recent successes in securing more appropriate levels of funding for home visiting programs, there is a continuing need for advocates to work both to maintain and to increase financial support at the local, state, and federal levels. Some particular ways in which these efforts might be accomplished are outlined in the next section.

Advocacy Action Steps

Disseminating Information

Individuals interested in becoming involved in advocacy should be aware that it is not necessary to engage in high level interactions with Congress to be an effective advocate for children. For example, simply disseminating scientifically sound information through means outside traditional academic channels furthers the goal of educating the general public and policymakers on child maltreatment prevention. Research on home visiting can be included in a wide range of presentations in not only classrooms but also professional training sessions and other community forums. Individuals with connections to agencies that provide services to children and families may have specific opportunities to disseminate this information to staff and/or clients through continuing education, public outreach, or other events sponsored by those organizations. During Child Abuse Prevention Month, in April of each year, many groups, including not only professional groups but also broader community groups, such as schools and churches, make an effort to offer related programming and would welcome an offer from a local expert to assist with that process. The key thing to keep in mind is that advocates should be proactive in identifying these educational opportunities. Whether it is an agency director, local official, or Congressional representative, individuals in positions to affect policy change typically have extremely busy schedules and are unlikely to approach experts for information. However, they and their staff are often very receptive to offers to provide training and information that is relevant to current issues.

The media is a potentially valuable, but often underutilized resource for advocates. Individuals can reach out to their local newspaper or other media outlets, including community newsletters and local magazines, with ideas for stories related to child abuse prevention. Sadly, local papers regularly report on individual incidents of child maltreatment, which can nonetheless provide an opportunity for advocates to stress the importance and promise of prevention efforts. Advocates can also submit letters to the editor, which often afford their author an opportunity to be more selective about the information that is included, as well as to present a more persuasive argument (in contrast with a news story, in which the reporter decides which information to include). Teachers may consider developing an assignment around composing and submitting a letter to the editor, and in that way also assist in training future advocates. In addition to newspapers, local television and/or radio stations are often required to devote a certain amount of air time to "public service programming," and will welcome offers to provide information on child maltreatment prevention; again, Child Abuse Prevention Month is a particularly good time to seek out these opportunities.

In connection with all of these efforts, advocates can not only disseminate their own work, but also leverage a wealth of resources that are readily available for just this purpose. Organizations such as Prevent Child Abuse America, the American Academy of Pediatrics, and the American Psychological Association, particularly its Division 37, the Society of Child and Family Policy and Practice, as well as independent policy research centers, such as Chapin Hall at the University of Chicago, and federal agencies, including the U.S. Department of Health and Human Services, have a large volume of high quality material on home visiting services available online. However, materials should be reviewed carefully prior to distribution to ensure that they are suitable for a particular audience.

Advocates may also leverage individual stories and anecdotes to personalize the issue for legislators and other decision makers. Combining memorable examples with scientific data on program effectiveness and the cost-benefit/cost-effectiveness of these programs is arguably the best strategy for ensuring that priority is given to child maltreatment prevention, particularly in regard to securing funding for programs.

Securing Funding

It is important to be aware that the most critical time to advocate for prevention programs is when budgets are being planned. While states typically bear primary responsibility for administering child and family service programs, severe budget cuts at the state level have resulted in local communities assuming increased responsibility for funding these programs, including home visitation. Regardless of whether an advocate is working at the local, state, or federal level, it is imperative that he or she ensures that policymakers have the information they need to include the necessary resources in the budget when that budget is being planned. This will always be well in advance of the time targeted for program implementation. For example, a county hoping to implement a home visitation program in the fall may be required to approve the budget for its fiscal year beginning October 1 and no later than July 1. In that case, advocacy efforts will need to commence at the first of the calendar year to ensure that program funds are available. Likewise, unless allocations for programs are included in state and federal budgets when they are submitted for approval, advocacy efforts can succeed in obtaining only statements of support for prevention programs rather than actual implementation, which necessarily requires an advance commitment of funds.

Collaboration

Effective advocacy is often the result of collaborative alliances between multiple groups working to protect children, at the local, regional, state, and/or national level. Individuals seeking to become involved in advocacy can typically find groups within their own community that bring together agencies and organizations serving children and families, and it is not uncommon for these groups to engage in organized advocacy efforts. For example, in Charlotte, North Carolina, the nonprofit Council for Children's Rights implemented a collaborative community process for selecting evidence-based parenting programs, which sought to engage experts from local universities. After the community narrowed its focus on the NFP model, the Council led advocacy efforts to start an NFP pilot site in Charlotte. Currently, the Council and its collaborative partners are working with private foundations to implement a statewide advocacy strategy to increase funding for the expansion of the program.

Joining and/or developing collaborative relationships with organizations that advocate for children can also provide opportunities for connecting directly with legislators. For example, the American Psychological Association (APA) regularly sponsors Congressional briefings that feature prominent experts in the field. Among the many groups with which APA has worked to address child maltreatment issues are the National Association for the Education of Young Children (NAEYC), the National Association of Social Workers (NASW), the American Pediatric

Association, and the American Bar Association (ABA). Note that working in partnership with other professional organizations also increases the number of potential points of contact for officials seeking to identify appropriate experts to participate in legislative hearings.

Notably, advocates can often advance their specific goals—in this case, child maltreatment prevention programs—by supporting related policies and programs that promise positive outcomes for children and families. For example, policies that improve parents' access to mental health and preventive medical services, support programs through which teen parents can complete their education, and initiatives that support affordable, quality child care and help parents to achieve financial stability, can all serve to prevent abuse (Abrams & Portwood, 2010). One prominent example of a broader policy that nonetheless advances home visiting programs is the Patient Protection and Affordable Care Act (P.L. 111-148), the primary health reform legislation signed into law by President Obama in 2010. Section 2951 of this law provides for a significant expansion of the federal funding available to support home visitation through the establishment of the Maternal, Infant, and Early Childhood Home Visiting Program (MIECHV).

Outcome and Next Steps

While this chapter was being written, the US Supreme Court heard oral arguments on the constitutionality of the Patient Protection and Affordable Care Act ("the Affordable Care Act") and later rendered its decision in DHHS v. Florida, Case No. 11-398, a process that serves to highlight how quickly the policy landscape can change for child advocates. At issue in the Supreme Court case were (1) the individual mandate and related provisions requiring most individuals to purchase health insurance coverage or to pay a penalty, and (2) those provisions of the Act that increase access to affordable health insurance by expanding eligibility for Medicaid. Much less discussed in the public domain (and not directly at issue in the case) were those provisions establishing the MIECHV. Under MIECHV, the Health Resources and Services Administration (HRSA) awarded $91 million in grants in fiscal year 2010 for planning and needs assessment, with the ultimate goal of supporting implementation of evidence-based home visiting models in targeted at-risk communities across the country. On September 22, 2011, U.S. Department of Health and Human Services Secretary Kathleen Sebelius announced $224 million in grants to support home visiting programs in 49 states. While these developments suggest a growing commitment to funding and, in fact, the Affordable Care Act provides $1.5 billion over 5 years to support maternal, infant, and early childhood home visitation programs (Pew Center on the States, 2010), the Supreme Court's ruling on the Affordable Care Act could have eradicated this progress. More specifically, had the Court found the individual mandate to be unconstitutional, the justices would then have addressed the issue of whether the mandate was severable, such that the balance of the Act would remain law, or whether all or a part of the entire Act must have been struck down, in effect abolishing the MIECHV.

Although the Court's ruling in regard to the constitutionality of the Affordable Care Act ended the immediate threat to MIECHV, it is important to note that advocates cannot simply assume that the issue is settled; many politicians remain eager to repeal "Obamacare," and the effect of future legislation on funding for home visiting programs cannot yet be ascertained. What is clear is that there will be a continued need for advocacy to ensure that appropriate and effective programs are available to all parents of young children in order to prevent child maltreatment. As the Affordable Care Act serves to illustrate, even the most favorable policy can change owing to a host of factors; such is the nature of the political process. To the extent that prevention can be "de-politicized" and bipartisan support obtained, funding for programs would appear to be more secure. For example, President Obama has advocated for home visiting programs as part of his "common ground" agenda, noting that such programs advance the shared goals of reducing the numbers of unintended pregnancies and women seeking abortions, increasing the number of adoptions, and providing more support and care for women who carry their children to term (Boonstra, 2009). Nonetheless, effective advocacy will necessarily require a long-term commitment.

As noted previously, prevention efforts have historically been grossly underfunded, and even with a continuation of current funding through MIECHV, significant additional resources will be required to ensure that all children are protected. While there is sound research to support the wide implementation of several models of home visiting programs, substantial work is still needed to ensure that high quality is maintained across programs, to improve the ability to reach all families at risk, to serve diverse ethnic and cultural groups effectively, to employ technology to enhance access and quality of services, and to achieve the right balance between providing formal services and strengthening the informal supports available to individuals and families (Child Welfare Information Gateway, 2011; Daro, 2009). In addition, there is increasing recognition that even when efforts to intervene with parents are successful, there is a need to improve the broader community environment to be supportive of children and families.

The key to ensuring that the necessary resources are available to address the challenges and opportunities for moving child abuse prevention forward is the commitment of those in the field to engage in activities that continue to educate policymakers and other decision makers, as well as their constituents, on the problems presented and the strategies available, with an emphasis on the scientific evidence regarding program effectiveness. Ideally, both scientists and practitioners can develop a solid understanding of the policymaking process and develop a level of comfort in dealing with its complexities. However, it is not necessary to be a law and policy expert to be an effective advocate. Every individual who contacts his or her legislator or who presents information to a local community leader makes a valuable contribution for children and families.

References

Abrams, L. P., & Portwood, S. G. (2010). Protecting children in their homes: Effective prevention programs and policies. In J. Lampien & K. Sexton-Radek (Eds.), *Protecting children from violence* (pp. 35–56). New York, NY: Psychology Press.

ACT against violence. (n.d.). Retrieved May 24, 2006, from www.actagainstviolence.org

Boonstra, H. D. (2009). Home visiting for at-risk families: A primer on a major Obama administration initiative. *Guttmacher Policy Review, 12,* 11–15.

Butchart, A., Harvey, A. P., Mian, M., Furniss, T., Kahane, T. (2006). *Preventing child maltreatment: A guide to taking action and generating evidence.* Geneva: World Health Organization and International Society for Prevention of Child Abuse and Neglect.

Centers for Disease Control and Prevention (CDC). (2009). *Parent training programs: Insight for practitioners.* Atlanta, GA: Centers for Disease Control and Prevention. Retrieved from http://www.cdc.gov/ViolencePrevention/pdf/Parent_Training_Brief-a.pdf

Chaffin, M. (2004). Is it time to rethink healthy start/healthy families? *Child Abuse & Neglect, 28,* 589–595.

Chaffin, M., & Friedrich, B. (2004). Evidence-based treatments in child abuse and neglect. *Children and Youth Services Review, 26,* 1097–1113.

Chaffin, M., Silovsky, J. F., Funderburk, B., Valle, L. A., Brestan, E. V., Balachova, T., et al. (2004). Parent-child interaction therapy with physically abusive parents: Efficacy for reducing future abuse reports. *Journal of Consulting and Clinical Psychology, 72*(3), 500–510.

Child Welfare Information Gateway. (2011). *Child maltreatment prevention: Past, present, and future.* Washington, DC: U. S. Department of Health and Human Services, Children's Bureau.

Corcoran, J. (2000). Family interventions with child physical abuse and neglect: A critical review. *Children and Youth Services Review, 22,* 563–591.

Culp, A. M., Culp, R. E., Anderson, J. W., & Carter, S. (2007). Health and safety intervention with first-time mothers. *Health Education Research, 22*(2), 285–294.

Culp, A. M., Culp, R. E., Hechtner-Galvin, T., Howell, C. S., Saathoff-Wells, T., & Marr, P. (2004). First-time mothers in home visitation services utilizing child development specialists. *Infant Mental health Journal, 25*(1), 1–15.

Culp, A. M., & Schellenbach, C. J. (2007). HFA research update. *Child and Family Policy and Practice Review, 3*(2), 15–18.

Daro, D. (1998). What is happening in the U.S.? *The Link (Newsletter of the International Society for Prevention of Child Abuse and Neglect), 7,* 6–7.

Daro, D. (2006). *Home visitation: Assessing progress, managing expectations.* Chicago, IL: Chapin Hall Center for Children and the Ounce of Prevention Fund.

Daro, D. (2009). *Embedding home visitation programs within a system of early childhood services.* Chicago, IL: Chapin Hall at the University of Chicago.

Daro, D. (2011). Prevention of child abuse and neglect. In J. E. B. Myers (Ed.), *The APSAC handbook on child maltreatment* (3rd ed., pp. 17–37). Thousand Oaks, CA: Sage.

Daro, D., & Connelly, A. (2002). Charting the waves of prevention: Two steps forward, one step back. *Child Abuse & Neglect, 26,* 731–742.

Daro, D., & Dodge, K. (2009). Creating community responsibility for child protection: Possibilities and challenges. *The Future of Children, 19*(2), 67–94.

Daro, D., & Gelles, R. J. (1992). Public attitudes and behaviors with respect to child abuse prevention. *Journal of Interpersonal Violence, 7,* 517–531.

Daro, D., & McCurdy, K. (1994). Preventing child abuse and neglect: Programmatic interventions. *Child Welfare, 73,* 405–430.

Daro, D., McCurdy, K., & Harding, K. (1998). *The role of home visiting in preventing child abuse: An evaluation of the Hawaii Healthy Start Program.* Chicago, IL: National Center on Child Abuse Prevention Research.

Dias, M. S., Smith, K., DeGuehery, K., Mazur, P., Li, V., Shaffer, M. L. (2005). Preventing abusive head trauma among infants and young children: A hospital-based, parent education program. *Pediatrics, 115*(4). Retrieved from www.pediatrics.org/cgi/content/full/115/4/e470

Dodgen, D. (2000). Public policy and intimate violence: Making the case for prevention and services. *University of Missouri Kansas City Law Review, 69*, 127–137.

Duggan, A., Caldera, D., Rodriguez, K., Burrell, L., Rohde, C., & Crowne, S. S. (2007). Impact of a statewide home visiting program to prevent child abuse. *Child Abuse & Neglect, 31*(8), 801–827.

Duggan, A., Fuddy, L., McFarlane, E., Burrell, L., Windham, A., Higman, S., et al. (2004). Evaluating a statewide home visiting program to prevent child abuse in at-risk families of newborns: Fathers' participation and outcomes. *Child Maltreatment, 18*, 3–17.

Duggan, A., McFarlane, E., Fuddy, L., Burrell, L., Higman, S. M., Windham, A., et al. (2004). Randomized trial of a statewide home visiting program: Impact in preventing child abuse and neglect. *Child Abuse & Neglect, 28*(6), 597–622.

DuMont, K., Mitchell-Herzfeld, S., Greene, R., Lee, E., Lowenfels, A., Rodriguez, M., & Dorabawila, V. (2008). Healthy Families New York (HFNY) randomized trial: Effects on early child abuse and neglect. *Child Abuse & Neglect, 32*, 295–315.

Fanga, X., Brown, D. S., Florence, C. S., & Mercy, J. A. (2012). The economic burden of child maltreatment in the United States and implications for prevention. *Child Abuse & Neglect, 36*, 156–165.

Finkelhor, D. (2008). *Childhood victimization: Violence, crime, and abuse in the lives of young people.* New York, NY: Oxford University Press.

Finkelhor, D., Ormrod, R. K., Turner, H. A., & Hamby, S. L. (2005a). The victimization of children and youth: A comprehensive, national survey. *Child Maltreatment, 10*(5), 5–25.

Finkelhor, D., Ormrod, R. K., Turner, H. A., & Hamby, S. L. (2005b). Measuring poly victimization using the JVQ. *Child Abuse & Neglect, 29*(11), 1297–1312.

Finkelhor, D., Turner, H., Ormrod, R., & Hamby, S. L. (2009). Violence, abuse, and crime exposure in a national sample of children and youth. *Pediatrics, 124*, 1411–1423.

Godenzi, A., & De Puy, J. (2001). Overcoming boundaries: A cross-cultural inventory of primary prevention programs against wife abuse and child abuse. *The Journal of Primary Prevention, 21*, 455–475.

Hahn, R. A., Mercy, J., Bilukha, O., & Briss, P. (2005). Letter to the editor. *Child Abuse & Neglect, 29*, 215–218.

Harding, K., Galano, J., Martin, J., Huntington, L., & Schellenbach, C. (2007). Healthy Families America effectiveness: A comprehensive review of outcomes. *Journal of Prevention & Intervention in the Community, 34*, 149–180.

Healthy Families America. (1994, October). *Violence Update, 5*(2), 1–4.

Hoefnagels, C., & Baartman, H. (1997). On the threshold of disclosure: The effects of a mass media field experiment. *Child Abuse & Neglect, 21*, 557–573.

Hoefnagels, C., & Mudde, A. (2000). Mass media and disclosures of child abuse in the perspective of secondary prevention: Putting ideas into practice. *Child Abuse & Neglect, 24*, 1091–1101.

Kempe, C. H., Silverman, F. N., Steele, B. F., Droegemueller, W., & Silver, H. K. (1962). The battered child syndrome. *Journal of the American Medical Association, 17*, 17–24.

Knox, M. S., Burkhart, K., & Hunter, K. E. (2011). ACT Against Violence Parents Raising Safe Kids Program: Effects on maltreatment-related parenting behaviors and beliefs. *Journal of Family Issues, 32*(1), 55–74.

Krug, E. G., Dahlberg, L. L., Mercy, J. A., Zwi, A. B., & Lozano, R. (Eds.). (2002). *World report on violence and health.* Geneva: World Health Organization.

Lalor, K., & McElvaney, R. (2010). Child sexual abuse, links to later sexual exploitation/high-risk sexual behavior, and prevention/treatment programs. *Trauma, Violence, & Abuse, 11*, 159–177.

Leeb, R. T., Paulozzi, L., Melanson, C., Simon, T., & Arias, I. (2008). *Child maltreatment surveillance: Uniform definitions for public health and recommended data elements.* Centers for Disease Control and Prevention, National Center for Injury Prevention and Control.

Long, N., Edwards, M. C., & Bellando, J. (2009). Parent-training interventions. In J. L. Matson, F. Andrasik, & M. L. Matson (Eds.), *Treating childhood psychopathology and developmental disabilities* (pp. 79–104). New York, NY: Springer.

Lundahl, B. W., Nimer, J., & Parsons, B. (2006). Preventing child abuse: A meta-analysis of parent training programs. *Research on Social Work Practice, 16*, 251–262.

MacMillan, H. L., Wathen, C. N., Barlow, J., Fergusson, D. M., Leventhal, J. M., & Taussig, H. N. (2009). Interventions to prevent child maltreatment and associated impairment. *Lancet, 373*, 250–266.

Miller-Perrin, C. L., & Perrin, R. D. (2013). *Child maltreatment: An introduction* (3rd ed.). Thousand Oaks, CA: Sage.

Nation, M., Crusto, C., Wandersman, A., Kumpfer, K. L., Seybolt, D., Morrissey-Kane, E., et al. (2003). *American Psychologist, 58*(6/7), 449–456.

Olds, D. L. (1997). The Prenatal/Early Infancy Project: Preventing child abuse and neglect in the context of promoting maternal and child health. In D. A. Wolfe, R. J. McMahon, & R. D. Peters (Eds.), *Child abuse: New directions in prevention and treatment across the lifespan* (pp. 130–154). Thousand Oaks, CA: Sage.

Olds, D. L., Eckenrode, J., Henderson, C. R., Kitzman, H., Powers, J., Cole, R., et al. (1997). Long-term effects of home visitation on maternal life course and child abuse and neglect: Fifteen-year follow up of a randomized trial. *Journal of the American Medical Association, 278*, 637–643.

Olds, D. L., Henderson, C. r., Cole, R., Eckenrode, J., Kitzman, H., Lucky, D., et al. (1998). Long-term effects of nurse home visitation on children's criminal and antisocial behavior: 15-year follow-up of a randomized controlled trial. *Journal of the American Medical Association, 280*, 1238–1244.

Olds, D. L., Henderson, C. R., Chamberlin, R., & Tatelbaum, R. (1986). Preventing child abuse and neglect: A randomized trial of nurse home visitation. *Pediatrics, 78*, 65–78.

Olds, D. L. (2006). The nurse-family partnership: An evidence-based preventive intervention. *Infant Mental Health Journal, 27*(1), 5–25.

Paulsell, D., Avellar, S., Sama Martin, E., & Del Grosso, P. (2011). *Home visiting evidence of effectiveness review: Executive summary*. Office of Planning, Research and Evaluation, Administration for Children and Families, U.S. Department of Health and Human Services. Washington, DC.

Peterson, L., Tremblay, G., Ewigman, B., & Saldana, L. (2003). Multilevel selected primary prevention of child maltreatment. *Journal of Consulting and Clinical Psychology, 71*, 601–612.

Pew Center on the States. (2010). *Maternal infant and early childhood home visiting program summary*. Retrieved from http://www.pewcenteronthestates.org/UploadedFiles/wwwpewcenteronthestates.org/Home_Visiting/Health_Care_Reform_Summary.pdf

Portwood, S. G. (2006). What we know—and don't know about preventing child maltreatment. *Journal of Aggression, Maltreatment, and Trauma, 12*, 55–80. co-published simultaneously in V. I. Vieth, B. L. Bottoms, & A. R. Perona (Eds.) *Ending child abuse: New efforts in prevention, investigation, and training*.

Portwood, S. G., & Dodgen, D. W. (2005). Influencing policymaking for maltreated children and their families. *Journal of Clinical Child and Adolescent Psychology, 34*, 628–637.

Portwood, S. G., Lambert, R. G., Abrams, L. P., & Nelson, E. B. (2011). An evaluation of the Adults and Children Together (ACT) Against Violence Parents Raising Safe Kids Program. *The Journal of Primary Prevention, 32*, 147–160.

Prinz, R. J., Sanders, M. R., Shapiro, C. J., Whitaker, D. J., & Lutzer, J. R. (2009). Population-based prevention of child maltreatment: The U.S. Triple P system population trial. *Prevention Science, 10*, 1–12.

Russell, B. S., Trudeau, J., & Britner, P. A. (2008). Intervention type matters in primary prevention of abusive head injury: Event history analysis results. *Child Abuse & Neglect, 32*(10), 949–957.

Sanders, M. R. (2008). The Triple P—Positive Parenting Program—A public health approach to parenting support. *Journal of Family Psychology, 22*, 506–517.

Sedlak, A. J. (1990). *Technical amendment to the study findings: National incidence and prevalence of child abuse and neglect: 1988*. Rockville, MD: Westat.

Sedlak, A. J., & Broadhurst, D. D. (1996). *Third National Incidence Study on child abuse and neglect*. Washington, DC: U.S. Department of Health and Human Services.

Sedlak, A. J., Mettenburg, J., Basena, M., Petta, I., McPherson, K., Greene, A., et al. (2010). *Fourth National Incidence Study of Child Abuse and Neglect (NIS–4): Report to Congress.* Washington, DC: U.S. Department of Health and Human Services, Administration for Children and Families.

Silva, J. (2007). *Parents raising safe kids: ACT 8-week program for parents.* Washington, DC: American Psychological Association.

Stevens, T. N., Ruggiero, K. J., Kilpatrick, D. G., Resnick, H. S., & Saunders, B. E. (2005). Variables differentiating singly and multiply victimized youth: Results from the National Survey of Adolescents and implications for secondary prevention. *Child Maltreatment, 10,* 211–223.

Turner, K. M. T., & Sanders, M. R. (2006). Dissemination of evidence-based parenting and family support strategies: Learning from the Triple P—Positive parenting program system approach. *Aggression and Violent Behavior, 11,* 176–192.

U.S. Department of Health and Human Services, Administration for Children and Families, Administration on Children, Youth and Families, Children's Bureau. (2010). *The Child Abuse Prevention and Treatment Act Including Adoption Opportunities & The Abandoned Infants Assistance Act.* Retrieved from http://www.childwelfare.gov/systemwide/laws_policies/federal.

U.S. Department of Health and Human Services, Administration for Children and Families, Administration on Children, Youth and Families, Children's Bureau. (2011). *Child Maltreatment 2010.* Retrieved from http://www.acf.hhs.gov/programs/cb/stats_research/index.htm#can.

Wang, C. T., & Holton, J. (2007). *Total estimated cost of child abuse and neglect in the United States.* Chicago, IL: Prevent Child Abuse America. Retrieved April 6, 2012, from http://Member.preventchildabuse.org/site/DocServer/cost_analysis.pdf?docID=144.

Webster-Stratton, C., & Reid, M. J. (2003). The incredible years parents, teachers, and children training series. In A. E. Kazdin & J. R. Weisz (Eds.), *Evidence-based psychotherapies for children and adolescents* (pp. 224–240). New York, NY: Guilford Press.

Weis, J. R., Sandler, I. N., Durlak, J. A., & Anton, B. S. (2005). Promoting and protecting youth mental health through evidence-based prevention and treatment. *American Psychologist, 60*(6), 628–648.

Wekerle, C., & Wolfe, D. A. (1993). Prevention of child abuse and neglect: Promising new reactions. *Clinical Psychology Review, 13,* 501–540.

Wekerle, C., & Wolfe, D. A. (1998). Windows for preventing child and partner abuse: Early childhood and adolescence. In P. K. Trickett & C. J. Schellenbach (Eds.), *Violence against children in the family and the community* (pp. 339–369). Washington, DC: American Psychological Association.

Wurtele, S. K., & Miller-Perrin, C. L. (2012). Global efforts to prevent sexual exploitation of minors. In H. Dubowitz (Ed.), *ISPCAN's world perspectives* (pp. 82-88). Colorado: International Society for Prevention of Child Abuse and Neglect.

Chapter 6
Strategies for Ending Homelessness Among Children and Families

Christina M. Murphy, Ellen L. Bassuk, Natalie Coupe, and Corey Anne Beach

Defining Child and Family Homelessness

The number of children and families experiencing homelessness in the United States has increased dramatically since the problem first emerged in the 1980s. Today, more than 1.6 million children, or one in 45, are homeless in a given year (The National Center on Family Homelessness, 2011d). Homelessness is a devastating experience for all family members and is especially traumatic for children. Permanent housing options in combination with ongoing supports and services must be implemented to prevent and end homelessness. This chapter describes a national and state-based advocacy effort—the Campaign to End Child Homelessness—launched by The National Center on Family Homelessness in 2009 to give a voice to homeless children and mobilize the political will to address this national tragedy. This chapter describes the extent and nature of child homelessness in America, discusses solutions, and details the Campaign's advocacy activities and outcomes.

Except during periods of economic depression, children and families were not a significant part of the homeless population until the mid-1980s. At that time, they comprised approximately 1 % of the overall homeless population (Bassuk, 2010), but their numbers have steadily climbed in the last 3 decades to 37 % in 2011 (United States Department of Housing and Urban Development, 2011). Between 2007 and 2010, financial speculation sparked collapse of the housing market and banking institutions, precipitating the Great Recession and a further spike in the numbers of homeless families. As a result, the number of homeless children increased by more than 448,000—a 38 % increase in just 3 years from 2007 to

C.M. Murphy, MM (✉) • E.L. Bassuk, MD • N. Coupe • C.A. Beach
The National Center on Family Homelessness, 200 Reservoir Street, Suite 200,
Needham, MA 02494, USA
e-mail: Christina.Murphy@familyhomelessness.org

A. McDonald Culp (ed.), *Child and Family Advocacy: Bridging the Gaps Between Research, Practice, and Policy*, Issues in Clinical Child Psychology,
DOI 10.1007/978-1-4614-7456-2_6, © Springer Science+Business Media New York 2013

2010—to a total of 1.6 million American children, or one in 45.[1] The number of homeless children in 2010 was more than 60,000 higher than after Hurricanes Katrina and Rita, which led to one of the greatest mass migrations in our nation's history. Given the impact of this historic natural disaster, it is startling that fallout from the man-made economic disaster between 2007 and 2010 has been even worse (The National Center on Family Homelessness, 2011d).

Homeless families are everywhere in our nation—in all states, most cities, and many communities. They number in the thousands, tens of thousands, and even hundreds of thousands. In smaller states, their numbers are in the low thousands. In larger states, child homelessness has become a catastrophic social problem. States with the highest percentage of homeless children are generally located in the South and Southwest—reflecting higher levels of poverty. States with the lowest percentage of homeless children are generally located in the North and Northeast (National Center for Homeless Education, 2011; United States Census Bureau, 2007)—where there is less poverty and stronger safety nets for children. However, between 2007 and 2010, only five states reported decreases in the numbers of homeless children— Louisiana, Michigan, Mississippi, Montana, and North Dakota (National Center for Homeless Education, 2011).

A typical sheltered homeless family comprises a mother in her late twenties with two children (Burt et al., 2000). Approximately 42 %of homeless children are under the age of six (Burt et al., 1999, 2000). Homeless families refer to a parent with a child who is up to 18 years old or a pregnant mother. Our counts and descriptions do not include unaccompanied children and youth (e.g., runaway or homeless children and youth who are on the streets alone without a parent). We use the definition of homelessness contained in federal legislation—Subtitle B of Part VII of the McKinney-Vento Homeless Assistance Act (Title X, Part C, of the No Child Left Behind Act of 2001) and adopted by the U.S. Department of Education (DOE) as well as several other federal departments. This definition includes children and youth who are: sharing the housing of other persons due to a loss of housing, economic hardship, or a similar reason (sometimes referred to as "doubled-up"); living in motels, hotels, trailer parks, or camping grounds due to a lack of alternative accommodations; living in emergency or transitional shelters; abandoned in hospitals; awaiting foster care placement; using a primary nighttime residence that is a public or private place not designed for, or ordinarily used as, a regular sleeping accommodation for human beings; living in cars, parks, public spaces, abandoned buildings, substandard housing, bus or train stations, or similar settings; and migratory children who qualify as homeless because they are living in circumstances described above.

---

[1] Each school year, Local Education Agencies identify and count the numbers of homeless children in their schools as mandated by the federal McKinney-Vento Homeless Assistance Act. These numbers are reported annually by school year (e.g., data reported from 2005 to 2006 are from the fall and spring semester of a single school year). To simplify our presentation of data, we use 2006 for the 2005–2006 school year, 2007 for the 2006–2007 school year, 2008 for the 2007–2008 school year, 2009 for the 2008–2009 school year, and 2010 for the 2009–2010 school year.

This definition of homelessness differs from the definition used by the U.S. Department of Housing and Urban Development (HUD), which includes people who are: living in a place not meant for human habitation; in emergency shelter; in transitional housing; exiting an institution where they temporarily resided; losing their primary nighttime residence, which may include a motel or hotel or a doubled-up situation, within 14 days and lack resources or support networks to remain in housing; families with children or unaccompanied youth who are unstably housed and likely to continue in that state; and fleeing or attempting to flee domestic violence, have no other residence, and lack the resources or support networks to obtain other permanent housing.

The major causes of homelessness for children and families are structural in nature. Poverty combined with our nation's lack of affordable housing push the most vulnerable families out of stable housing onto a path towards homelessness (Bassuk, 2010; Bassuk et al., 1996). Other reasons for family and child homelessness include unemployment, limited access to resources and supports, health and mental health issues, and experiences of violence. The process of becoming homeless involves the loss of belongings, sense of safety, reassuring routines, and community. Before turning to emergency shelter, most families double up in overcrowded apartments with relatives or friends (Bassuk, 2010). Others stay in motel rooms or sleep in cars or campgrounds (The National Center on Family Homelessness, 2009). Families are often forced to split up—with children placed with extended family, friends, or in foster care (Barrow & Lawinski, 2009). When families turn to homeless shelters—often as a last resort—they must quickly adjust to noisy, chaotic, overcrowded, and sometimes unsafe situations.

Homelessness is a devastating experience that significantly impacts the health and wellbeing of adults and children (Rog & Buckner, 2007). The rates of traumatic stress in the lives of families who are homeless are extraordinarily high (Guarino & Bassuk, 2010). Often, members of homeless families have experienced ongoing trauma in the form of childhood abuse and neglect, domestic violence, and community violence, as well as the trauma associated with poverty and the loss of home, safety, and sense of security. A staggering 92 % of homeless women report having experienced severe physical and/or sexual assault at some point in their lives. Upwards of 50 % of all homeless women report that domestic violence was the immediate cause of their homelessness. By age 12, 83 % of homeless children have been exposed to at least one major violent event (Bassuk et al., 1996). These experiences impact how children and adults think, feel, behave, relate to others, and cope. Traumatic stresses are cumulative and increase the risk of children developing health, behavioral, and social problems as adults (Brown et al., 2009).

Homeless children often live in chaotic and unsafe environments. Dramatic life changes such as moving from place to place, family separations, and placement in foster care are common. The level of fear and unpredictability in the lives of homeless children can be extremely damaging to their growth and development. Children experiencing homelessness are 4 times more likely to show delayed development and twice as likely to have learning disabilities (The National Center on Family Homelessness, 1999). Many homeless children manifest delays in gross and fine motor skills, and social and personal growth (Bassuk & Rosenberg, 1990) that may affect their ability to function and form sustaining, supportive adult relationships.

Each year, 97 % of homeless children move up to 3 times, 40 % attend two different schools, and 28 % attend three or more different schools. One-third repeat a grade (The National Center on Family Homelessness, 1999). It is not surprising that 16 % are less proficient at reading and math than their peers. Fewer than 25 % of homeless children graduate from high school (The National Center on Family Homelessness, 2009). The constant barrage of stressful and traumatic experiences has profound effects on their development and ability to learn, ultimately affecting their success in life.

Children experiencing homelessness are more likely than other children to suffer from acute and chronic illnesses. Homeless children go hungry at twice the rate of other children (The National Center on Family Homelessness, 1999). Not surprisingly, children who are homeless have 3 times the rate of emotional and behavioral problems, including high rates of anxiety, depression, sleep problems, shyness, withdrawal, and aggression. Many worry that something bad will happen to their family members (The National Center on Family Homelessness, 2009). These factors combine to create a life-altering experience that inflicts profound and lasting scars.

Homeless children depend on their mothers for nurturance, protection, and support. However, homeless mothers struggle more often from poor physical health and emotional issues compared to the general population. Over one-third have a chronic physical health condition. For example, mothers who are homeless have higher rates of asthma, anemia, ulcers, and hypertension than in the general population (Bassuk et al., 1996). Mothers experiencing homelessness struggle with mental health and substance use issues (Bassuk et al., 1997). High rates of posttraumatic stress disorder (PTSD) among homeless and extremely poor women are well-documented (Bassuk et al., 1996). In addition, current rates of depression in homeless mothers (52 %) are 4–5 times greater than women overall (12 %) (Knitzer, Theberge, & Johnson, 2008). As a result, these women have considerable difficulty accessing help and support for themselves and their children.

The social costs of child and family homelessness are high. These include the immediate costs of shelters, Medicaid, or health care for treating acute and chronic health conditions; mental health care and substance abuse treatment; police intervention; incarceration; and foster care. It costs taxpayers more money to place a family in emergency shelter than in permanent homes (National Alliance to End Homelessness, 2006a). There are also "opportunity costs," representing the lost opportunities that stable housing would provide in terms of greater educational attainment, better health, stable employment, higher wages, and increased income. These carry not only personal, but social benefits through increased productivity, increased ability to purchase goods and services, and decreased unemployment and disability compensation. In addition, according to a study that examined categories of adverse childhood experiences and use of services among people experiencing homelessness, the long-term costs are high (Larkin & Park, 2012). Adverse childhood experiences are strongly associated with health and social problems later in life (Felitti et al., 1998) that increase the chance of becoming homeless.

Solutions to Child and Family Homelessness

Moving out of homelessness and into permanent housing requires resources beyond the reach of many families. We believe that we can end this urgent problem if national, state, and local political leaders, service providers, advocates, businesses, and philanthropic communities work together and there is the political will to develop coordinated and strategic plans. All levels of government and the private sector must create an efficient, integrated, fully funded, and high quality system of housing and services for children and their families.

Homelessness is fundamentally a housing crisis. Nowhere in America can a full-time worker earning minimum wage afford to rent a two-bedroom unit priced at fair market value. Even with two full-time minimum wage earners, decent housing is barely attainable (National Low Income Housing Coalition, 2012). Any solution to child and family homelessness must have safe, affordable housing and ongoing residential stability as its foundation.

The need for increased numbers of affordable housing units is urgent. Given the backlog and waitlists for government funded housing voucher programs like Section 8, we need more affordable housing options. Creating housing trust funds that support new construction, rehabilitation, preservation, acquisition, permanent supportive housing, and services for special populations is a critical strategy. Many also use these trust funds for transitional housing and emergency rental assistance. Housing trust funds are established by ordinance or legislation on a state, county, or city level, and target low-income households. They rely on public revenue sources (e.g., real estate transfer taxes, interest from state-held funds, document recording fees) that vary depending on the community's resources (Brooks, 2007).

The Housing and Economic Recovery Act of 2008 established a National Housing Trust Fund (NHTF), creating our nation's first new production program specifically targeted to extremely low-income households since the inception of the Section 8 program in 1974. The National Housing Trust Fund is needed to help address the severe shortage of rental homes that are affordable for the lowest income families. Unfortunately, due to the recent housing market crash and subsequent Congressional efforts to reconfigure, and in some cases, dismantle the intended funding sources, Fannie Mae and Freddie Mac (government sponsored enterprises that expand the secondary mortgage market by increasing the number of lenders and money available for mortgage lending and new home purchases), the National Housing Trust Fund has yet to secure funding.

In addition to more available housing stock, families experiencing homelessness often need help affording high rents. Section 8 vouchers pay for a portion of housing; the remaining portion is paid for by the family. However, there are more families who need vouchers than the number available. To increase the number of Section 8 vouchers, new federal funding is necessary.

Housing is an essential component of the solution, but for many families and children, it is not sufficient. If we are concerned about the wellbeing of our nation's children, services and supports must be part of the solution. As children and families move from homelessness into housing, services and supports are necessary to achieve the transition back to the community, maintain long-term housing, and progress towards independence. In addition to affordable housing, we must address the need for education, jobs that pay a livable wage, child care, transportation, health and mental health, hunger, violence, family supports, and basic services for children.

The U.S. Department of Housing and Urban Development is committed to implementing programs that move families into housing quickly, thus supporting a "Housing First" model. Instead of moving homeless individuals and families through different levels of housing, getting closer to independent housing with each move (e.g., from a public shelter to transitional housing and then to an independent apartment), as has been the practice for many years, Housing First moves homeless families immediately from the streets or shelters into their own apartments. Various services are also delivered to promote housing stability and wellbeing—mostly after the housing placement (National Alliance to End Homelessness, 2006b).

Studies investigating the impact of housing and services on families are limited. Most of the existing research does not carefully define the nature, duration, and intensity of services necessary to support families and children. However, both research and feedback from the field strongly suggest the importance of supports and services for ensuring long-term housing stability for families (Bassuk & Geller, 2006; Bassuk, Volk, & Olivet, 2010).

A review of studies investigating the role of housing and services in ending family homelessness found that access to housing vouchers seems to increase residential stability and that case management and other services also contribute to residential stability and other desirable outcomes, including family preservation and reunification (Bassuk & Geller, 2006; Bassuk et al., 2010; National Scientific Council on the Developing Child, 2004,2005; Nolan, Broeke, Magee, & Burt, 2005; Philliber Research Associates, 2005; Rog & Gutman, 1997; Weitzman & Berry, 1994).

All families are interdependent and cannot survive in a society as complex as ours without the help and support of others. Many families have an economic and social margin that helps ensure access, availability, and robustness of support networks and services. For example, in a middle class family, it is less likely that expending resources on a medical illness of a family member will destabilize the family. In addition, many middle-income families access supports and services such as counselors, specialized health care, and educational resources in raising their children (Bassuk et al., 2010).

The service needs of families who are homeless are similar to the needs of all families and fall on a continuum, best illustrated in the shape of a bell-shaped curve. Ninety percent of families experiencing homelessness need some ongoing infusion of supports and services. The average homeless family—approximately 80 % of all homeless families—has ongoing needs that may wax and wane over time; may be episodic in nature; and vary in intensity with life circumstances, transitions, and stressors. These families need ongoing supports and a variable level of services over time. On either side of the bell curve are a small number of families—on the left approximately 10 % who need only basic services and transitional supports. By contrast, on the right side of the curve, another 10 % of families may need lifetime income supports and high levels of intensive services in order to maintain their families in permanent housing (Bassuk et al., 2010).

Ending child homelessness in the United States is urgent and possible. There must be a stable, fully funded continuum of housing options and high quality services for children and their families. Strong, ongoing coordination and collaboration among all stakeholders is required to ensure that resources are distributed effectively and strategically. These efforts must be coordinated across traditional areas of practice and government structures to provide a robust support network as well as opportunities for children and families, so that not one child will be homeless in America for even one night.

Goals of the Advocacy Effort

Throughout the 1990s and much of the 2000s, the federal government and many state governments focused on solving the problems of chronically homeless, single adults with a long duration of homelessness and a disability (e.g., substance abuse). Plans were developed, solutions were implemented, progress was made, and the number of chronically homeless, single adults decreased (National Alliance to End Homelessness, 2010). However, during this period, the number of homeless families increased from approximately 1 % of the overall homeless population in the 1980s to 37 % in 2011 (United States Department of Housing and Urban Development, 2011). Solutions that address homelessness for chronically single adults do not take into account the unique needs of homeless children and their families. To end child homelessness, we must focus on solutions that set families on a path to long-term residential stability, self-sufficiency, and improved wellbeing.

The advocacy work of the Campaign to End Child Homelessness described in this chapter is an initiative of The National Center on Family Homelessness (The National Center), a 501(c)(3) nonprofit organization funded by grants and private donations. The National Center conducts state-of-the-art research, develops and shares innovative solutions, and creates public awareness about the unique needs of homeless families and children. The mission of The National Center is to end family homelessness across America and give every child a chance.

In order to raise public awareness about child homelessness and to move federal, state, and local policymakers to action, in 2009, The National Center released *America's Youngest Outcasts: State Report Card on Child Homelessness*. Updating a study The National Center released in 1999, the report provided a comprehensive snapshot of child homelessness in the U.S. *America's Youngest Outcasts* documented that one in 50 children were homeless over the course of a year (based on 2006 numbers) and reported data for each state in 4 areas: extent of child homelessness, child wellbeing, structural risk factors for homelessness, and state level policy and planning activities (The National Center on Family Homelessness, 2009).

Each state was ranked in the 4 areas and then given an overall rank. The report also included recommendations for solutions at the federal and state level. The National Center's leadership and staff wanted the report to have lasting impact; therefore, following the release of the report, launched a national Campaign to End Child Homelessness (Campaign) with the aim of galvanizing the public and political will necessary to end this crisis. Because it is unacceptable for any child to be homeless for even one night, the Campaign is a call to action with the following goals:

- Increase public awareness of the extent and impact of homelessness on children and families.
- Inform policies and plans to better address the needs of homeless children and families.
- Improve programs and services to meet the unique needs of homeless children and families.

The Campaign connects families, communities, service providers, advocates, religious organizations, policymakers, state and local officials, and the media to address child and family homelessness through an array of coordinated local, state, and national efforts. The Campaign seeks to discover and share solutions that strengthen our nation's capacity to help families and children and leads the effort to galvanize action to ensure stable housing and wellbeing for all families.

Advocacy Action Steps

In March 2009, The National Center released *America's Youngest Outcasts* at a briefing sponsored by Senator Robert P. Casey, Jr. from Pennsylvania with more than 50 Congressional staff, federal government employees, service providers, consumers, and advocates in attendance. In an effort to increase awareness, The National Center staff delivered the report to approximately 350 key Senators and Representatives and mailed it to White House staff, Secretaries and staff at federal agencies, all 50 Governors, national and state advocates, state homeless coalitions, homeless shelters, service providers, the philanthropic community, and other stakeholders. The National Center staff also sent information about the report to media outlets throughout the country to increase awareness among the general public, which resulted in over 3,000 articles from national and local outlets such as daily and weekly newspapers, television shows, radio shows, Internet-based political and news sites, and blogs. These reports primarily focused on the large numbers of children who are homeless each year: in 2009, approximately 1 in 50. Increased public awareness generated by the resounding media response following the release of *America's Youngest Outcasts* helped generate local and state interest in the goals of the Campaign and set The National Center on a path towards creating local and national buy-in into the Campaign goals.

Federal Activities

The attention of national policymakers to the plight of homeless children and families increased significantly after the release of the report. At President Barack Obama's first nationally televised press conference two and a half months into his first term, a reporter from *Ebony* magazine asked about the data in *America's Youngest Outcasts*. The President replied that he was heartbroken that any child in America is homeless, declared that it was not acceptable for children and families to be without a roof over their heads, and pledged that his Administration would be initiating a range of programs to end homelessness. After the press conference, The National Center staff members were invited to a meeting with White House staff and other homeless advocacy organizations to discuss policy solutions to child and family homelessness. Five White House staff members as well as staff from three federal agencies expressed interest in working on initiatives to address the problem of family homelessness. The U.S. Interagency Council on Homelessness (USICH), a federal agency consisting of 19 Cabinet Secretaries that coordinates the federal response to homelessness, took the lead on this effort.

In 2010, the USICH began to develop a federal plan to prevent and end homelessness, including child and family homelessness. The National Center staff developed and submitted written recommendations to the USICH about how to end homelessness for families with children and for veteran families. The recommendations were based on knowledge gained by The National Center's research about how to end homelessness and experience overseeing and evaluating programs that serve homeless families and children. The National Center staff also participated in two workgroup meetings to strategize with federal staff about ending family homelessness, and met with USICH Executive Director and Deputy Director to discuss how to include the needs of children, youth, and families in federal efforts to end homelessness.

In June 2010, the USICH released *Opening Doors: Federal Strategic Plan to Prevent and End Homelessness* (United States Interagency Council on Homelessness, 2010). For the first time, it addresses the needs of children, youth, and families as well as veteran families. It also represents an unprecedented opportunity for the federal government to address homelessness in a coordinated and strategic way. The plan sets goals to end child, youth, and family homelessness in 10 years and chronic and veteran homelessness in 5 years. It includes objectives and strategies under the following themes: increase leadership, collaboration, and civic engagement; increase access to stable and affordable housing; increase economic security; improve health and stability; and retool the homeless crisis response system. Since homeless families and children had been relatively excluded from national policy before these efforts, this outcome represents significant progress.

With *Opening Doors* in place, leadership at The National Center felt that it was a critical time to invest additional resources in influencing federal policy. The National Center's home base is in Massachusetts; without a dedicated policy expert in Washington, DC, the Campaign would not be able to influence federal policy solutions that would prevent and end child and family homelessness. As a result, in

January 2011, the Campaign hired a Policy Director and opened an office in Washington, DC. The Policy Director's work is supported by two Massachusetts-based Campaign staff members and responsibilities include: developing and implementing a national policy agenda to end child homelessness; raising public awareness of and engagement in the issue of child and family homelessness; and educating policymakers about the needs of homeless children and effective responses.

To define priorities for The National Center's federal work, staff completed a comprehensive environmental scan of current policies related to child, youth, and family homelessness. The Policy Director interviewed national advocacy organizations as well as Congressional and federal staff and reviewed national advocacy, federal government, and Congressional websites. From information and insights gathered during the environmental scan, the Campaign developed and released a *Federal Policy Agenda* for 2011–2012 that offers federal recommendations and policy solutions to the significant issues faced by homeless children and their families—housing, supportive services, domestic violence, health and mental health, hunger, early childhood education, education, income, and planning, research, and data collection. Examples of the type of recommendations include increasing funding for housing assistance programs; increasing the enrollment of homeless families in supportive programs like Medicaid, Temporary Assistance for Needy Families, the Supplemental Nutrition Assistance Program (formerly food stamps), and substance abuse and mental health programs; increasing access to early childhood programs for young homeless children; promoting school stability for homeless children and youth; expanding workforce development programs to include homeless youth and parents; and ensuring that all federal studies and data collection efforts include questions about residential status and stability (The National Center on Family Homelessness, 2011a).

The *Federal Policy Agenda* was mailed to members of Congress in the states where the Campaign is doing some targeted work along with a copy of the state's plan (see State Activities section for more information) and distributed electronically to all relevant members of Congress and the Administration. To continue to promote the policies delineated in the *Federal Policy Agenda*, the Campaign hosted a webinar attended by more than 400 individuals; about half were Congressional and Administration staff (including staff from the USICH). Over the course of the next 6 months, Campaign staff visited over 50 Congressional and Administration staff to share recommendations from the *Federal Policy Agenda* and *America's Youngest Outcasts*. The implementation of recommendations in the *Federal Policy Agenda* will go far in putting the federal government on track to accomplish its goal of ending family homelessness in 10 years.

State Activities

After releasing *America's Youngest Outcasts* and launching the Campaign to End Child Homelessness, one of The National Center's goals was to initiate work in various states that were ranked among the bottom ten in the report. Based on relationships The National Center had from previous projects, staff decided to develop state-based Campaigns in four of the bottom ten ranked states: Florida, Georgia, Mississippi, and New Mexico.

Staff felt the critical first step in working in states was to develop partnerships with local organizations dedicated to working with homeless children and families in each state. As a national organization, it is important for us to partner with those that have in-depth knowledge of local and regional needs, challenges, and strengths within the homeless service system which vary across the country. There are also many organizations serving homeless families directly and working to end homelessness, making collaborations and relationships critical in order to achieve the best possible outcomes. For example, two of the Campaign's partner organizations are the Florida Coalition for the Homeless and the Georgia Alliance to End Homelessness—both state-based organizations whose members include homeless service providers and advocates committed to ending homelessness. Two Massachusetts-based Campaign staff work with the state partner organizations to build collaborations with and seek input from key stakeholders who can share information about the needs and dynamics on the ground, which differ across states and regions within each state. In Mississippi, a full-time, Jackson, MS-based staff person oversees Campaign activities because a funder was specifically interested in supporting local activities.

To ensure the Campaign's work was locally relevant, staff needed to identify the following in each region: (1) key issues facing homeless children and their families; (2) services, programs, and policies that support children and families who are homeless; and (3) community leaders and stakeholders involved who have influence over relevant programs and policies in each state. To collect this information, The National Center staff met with community leaders, service providers, advocates, and policymakers in each state over the course of several months. In Georgia, staff gave presentations about the report and the Campaign at three meetings attended by homeless and social service providers. In Florida, the Campaign sponsored seven community meetings around the state and presented a workshop at a statewide housing and homelessness conference. In Mississippi, staff facilitated five community meetings around the state and met individually with many homeless and social service organizations to get their feedback. In New Mexico, staff collaborated with several partner organizations to sponsor a 2-day, statewide summit with workshops and opportunities for discussion and input. Within each state, staff collected additional information about local circumstances and spoke with parents who were homeless to learn about how they became homeless and their family's experiences while homeless.

The Campaign used the information staff learned within each region and the knowledge The National Center and the Campaign's local partners have gained over the years to develop state-specific recommendations to end child homelessness. With partner organizations, the Campaign reviewed feedback and data collected, identified key issues and gaps in services, and proposed solutions. These solutions were reviewed by additional local organizations who offered feedback. The recommendations were then published—along with data from *America's Youngest Outcasts* and summaries of information collected from people around the state, homeless parents, and our research—in state-specific plans: *Florida Plan to End Child Homelessness, Georgia Plan to End Child Homelessness, Mississippi Plan to End Child Homelessness*, and *Ending Child Homelessness in New Mexico*. Each Plan addresses how to increase public awareness about the extent and impact of homelessness on children and families, inform state and local policies and plans to address the needs of homeless children and families, and improve programs and services to meet the unique needs of this population—the three main goals of the national Campaign and the state Campaigns (The National Center on Family Homelessness, 2010, 2011b, 2011c; New Mexico Children, Youth, and Families Department and the New Mexico Campaign to End Child Homelessness, 2010).

The Campaign and local partners released the state Plans at public events and to local media outlets. The Florida Plan was released by the Florida Coalition for the Homeless during a homeless advocacy day event at the State Capitol in Tallahassee. The Georgia Plan was released at a statewide conference on homelessness sponsored by the Georgia Alliance to End Homelessness. In Mississippi, the Plan was released at an event in Jackson in conjunction with the chair of the Mississippi State Senate Housing Committee. In New Mexico, the Plan was presented at a hearing of the Legislative Health and Human Services Committee in conjunction with the state's Children, Youth and Families Department. Similar to the inclusion of the needs of children and families in *Opening Doors*, these state-specific plans represented significant steps forward in Florida, Georgia, Mississippi, and New Mexico. Prior to their release, none of the states had plans to end homelessness that specifically addressed the needs of children and families.

Outcomes of our Advocacy Efforts

Federal Outcomes and Successes

Since the release of the *Federal Policy Agenda*, the Campaign has been working to implement strategies to meet its goals. Many programs and policies contribute to preventing and ending child and family homelessness, so it is necessary to work across multiple federal agencies, Congressional committees, with states and locales, and the public and private sectors. The Campaign aims most of its efforts towards opportunities that arise and policies that have traction with Congress and/or the Administration. Strategies include: partnering with other advocacy groups and collaborating on mutual goals; building relationships with staff from Capitol Hill, USICH, and the Administration and working together on issues that affect homeless children and their families; educating policymakers through the creation and dissemination of policy briefs, webinars, and other educational materials; drafting legislation; and building grassroots support through regular e-newsletter updates, action alerts, Facebook updates, and Twitter postings.

Thus far, the Campaign has focused on federal appropriations to protect and strengthen funding for programs serving homeless children and families. Staff members have also worked to develop and move legislation forward on issues including: the National Housing Trust Fund, Violence Against Women Act Reauthorization, the Homeless Children and Youth Act, and Workforce Investment Act Reauthorization. In addition, the National Center staff members have been working with the USICH to implement *Opening Doors* and to add recommendations where there are gaps in the original plan, particularly in the areas of early childhood education, overall education, and youth. During 2012, 2 years after releasing *Opening Doors*, the USICH released an update to the plan that included more specific recommendations in these areas.

The Campaign's current success can partly be traced to staff ability to build collaborations around policy issues. In June 2011, the Campaign led efforts with two major coalitions to sponsor a joint meeting of national child and youth development organizations and homeless advocacy groups. Attendees discussed how to increase collaboration between these two fields. Coming out of the meeting, the Campaign and partners released *Improving Federal Collaboration for Homeless Children and Youth*. The brief highlights recommendations on improving federal coordination and collaboration among agencies and programs, and was electronically distributed to relevant White House staff, members of Congress, and advocates.

Another key component of the Campaign's success has been staff ability to raise awareness and educate policymakers. To accomplish this goal, staff members arrange events showcasing policies in the *Federal Policy Agenda*. In November 2011, the Campaign held a federal policy briefing on child and family homelessness and launched *Looking Into Light* at HUD, a photo exhibit documenting the experience of family homelessness and highlighting the solutions. The National Center developed this exhibit to raise awareness. The photos were selected from an archive of 20,000 images of homeless families and children taken during the late 1980s and early 1990s and donated by the photographer. The briefing and exhibit commemorated National Homelessness Awareness Month. More than 90 national advocates, federal agency and Congressional staff attended the events in person. The briefing was live broadcasted online by HUD to media outlets and advocates across the nation. Speakers included USICH's Executive Director and HUD's Assistant Secretary for Community Planning and Development along with staff from the National Center, a member of the National Center's Consumer Advisory Board, and leaders from the national homeless advocacy community. The *Looking Into Light* exhibit was displayed at HUD throughout National Homeless Awareness Month. The exhibit is now touring the country educating and inspiring viewers to take action to end child homelessness.

State Outcomes and Successes

Since the release of the state plans, the Campaign has been working in each state to implement various recommendations.

The *Florida Plan to End Child Homelessness* was included in the Florida Council on Homelessness' Annual Report to the Governor and distributed to state senators and representatives. Following the release of the *Florida Plan*, staff invited the local homeless coalitions to join two conference calls to discuss and provide input on implementing the Plan's recommendations. To highlight National Homelessness Awareness Month in November, the Florida Campaign also wrote an opinion piece that was distributed to media outlets across the state.

The New Mexico Plan—*Ending Child Homelessness in New Mexico*—recommends establishing a New Mexico Interagency Council on Homelessness (NMICH). During the 2011 legislative session, a key partner of the New Mexico Campaign Steering Committee introduced legislation requesting that the Governor and Legislative Council create an NMICH. Both the New Mexico House and Senate voted to pass the legislation, but the Governor and Legislative Council have yet to act on it.

The Mississippi Campaign has worked to increase awareness of the scope and impact of child homelessness among state legislators and policymakers and to inform the state's policies and plans by advocating for a Mississippi Interagency Council on Homelessness (MSICH). Towards this end, the Mississippi Campaign worked to introduce legislation in the state House and Senate during the 2011 session that would establish a MSICH. The legislation did not make any progress in 2011. It was reintroduced during the 2012 session and passed from the House Youth and Family Affairs Committee to the Public Health and Human Service Committee, but did not progress further. Between the 2011 and 2012 legislative sessions, the chairs of the committees where the legislation was referred changed hands, causing a setback for the Mississippi Campaign. Although the Mississippi Campaign has increased awareness of the need for an MSICH and mobilized some support, more work needs to occur before this legislation is officially enacted.

As part of the Mississippi Campaign's advocacy strategy, staff members are continuously educating members of the Mississippi Legislature about the benefits of creating an MSICH. Staff presented the *Mississippi Plan to End Child Homelessness* in 2011 to the state's Select Committee on Poverty and held an educational event at the State Capitol that was covered by Jackson area media outlets. In the fall of 2011, the Mississippi Campaign also testified at a hearing of the Mississippi House of Representatives Committee on Public Health and Human Services about establishing an MSICH. Members of the House Committee on Public Health and Human Services, House Select Committee on Poverty, and Senate Committee on Housing attended the hearing, which was called by the chair of the House Committee on Public Health and Human Services, and covered by Jackson area media outlets. In February 2012, the Mississippi Campaign hosted another educational event at the State Capitol—also covered by local media.

Next Steps

In December 2011, the Campaign released an updated version of *America's Youngest Outcasts* with data through 2010, state rankings, and a federal call to action. The new report documented that child homelessness in the United States has increased from 1 in 50 to 1 in 45 children annually (The National Center on Family Homelessness, 2011a, 2011b, 2011c, 2011d). Once again, the report received a significant amount of attention from the media, policymakers, and homeless service providers and advocates from around the country. The Campaign will use this updated report as we used the original—as a call to action for work moving forward.

The current economic recession has compounded the challenges faced by the Campaign and partners on the ground throughout the country. The number of homeless families continues to grow dramatically. Although this has led to an increased demand for shelter and support services, budgets have been severely cut, compounding the financial strain on homeless service providers. Given the economic downturn coupled with the challenging political climate, finding additional resources to address child and family homelessness is a formidable challenge. Within this context, policy change has become more difficult and protracted; attention has shifted to maintaining and maximizing existing resources.

Still, Campaign staff members continue to work to implement goals to increase awareness about child homelessness, galvanize public and political will for decisive action, inform policy solutions, and improve programs and services. The Campaign continues to work in Washington, DC and in the four states to implement the federal and state policy priorities laid out in *America's Youngest Outcasts 2010*, the *Federal Policy Agenda,* and the state plans to end child homelessness. Staff members also continue efforts to provide training and technical assistance to homeless service providers throughout the country in order to ensure high quality programs and services for homeless children and their families. Although progress is incremental albeit slow, the increase in numbers of homeless families continues to draw attention to the problem and makes eventual change probable. With this in mind, the National Center hopes to expand the work of the Campaign into more states, continuing with the states ranked in the bottom ten in *America's Youngest Outcasts 2010*. To read reports, plans, and other resources from the Campaign and the National Center, and to stay updated on the work of the Campaign, visit www.HomelessChildrenAmerica.org and www.familyhomelessness.org and find the National Center on Facebook and Twitter.

References

Barrow, S. M., & Lawinski, T. (2009). Contexts of mother-child separations in homeless families. *Analyses of Social Issues and Public Policy, 9*(1), 157–176.

Bassuk, E. L. (2010). Ending child homelessness in America. *The American Journal of Orthopsychiatry, 80*(4), 496–504.

Bassuk, E. L., Buckner, J. C., Weinreb, L. F., Browne, A., Bassuk, S. S., Dawson, R., et al. (1997). Homelessness in female-headed families: Childhood and adult risk and protective factors. *American Journal of Public Health, 87*(2), 241–248.

Bassuk, E. L., & Geller, S. (2006). The role of housing and services in ending family homelessness. *Housing Policy Debate, 17*(4), 781–806.

Bassuk, E. L., & Rosenberg, L. (1990). Psychosocial characteristics of homeless and children without homes. *Pediatrics, 85*(3), 257–261.

Bassuk, E. L., Volk, K. T., & Olivet, J. (2010). A framework for developing supports and services for families experiencing homelessness. *The Open Health Services and Policy Journal, 3*, 34–40.

Bassuk, E. L., Weinreb, L. F., Buckner, J. C., Browne, A., Salomon, A., & Bassuk, S. S. (1996). The characteristics and needs of sheltered homeless and low-income housed mothers. *Journal of the American Medical Association, 276*(8), 640–646.

Brooks, M. E. (2007). *Housing trust fund progress report 2007*. Frazier Park, CA: Housing Trust Fund Project, Center for Community Change.

Brown, D. W., Anda, R. F., Tiemeier, H., Felitti, V. J., Edwards, V. J., Croft, J. B., et al. (2009). Adverse childhood experiences and the risk of premature mortality. *American Journal of Preventive Medicine, 37*(5), 389–396.

Burt, M. R., Aron, L. Y., Douglas, T., Valente, J., Edgar, L., & Britta, I. (1999). *Homelessness: Programs and the people they serve: Summary report-findings of the National Survey of Homeless Assistance Providers and Clients*. Washington, DC: The Urban Institute.

Burt, M. R., Aron, L. Y., Douglas, T., Valente, J., Edgar, L., & Britta, I. (2000). *America's homeless II: Populations and services*. Washington, DC: The Urban Institute.

Felitti, V. J., Anda, R. F., Nordenberg, D., Williamson, D. F., Spitz, A. M., Edwards, V., et al. (1998). Relationship of childhood abuse and household dysfunction to many of the leading causes of death in adults: The adverse childhood experiences (ACE) study. *American Journal of Preventive Medicine, 14*(4), 354–364.

Guarino, K., & Bassuk, E. L. (2010). Working with families experiencing homelessness. *Journal of Zero to Three: National Center for Infants, Toddlers, and Families, 30*(3), 11–20.

Knitzer, J., Theberge, S., & Johnson, K. (2008). *Reducing maternal depression and its impact on young children: Toward a responsive early childhood policy framework*. New York, NY: National Center for Children in Poverty.

Larkin, H., & Park, J. (2012). Adverse childhood experiences (ACEs), service use, and service helpfulness among people experiencing homelessness. *Families in Society: The Journal of Contemporary Social Services, 93*(2), 85–93.

National Alliance to End Homelessness. (2006a). *Promising strategies to end family homelessness*. Washington, DC: Author.

National Alliance to End Homelessness. (2006b). *What is housing first*. Washington, DC: Author.

National Alliance to End Homelessness. (2010). *Chronic homelessness policy solutions*. Washington, DC: Author.

National Center for Homeless Education. (2011). *Education for homeless children and youth program data collection summary: From the school year 2009-10 federally required state data collection for the McKinney-Vento Education Assistance Improvements Act of 2001 and comparison of the SY 2007-08, SY 2008-09, and SY 2009-10 data collections*. Greensboro, NC: Author.

National Low Income Housing Coalition. (2012). *Out of reach 2012: America's forgotten housing crisis*. Washington, DC: Author.

National Scientific Council on the Developing Child. (2004). *Young children develop in an environment of relationships: Working paper no. 1*. Cambridge, MA: Author.

National Scientific Council on the Developing Child. (2005). *Excessive stress disrupts the architecture of the developing brain: Working paper no. 3*. Cambridge, MA: Author.

New Mexico Children, Youth, and Families Department and the New Mexico Campaign to End Child Homelessness. (2010). *Ending child and family homelessness in New Mexico*. Santa Fe, NM: Author.

Nolan, C., Broeke, C., Magee, M., & Burt, M. R. (2005). *The family permanent supportive housing initiative: Family history and experiences in supportive housing*. Washington, DC: Urban Institute and Harder & Company Community Research.

Philliber Research Associates. (2005). *Supportive housing for families' evaluation: Accomplishments and lessons learned*. Accord, NY: Corporation for Supportive Housing.

Rog, D. J., & Buckner, J. C. (2007). *Homeless families and children*. Paper presented at the 2007 National Symposium on Homelessness Research, Washington, DC. Retrieved May 12, 2010 from http://aspe.hhs.gov/hsp/homelessness/symposium07/rog/index.htm

Rog, D. J., & Gutman, M. (1997). The homeless families program: A summary of key findings. In S. L. Isaacs & J. R. Knickman (Eds.), *The Robert Wood Johnson Foundation Anthology: To improve health and health care* (pp. 209–231). San Francisco: Jossey-Bass.

Subtitle B of Title VII of the McKinney-Vento Homeless Assistance Act within the No Child Left Behind Act of 2001 (Title X, Part C, Public Law 107-110).

The National Center on Family Homelessness. (1999). *Homeless children: America's new outcasts*. Newton Centre, MA: Author.

The National Center on Family Homelessness. (2009). *America's youngest outcasts: State report card on child homelessness*. Newton Centre, MA: Author.

The National Center on Family Homelessness. (2010). *Mississippi plan to end child homelessness*. Needham, MA: Author.

The National Center on Family Homelessness. (2011a). *Federal policy agenda*. Needham, MA: Author.

The National Center on Family Homelessness. (2011b). *Florida plan to end child homelessness*. Needham, MA: Author.

The National Center on Family Homelessness. (2011c). *Georgia plan to end child homelessness*. Needham, MA: Author.

The National Center on Family Homelessness. (2011d). *America's youngest outcasts: 2010*. Needham, MA: Author.

Title I of the Housing and Economic Recovery Act of 2008 (Section 1338, Public Law 110-289).

United States Census Bureau. (2007). *Table S1703: Selected characteristics of people at specified levels of poverty in the last 12 months* [Data file]. Retrieved from http://factfinder.census.gov/servlet/STTable?_bm=y&-context=st&-qr_name=ACS_2007_1YR_G00_S1703&-ds_name=ACS_2007_1YR_G00_&CONTEXT=st&-tree_id=307&-redoLog=true*-_caller=geoselect&-geo_id=01000US&-format=&-_lang=en

United States Department of Housing and Urban Development. (2011). *HUD's 2011 CoC homeless assistance programs—Homeless populations and subpopulations* [Data file]. Retrieved from http://www.hudhre.info/index.cfm?do=actionHomelessrptsSearch

United States Interagency Council on Homelessness. (2010). *Opening Doors: Federal strategic plan to prevent and end homelessness*. Washington, DC: Author.

Weitzman, B. C., & Berry, C. (1994). *Formerly homeless families and the transition to permanent housing: High-risk families and the role of intensive case management services*. New York: Edna McConnell Clark Foundation.

Chapter 7
Lessons Learned About the Impact of Disasters on Children and Families and Post-disaster Recovery

Joy D. Osofsky and Howard J. Osofsky

Disasters affect the lives of millions of children each year causing immense hardship and suffering. Traumatic experiences for children and their families caused by natural disasters (earthquakes, hurricanes, tornadoes, floods, tsunamis, fires) and human made disasters (industrial accidents, nuclear fall-out, armed conflict, terrorism, disease outbreaks) are often cumulative. When children and families are unpacked by disasters, they frequently are displaced, lose their homes and property, suffer economic hardship, loss of community and social supports, and, at times, experience injury and death of loved ones.

Children of all ages are impacted by disasters with differential reactions depending on developmental level (Masten & Osofsky, 2010; Osofsky, Osofsky, & Harris, 2007). However, young children are particularly vulnerable to being traumatized by disasters because their experiences are dependent on and mediated through the responses and experiences of parents, caregivers, and other adults in their environment who may also be traumatized. Adolescents are vulnerable in other complex ways. Because of their increasing independence from family and dependence on peers, they are at risk for negative influences such as risky behaviors, substance abuse, and other maladaptive behaviors. Although exposure to disasters is negative for all children and families, it is important to recognize that with protection and support, most children will be resilient (Masten & Narayan, 2012; Masten & Osofsky, 2010). At the same time, because the environment during and after a disaster may be very confusing for young children, it is common for them to appear numb, unresponsive, and anxious. The behaviors and emotions that may follow

J.D. Osofsky, Ph.D. (✉)
Departments of Pediatrics and Psychiatry, Louisiana State University Health Sciences Center, 1542 Tulane Avenue, 2nd Floor, New Orleans, LA 70112, USA
e-mail: josofs@lsuhsc.edu

H.J. Osofsky, M.D., Ph.D.
Department of Psychiatry, Louisiana State University Health Sciences Center, New Orleans, LA, USA

A. McDonald Culp (ed.), *Child and Family Advocacy: Bridging the Gaps Between Research, Practice, and Policy*, Issues in Clinical Child Psychology, DOI 10.1007/978-1-4614-7456-2_7, © Springer Science+Business Media New York 2013

reflect their anxiety with frequent behavioral and emotional dysregulation often interpreted by adults as misbehavior and leading to parental impatience and even, at times, harsh punishment. Too often, disaster preparedness and responses have given little emphasis to the needs of children. Preparedness, planning effectively for responding to children's needs, and responding sensitively to support both children and families are very important to build resilience and aid recovery.

Massive disasters such as hurricanes, earthquakes, tsunamis, tornadoes, flooding, and fires impact both physically and psychologically on children and families. Damage includes physical destruction, loss of homes, property, toys, pets, and, for many, separation from or loss of family members and community. Disasters with slow recovery and multiple complexities (a combination of natural and technological disasters) can be especially difficult for children and families resulting in acute and chronic psychological effects (Kessler, Galea, Jones, & Parker, 2006; Kronenberg et al., 2010; Osofsky, Osofsky, Kronenberg, Brennan, & Hansel, 2009; Weems et al., 2007, 2009) that negatively impact the child's normal developmental trajectory (Pynoos, Steinberg, & Piacentini, 1999; Shaw, 2000). Families in the Gulf region have had to cope with multiple disasters being impacted by Hurricane Katrina and approximately 41/2 years later the devastation caused by the Deepwater Horizon Incident (Gulf Oil Spill) resulting in cumulative traumatization and indications of community corrosion (Palinkas, 2009; Palinkas, Petterson, Russell, & Downs, 1993; Picou, Marshall, & Gill, 2004). Another example of the interaction of complex natural and technological disasters is the 2011 earthquake, tsunami, and nuclear fall-out in Japan. The initial earthquake and tsunami resulted in a severe natural disaster that was compounded by the technological nuclear disaster resulting in both immediate and long-lasting individual, family and community impacts with continual concerns about keeping children and families safe due to the nuclear fall-out (Watanabe, 2012). Large-scale disasters, such as Hurricane Katrina combined with the Gulf Oil Spill and the Japanese earthquake, tsunami, and nuclear disaster are of particular importance related to children's development as they affect not only individuals but also multiple systems, including microsystems and exosystems, in which children develop (Bronfenbrenner, 1986; Goldstein, Osofsky, & Lichtveld, 2011; Masten & Narayan, 2012; Masten & Obradović, 2008; Osofsky, Palinkas, & Galloway, 2010). For children experiencing such disasters, their once-thriving communities including homes, neighborhoods, grocery stores, and playgrounds are no longer functional; many children experience multiple moves and changes in schools, separation from friends and family members, and much parental stress resulting from family disruption and unemployment (Osofsky et al., 2007a, 2007b, 2009; Watanabe, 2012). Families impacted by such disasters are threatened with severe economic difficulties as well as loss of traditional supports and even their identities as they must learn to live and thrive in other communities often with lessened economic resources. For those communities living by the water and depending on fishing for their economic survival as well as their identity, the tsunami and nuclear disaster in Japan and the oil spill in Louisiana have threatened the tranquil fishing and wildlife areas on the coast. If it is possible to draw from other disaster data, information from the Exxon-Valdez Oil Spill (www.onearth.org/

article/lessons-from-the-exxon-valdez; Palinkas, 2009; Picou & Gill, 1996) showed the significant vulnerability of children over time with much impact on individual, family, and community identity. Long-term outcomes for young children who are still developing are still in question, and such uncertainties are common for all children exposed to a disaster with slow recovery.

What We Know About the Impact of Disasters on Children

Disaster research indicates that the impact on children depends upon the nature of the disaster, the age and vulnerability of the child, the types of resources available to the child, and family and community supports (Masten & Osofsky, 2010). While young children are more vulnerable, there is more research on older children that can provide a perspective for an understanding of developmental issues. Child-focused disaster studies most often focus on post-disaster symptomatology. For example, most of the research on the impact of exposure to hurricanes indicates that children are at a high risk for symptoms of depression, anxiety, and posttraumatic stress (PTSD) (Goenjian et al., 2001; Kessler et al., 2006; Osofsky et al., 2007a, 2007b; Osofsky, Osofsky, Kronenberg, Brennan, & Hansel, 2009) and studies on the impact of other natural disasters such as earthquakes and tsunamis indicate children show symptoms of PTSD (Goenjian et al., 2005; John, Russell, & Russell, 2007; La Greca, Silverman, Vernberg, & Prinstein, 1996; Lonigan, Shannon, Taylor, Finch, & Sallee, 1994; Pfefferbaum, 1997; Piyasil et al., 2007; Pynoos et al., 1993).

Overall, the relation between PTSD symptoms and disaster-specific aspects of trauma has been well documented in the literature. For example, a study of 16- and 17-year-old children following a 1999 earthquake in Greece (Roussos et al., 2005) as well as studies of 13-year-olds following Hurricane Mitch in Nicaragua (Goenjian et al., 2001, 2005) showed that exposure to a natural disaster was consistently related to increases in the severity of PTSD symptoms. In a study of over 5,000 children ages 9–19 who experienced displacement and damage to their homes as a result of Hurricane Hugo, PTSD was associated with traumatic experiences (Lonigan et al., 1994). Similarly, Russoniello et al. (2007) found that 9–12-year-old children, whose homes were flooded as a result of Hurricane Floyd, were 3 times more likely to have symptoms of PTSD compared to those whose homes did not flood. Hamada, Kameoka, Yanagida, and Chemtob (2003) reported that 6–12-year-old children who experienced Hurricane Iniki were more likely to report posttraumatic symptoms if they felt that their lives or the lives of others were threatened at the time of the hurricane.

The issue of cumulative traumatic experience is important in understanding the severity of symptoms. For example, Neuner, Schauer, Catani, Ruf, and Elbert (2006) assessed 64 tsunami survivors in Sri Lanka, ages 8–14, and found that previous traumas, including exposure to war, domestic violence, community violence, medical treatment, physical abuse, and natural disaster, were associated with increased posttraumatic stress symptoms. Similarly, Garrison, Weinrich, Hardin, Weinrich, and Wang (1993) assessed 1,264 children, ages 11–17, following Hurricane Hugo and found that experiencing previous violent, traumatic events was associated with increased likelihood of PTSD.

Many of these studies indicate that children have reported comorbid symptoms of depression following natural disasters. The studies have shown the presence of each disorder following disasters despite the overlap in symptomatology of PTSD and depression, including anhedonia, sleep difficulties, problems with concentration, irritability, and a restricted range of affect (Goenjian et al., 2001; Kolaitis et al., 2003; Roussos et al., 2005). For example, a study of PTSD and depression in children between the ages of 7 and 17 who were affected by a super-cyclone in India showed that, although PTSD and depression were significantly correlated, most children with PTSD did not meet criteria for depression, and 55.7 % of children with a diagnosis of depression did not meet criteria for PTSD (Kar et al., 2007). Unlike symptoms of PTSD, depression has not been found to be consistently related to level of disaster exposure or proximity. Depression has been associated with several different factors including reported difficulties at home following the disaster (Roussos et al., 2005), death of a family member (Goenjian et al., 2001), and feeling that one's own life or the lives of family members were in danger (Thienkrua et al., 2006).

Research regarding how children express traumatic responses has been well established. Commonly observed traumatic reactions in school-age children include: specific fears, separation difficulties, sleep problems, reenactment of the trauma in play, regression, somatic complaints, irritability, decline in academic performance, fear of recurrence of the trauma, and trauma-related guilt (Steinberg, Brymer, Decker, & Pynoos, 2004; Vogel & Vernberg, 1993). Adolescents, on the other hand, often express difficulties through individuation and identity development processes. Pynoos (1993) stated that "a trauma-induced sense of discontinuity can give a disrupting influence on the adolescent task of integrating past, present, and future expectations into a lasting sense of identity" (p. 222). Pynoos (1993) reaffirmed Blos (1967) who described adolescence as is a period of individuation and elaborated that any threat to this process as a result of traumatic experiences can potentially disrupt the developmental focus of this important period.

Response, Recovery, and Resilience Following Disasters

Systematic longitudinal research on children in disasters, response and recovery, can be extremely helpful in developing more sensitive and efficient responses to their needs. In order to be most effective, however, planners and responders need to be mindful of the developmental needs of children of all ages. In addition to federal organizations such as Red Cross, Save the Children, SAMSHA, Federal Emergency Management Agency (FEMA), and materials developed by the National Child Traumatic Stress Network and the National Center for PTSD, trauma-informed experts on developmental needs of children of different ages can contribute significantly to disaster response and recovery. "Understanding children's responses to different disaster situations across age and post-disaster circumstances can help us learn which children are most at risk and what supports are most important to consider in recovery" (Children and Disasters, Child Development Research in Brief, www.srcd.org, 2010).

Recent theoretical research has focused on examining patterns of resilience and recovery as it relates to developmental theories and trajectories for children. Important factors that support resilience in preparation for and following disasters include promotive and protective influences (Bonanno, 2004; Bonanno & Mancini, 2008; Layne et al., 2009; Masten & Obradović, 2008). Masten and Narayan (2012) and Masten and Osofsky (2010) discussed promotive factors as those predicting better outcomes at all levels of risk or adversity and protective factors that are more important when risk or adversity if high. These two perspectives are extremely important in understanding the effect of disasters on children. The impact of disasters and developmental issues that follow are influenced by the nature and severity of the exposure, the importance of pre- and post-disaster context for understanding disaster response and recovery, protective factors for positive recovery such as strengths and individual characteristics, and the possible role of children's age, and gender (Masten & Osofsky, 2010). Pynoos (1993) discussed factors that influence poor long-term outcomes following disasters including extended periods of high cumulative adversity related to breakdown of infrastructure, ongoing economic consequences, family stress, loss of life and property, and other aspects of slow recovery.

While parents play a key protective role for children of all ages related to preparedness, safety, communication, and role-modeling adaptive behaviors, parents are particularly important for younger children who are more vulnerable and dependent on adults. To ensure the protection of children during and following disasters, it is important to be cognizant of parental stresses as well as the need for parental education and information in order for parents/caregivers to carry out their caring roles most effectively. While relatively few studies are available for parents related to factors that support resilience in children, a recent study by Kithakye et al. (2010), which also includes pre-disaster adjustment, shows that self-regulation skills in preschoolers were associated with prosocial behavior in general and had an moderating effect on the impact of exposure severity on prosocial outcomes. Masten (2007) also found that self-regulation skills can support a protective role for children.

An important part of disaster preparedness for children must involve parents and caregivers to effectively plan and carry out the roles of protection, communication, and safeguarding children under very difficult circumstances. As mentioned above, an additional risk factor for children is prior traumatic experiences and losses that play a key role in how young children (or children and adults of any age) will react to and cope with disasters. Children with prior difficulties and those who have experienced previous trauma or loss, and continue to experience post-disaster trauma and adversities, are at higher risk for mental and behavioral health problems than those without these compounding difficulties (Bowlby, 1973; Laor et al., 1997; Osofsky, 2004; Osofsky, Osofsky, Hansel, & Reuther, 2011; Pynoos, 1993; Pynoos, Steinberg, & Goenjian, 1996; Vogel & Vernberg, 1993).

Understanding how resilience and self-efficacy may operate in individuals, families, and groups following disasters can contribute a great deal to an understanding of responses and ways to support recovery. In the aftermath of disasters, it may be very difficult to maintain the crucial components of Masten's "short list" that supports resilience and contributes to individual self-efficacy (Masten & Obradovi , 2008). For example, with evacuations and displacements, families and friends may be separated due to circumstances of the evacuation including separations for reasons of safety, living in crowded shelters, and economic necessity. Further, parents are dealing with additional stresses such as loss of homes, employment, and services as well as uncertainties about the future. Other usual supports from community services are also frequently disrupted when caregivers such as teachers, clergy, and clinicians are also dealing with personal and community losses. These factors can interfere with effective caregiving and gaining support from family, friends, and community. Supportive schools and teachers are a protective factor; however, with displacement, children will often be in new schools with different teachers. For example, following Hurricane Katrina, children who evacuated from areas heavily impacted by the storm attended an average of two schools with some children attending as many as nine schools in 1 year (Osofsky, 2011a, 2011b; Osofsky et al., 2009). Faith and hope are important protective factors that can be significantly disrupted by disaster; however, with spirituality, this positive force for recovery is frequently present even in the midst of destruction following disasters. Self-regulation skills, another important protective factor for resilience and component of self-efficacy, are also frequently disrupted in the aftermath of disasters due to the lack of routines, continual changes in living arrangements, school, and caregiving. However, for those children are able to adapt more easily, these skills are often present. For children and adolescents to show resilience and self-efficacy following disasters, there must be either some protective factors in place despite the disruption or confusion, or adults in the environment who, even with the uncertainty, can create a reasonably amount of stability and support.

In order to achieve positive outcomes, support from adults and an environment that can create a sense of "normalcy" in an abnormal environment are very important (see Osofsky et al., 2007a, 2007b). While there is a great deal of literature on trauma experiences and negative mental and behavioral health symptoms, relatively little is known about how resilience following disasters or trauma contributes to a child's perceived ability to achieve future goals. Yet the St. Bernard Parish School System, located about 10 miles from the city of New Orleans, whose school buildings were totally destroyed by Hurricane Katrina and the breaching of the levees, intuitively knew that focus should not only be on current recovery following a major disaster but also on the importance of rebuilding schools to help develop a sense of community and what the future holds for affected children and their families. We approached the St. Bernard Parish Superintendent and Assistant Superintendent, first in Baton Rouge where we had all evacuated and were working to find families and respond to the disaster, and later in September 2005 on the second level of the St. Bernard School Administration Building—the first level was still covered with muck with efforts being made to start cleaning and rebuilding. At that time, most of the school administrators, principals, and teachers were living in FEMA trailers near the administration building and one remaining high school building where only the second level was usable. The St. Bernard Parish School Board opened the St. Bernard Unified School in temporary structures less than 3 months after Hurricane Katrina, becoming the first school to open in the flood zone in an effort to create a sense of normalcy for the children and families. The rapid planning and reopening of the school made it possible for many residents who worked at the school and in factories nearby to return and begin rebuilding their homes without having to send their children away to school. The LSU Health Sciences Center mental health team worked hand-in-hand with the school when they reopened and continued to provide services for children and support to counselors, teachers, and parents in the now 11 rebuilt schools. The level of reported mental health symptoms—posttraumatic stress and depression—were high in heavily impacted areas and there was a need to develop creative ways to support resilience in children. To accomplish this objective, the St. Bernard Unified School System collaborated with the Louisiana State University Health Sciences Center Department of Psychiatry and developed the, St. Bernard Family Resiliency Project (SBFRP). This program was part of the school system's mission in promoting a positive and healthy recovery environment for their students. The Youth Leadership Program established for "ordinary" children as part of SBFRP has led to students developing helpful school, family, and community projects as well as demonstrating increased and lasting self-efficacy and leadership skills. What we learned together with this remarkable public school system about the process of recovery following disasters is that rebuilding schools as soon as possible and school resilience programs are an important part of the solution.

The Need for Advocacy: Lessons Learned About Disaster Response

Disasters of all kinds occur far too frequently, be they hurricanes, typhoons, earthquakes, fires, flooding or technological disasters. The potential for children to be impacted is great because, even with preparedness, it is not possible to anticipate when a disaster may occur. When a disaster occurs, not only are children affected but also parents and other caregivers who are so important in keeping children safe and providing both protection and nurturance. Further with displacement, there is disruption and loss of property, sometimes lives, and ordinary routines that are so helpful for the stability and positive growth of children. Children who lack the cognitive and emotional capacity and skills to cope with the traumatic experience and uncertainties can be profoundly impacted by disasters. Children of all ages are more or less dependent upon parents and other caregivers to support their development and meet their needs and parents/caregivers may not have the physical or emotional resources available to be able to meet their children's needs. For all children separation from significant caregivers, loss of homes, toys, pets, and normal routines affect their response and recovery. With displacements, there may be a dramatic impact on the established relationship between the child and his or her parents as well as extended family and other trusted adults. Disaster response can be much improved with more attention to the developmental needs of children of different ages. Older children and adolescents also can play key roles in the rebuilding while they build their own resilience. These activities provide the opportunity for older children to contribute to rebuilding and helping the community and supporting younger children as a way to build their resilience and support self-efficacy and to prevent risk-taking behaviors that are common after disasters when teenagers have lost their usual support structures. Cultural and spiritual practices, even without the physical structures that may have supported them are also crucial for building both individual and community resilience. With better preparation and acknowledgement of difficulties, it is anticipated that children will be able to be provided with much more support during and in the aftermath of disasters.

Goal: Provide Disaster Relief for Children in Hurricane Katrina

Perhaps it is worth sharing one experience among many following Hurricane Katrina. Working on disaster response and recovery, with our Louisiana State University Health Sciences Center (LSUHSC) team, we had the opportunity to implement a "disaster recovery plan" on the two cruise ships that were sent to New Orleans and docked at Julia Street Harbor 2 weeks after Hurricane Katrina to house first responders (police, firefighters, emergency medical services) and city workers, 80 % of whom had lost their homes. Our LSUHSC team had already been working with many first responders at the Emergency Response Staging area. At the request of local, state, and federal authorities, when the ships arrived, we reached out to New Orleans Police Department (NOPD), the New Orleans Fire Department (NOFD), the Coast Guard, FEMA, and other authorities encouraging family members, including children, most of whom were still displaced, to join first responders living on the boats. In this safe environment, we were able to help individuals and families solve problems and cope better, thus contributing to individual, family, and community resilience. Our LSUHSC team was available to provide support for children and families and respond to developmental needs and promote strengths. The work included reaching out to the Red Cross, facilitating access to FEMA and insurance companies, and connecting with the State Board of Education and principals of schools that were open in nearby parishes to place the children in schools while they were living on the boat. We also arranged with the school systems and administration for after-school tutoring on the boat as so many children had missed weeks of school because of their displacement. Our LSUHSC team also worked with the Substance Abuse and Mental Health Services Administration (SAMHSA) volunteers and the cruise ship personnel to set up child care centers on the boats to give the children places to play and provide some respite for the parents who had so many issues to deal with at that time.

Advocacy Steps: Hurricane Katrina

Advocacy efforts for children and families in the aftermath of Hurricane Katrina are listed as steps that the LSUHSC team took to work with different agencies and state and federal entities to ensure children's safety and emotional and physical wellbeing. The steps below allowed us to reunite children with their parents if at all possible, return children into school settings, establish routines, and provide calm atmospheres among the chaos.

1. Visited Red Cross shelters and worked with staff to attend to needs of children and families for family space, play areas for young children, toys for children, basic needs for privacy and bringing families together, understanding of the traumatic experiences they went through during the hurricane, evacuation, and displacement losses.
2. Contacted and trained first responders—police, firefighters, and emergency workers related to trauma and the impact on children and families, survivors and issues of vicarious traumatization especially for first responders with so much loss themselves.
3. Contacted and trained nontraditional first responders—teachers, head start providers related to the effects of trauma and the impact on children and families, survivors, and issues of vicarious traumatization. For these nontraditional first responders, it was very difficult for them to be emotionally available to the children when they were suffering so much loss personally.
4. Worked with Office of Mental Health collaborating on obtaining funding for Crisis Counseling Program and Specialized Counseling Services Program to meet the needs of children and families following Hurricane Katrina.
5. Met with crisis counselors in collaboration with Office of Mental Health and Crisis Counseling Program to provide training and consultation related to trauma and the impact on children and families including issues of vicarious traumatization.
6. Worked on two boats brought into New Orleans to house first responders (policy, firefighters, emergency management services, city workers) all of whom had lost their homes.

   (a) Received permission from FEMA and NOPD to allow us and a social worker to live on the boat with the first responders in order to allow us to be more available and provide additional support. Notably, the social worker had lost her home and many of us had temporary living quarters in Baton Rouge.
   (b) Worked with FEMA, Coast Guard, NOPD, and others to allow and encourage families to join first responders on the boats to support a sense of community after such loss.
   (c) Communicated and worked side by side with State Board of Education and outlying school superintendents to create space in their schools for children housed on the boats and to register them for school on the docks where the

boats were docked. This entailed requesting the President of New Orleans School Board to allow the children in New Orleans to attend out-of-parish schools and receive credit. This also meant that we helped develop new community-based schools in destroyed areas with school-based clinic for younger children and families and that we worked with the transportation department to provide school buses to pick up children at the dock to go to school.

(d) Set up child care centers on the boats by working with FEMA, Coast Guard, and SAMHSA.

(e) Sent professional volunteers to the boats who were trained in working with children. We collaborated with SAMSHA to ensure that professionally trained volunteers were helping the children.

(f) Supported the schools to open up their after-school programs and other community activities on the boats by working with FEMA and the Coast Guard.

7. Provided mental and behavioral health providers in temporary school settings when they opened with the support of the administration of St. Bernard Schools. All the schools in St. Bernard parish were totally destroyed.

8. Talked directly with the US Senators to establish priority of the Gulf South for National Child Traumatic Stress Network funding following Hurricane Katrina to be mandated by Congress.

9. Coedited Special Issue of Child Development on Disasters and Child Development with Dr. Ann Masten including international contributions to raise awareness of issues.

10. Testified before National Commission on Children and Disasters with Dr. Ann Masten sponsored by Society for Research in Child Development.

Outcomes of the Disaster Relief

The outcomes of our efforts in New Orleans were felt both locally and nationally. For example, the Gulf South region was established as a priority area for the National Child Traumatic Stress Network funding following Hurricane Katrina. The positive outcomes of the disaster relief efforts in New Orleans at the local level are best illustrated by describing scenarios of individual children and families.

• A 5-year-old developmentally disabled child on the boat was being pushed in his wheel chair by his 8-year-old brother. His mother was distraught and barely able to communicate with our staff. Although she did not believe it was possible, we arranged for special needs services to be provided to her child in a school in a nearby parish. She then began to smile for the first time and think positively about the future.

• A 6-year-old boy was being cared for by his grandparents on the boat, one of whom had a debilitating medical illness. They were very concerned because this lively, happy youngster had become withdrawn and noncommunicative. When we sat down with him, he cried because his father, a police officer, who he did not know was stranded at the Convention Center, did not come to the Superdome where he had been evacuated and bring him a cake for this birthday. We not only explained that his father loved him, but also worked with the police department to unite him with his father. He again became a happy, outgoing child.

- Three teenagers were very concerned because they could not complete their college entrance requirements and did not have the documents from their school that was totally flooded. They and their parents believed that they would not be able to go to college and room on campus with peers. We were able to work with the school system and the college to waive some of the requirements and allow them to be accepted as planned with needed financial support.
- Preadolescent children were drawing pictures in their time on the boat of their threatening experiences during the hurricane that were violent and upsetting to them. Their parents and the volunteers from out-of-town were worried and wanted them to stop drawing. We explained that it is important for children and adolescents to be supported in expressing their reactions to traumatic experiences as part of their recovery.
- Our LSUHSC team joined with NOPD and SAMHSA volunteers to plan special child and family events with the parents where they could sing songs and perform as groups in front of an audience. An example of such a fun event was the Halloween Party on the boat where we were able to provide costumes for the children and allow them play "trick or treat," laugh, and play.

We experienced a "new normal" on the cruise ships where first responders lived with their families for many months and developed new relationships and ways of supporting themselves and their families after experiencing so much loss. Having learned much first-hand about disaster response and recovery, what works and what doesn't we had the opportunity to share that knowledge in Chile, China, and Japan following earthquakes, typhoons, tsunamis, and the Fukushima Daiichi nuclear disaster.

Conclusion

By definition, it is not possible to be fully "prepared" when disasters occur. It is important to apply scientific developmental psychology knowledge to the response to disaster recovery in order to create environments that can provide the most sensitive support for children of all ages and their families. While support appropriately should be given to adults and individuals with special needs, inadvertently the important needs of children and families receive relatively less attention. There can be the well-meaning, but mistaken, assumption that children are less impacted by these traumatic experiences and that they will just "bounce back" quickly. Individuals and communities can and should plan and prepare in ways that will be supportive of children, families, and communities and promote resilience. In response to disasters, it is crucial to understand developmental needs and include in planning ways to respond in developmentally sensitive manner including protection and restoration of attachment relationships (parent/caregiver–child) relationships as soon as possible. While recognizing evacuations and relocations may be needed, careful preparations need to be made mindful of children's needs to be kept together with their caregivers. In shelters and other emergency sites, it is important to think about and plan for the needs of children of different ages and their caregivers. Special support needs to be provided to the children including reunification with parents and caregivers as rapidly as possible.

Recognizing the importance of relationships between parents/caregivers, if injury or loss of a parent occurs, nurturing consistent care by responders is crucial. Recognizing the importance of the relationships between children and parents/caregivers, if there is a loss of a caregiver which unfortunately happens with disasters, nurturing, consistent care is needed for children who have experienced such losses. One of the important ways to achieve these objectives is to train all who respond to disasters including both traditional (police, firefighters, emergency personnel) and nontraditional first responders (parents, school administrators, teachers, child care providers) about the developmental responses to trauma including the unanticipated traumas associated with disasters that can be expected for children of different ages. It is important in disaster response for mental health providers and others to partner with all of the institutions in the local community that will come into contact with children including designated responders, volunteer agencies, the faith-based community, the police and sheriff's departments, school administration, and teachers to be able to support the recovery of individuals and support the community.

An important part of training and outreach is to recognize that vicarious traumatization and compassion fatigue may impact on those who work with and are exposed to traumatized children. Traumatized children, especially those who are young, can affect adults in different ways, but most often pull extreme reactions ranging from empathy to anger. Such feelings can be an integral part of the work with traumatized children. Individuals find their own ways to cope with these overwhelming feelings; regular support for individuals and by institutions is necessarily accompanied by self-care and reflective supervision if available.

One of the most important organizing principles that help children grow and develop behavioral and emotional regulation skills is normal routines and activities, all of which are drastically disrupted during and after disasters. Children need opportunities to play and learn, be with their friends, participate in school, and in the community. With disasters, major disruptions occur in all of these areas and responders and helpers need to support the establishment of routines and what we have called a "new normal."

In disaster response and recovery, it is important to "think out of the box" to support and advocate for children. In the past 7 years we have had the opportunity to learn so much about what can make a difference for children and families after disasters. Advocacy related to response, recovery, and resilience can make a significant difference for outcomes.

References

Blos, P. (1967). *The adolescent passage*. New York: International Universities Press.

Bonanno, G. A. (2004). Loss, trauma, and human resilience: Have we under-estimated the human capacity to thrive after extremely aversive events? *American Psychologist, 59*, 20–28.

Bonanno, G. A., & Mancini, A. D. (2008). The human capacity to thrive in the face of potential trauma. *Pediatrics, 121*, 369–375.

Bronfenbrenner, U. (1986). Ecology of the family as a context for human development: Research perspectives. *Developmental Psychology, 22*, 723–742.

Bowlby, J. (1973). Attachment and loss: Vol. 2. Separation: Anxiety and anger. New York: Basic Books.

Children and Disasters. (2010). *Child development research in brief.* www.srcd.org. Accessed 10 oct 2012.

Garrison, C. Z., Weinrich, M. W., Hardin, S. B., Weinrich, S., & Wang, L. (1993). Post-traumatic stress disorder in adolescents after a hurricane. *American Journal of Epidemiology, 138*, 522–530.

Goenjian, A., Molina, L., Steinberg, A., Fairbanks, L., Alvarez, M., Goenjian, H., et al. (2001). Posttraumatic stress and depressive reactions among Nicaraguan adolescents after hurricane Mitch. *The American Journal of Psychiatry, 158*, 788–794.

Goenjian, A., Walling, D., Steinberg, A., Karayan, I., Najarian, L., & Pynoos, R. (2005). A prospective study of posttraumatic stress and depressive reactions among treated and untreated adolescents 5 years after a catastrophic disaster. *The American Journal of Psychiatry, 162*, 2302–2308.

Goldstein, B. D., Osofsky, H. J., & Lichtveld, M. D. (2011). The gulf oil spill. *The New England Journal of Medicine, 364*, 1334–1348.

Hamada, R., Kameoka, V., Yanagida, E., & Chemtob, C. (2003). Assessment of elementary school children for disaster-related posttraumatic stress disorder symptoms: The Kauai recovery index. *The Journal of Nervous and Mental Disease, 191*, 268–272.

Kar, N., Mohapatra, P., Nayak, K., Pattanaik, P., Swain, S., & Kar, M. (2007). Post-traumatic stress disorder in children and adolescents one year after a super-cyclone in Orissa, India: Exploring cross-cultural validity and vulnerability factors. *BMC Psychiatry, 14*, 8.

Kessler, R. C., Galea, S., Jones, R. T., & Parker, H. A. (2006). Mental illness and suicidality after Hurricane Katrina. *Bulletin of the World Health Organization, 84*, 930–939.

Kithakye, M., Morris, A. S., Terranova, A. M., & Myers, S. S. (2010). The Kenyan political conflict and children's adjustment. *Child Development, 81*, 1113–1127.

Kolaitis, G., Kotsopoulos, J., Tsiantis, J., Haritaki, S., Rigizou, F., Zacharaki, L., et al. (2003). Posttraumatic stress reactions among children following the Athens earthquake of September 1999. *European Child and Adolescent Psychiatry, 12*, 273–280.

Kronenberg, M. E., Hansel, T. C., Brennan, A. M., Lawrason, B., Osofsky, H. J., & Osofsky, J. D. (2010). Children of Katrina: Lessons learned about post-disaster symptoms and recovery patterns. *Child Development, 81*, 1241–1259.

La Greca, A., Silverman, W., Vernberg, E., & Prinstein, M. (1996). Symptoms of posttraumatic stress in children after Hurricane Andrew: A prospective study. *Journal of Consulting and Clinical Psychology, 64*, 712–723.

Laor, N., Wolmer, L., Mayes, L. C., Gershon, A., Weizman, R., & Cohen, D. J. (1997). Israeli preschools under Scuds: A 30-month follow-up. *Journal of American Academy of Child and Adolescence Psychiatry, 36*, 349–356.

Layne, C. M., Beck, C. J., Rimmasch, H., Southwick, J. S., Moreno, M. A., & Hobfoll, S. E. (2009). Promoting "resilient" posttraumatic adjustment in childhood and beyond: "Unpacking" life events, adjustment trajectories, resources, and interventions. In D. Brom, R. Pat-Horenczyk, & J. Ford (Eds.), *Treating traumatized children: Risk, resilience, and recovery* (pp. 13–47). New York: Routledge.

Lessons from the Exxon-Valdez: Oil spills shatter relationships and communities. Accessed from http://www.onearth.org/article/lessons-from-the-exxon-valdez

Lonigan, C. J., Shannon, M. P., Taylor, C. M., Finch, A. J., Jr., & Sallee, F. (1994). Children exposed to disaster: II. Risk factors for the development of post-traumatic symptomatology. *Journal of the American Academy of Child and Adolescent Psychiatry, 33*, 94–105.

Masten, A. S. (2007). Resilience in developing systems: Progress and promise as the fourth wave rises. *Development and Psychopathology, 19*, 921–930.

Masten, A. S. (2013). Risk and resilience in development. In P. D. Zelazo (Ed.), *Oxford handbook of developmental psychology, 2*, 579–607. New York: Oxford University Press.

Masten, A. S., & Narayan, A. J. (2012). Child development in the context of disaster, war and terrorism: Pathways of risk and resilience. *Annual Review of Psychology, 63*, 227–257.

Masten, A. S., & Obradović, J. (2008). Disaster preparation and recovery: Lessons from research on resilience in human development. *Ecology and Society, 13*(1), 9 [Online] URL: http://www.ecologyandsociety.org/vol13/iss1/art9/

Masten, A. S., & Osofsky, J. D. (2010). Disasters and their impact on child development: Introduction to the Special Section. *Child Development, 81*, 1029–1039.

Neuner, F., Schauer, E., Catani, C., Ruf, M., & Elbert, T. (2006). Post-tsunami stress: A study of posttraumatic stress disorder in children living in three severely affected regions in Sri Lanka. *Journal of Traumatic Stress, 19*, 339–347.

Osofsky, H., Osofsky, J., Kronenberg, M., Brennan, A., & Hansel, T. (2009). Posttraumatic stress symptoms in children after Hurricane Katrina: Predicting the need for mental health services. *The American Journal of Orthopsychiatry, 79*, 212–220.

Osofsky, H. J., Palinkas, L. A., & Galloway, J. A. (2010). Mental health effects of the gulf oil spill. *Disaster Medicine and Public Health Preparedness, 4*, 273–276.

Osofsky, J. D. (Ed.). (2004). *Young children and trauma: Interventions and treatment*. New York: Guilford.

Osofsky, J. D. (2011a). Young children and disasters: Lessons learned from Hurricane Katrina about the impact of disasters and postdisaster recovery. In J. D. Osofsky (Ed.), *Clinical work with traumatized young children* (pp. 295–312). New York: Guilford Publishers.

Osofsky, J. D. (2011b). Vicarious traumatization and the need for self-care in working with traumatized young children. In J. D. Osofsky (Ed.), *Clinical work with traumatized young children* (pp. 336–348). New York: Guilford Publishers.

Osofsky, J. D., Osofsky, H. J., Hansel, T. C., & Reuther, E. (2011, October). *Mental health impacts of the gulf oil spill*. National Child Traumatic Stress Network Webinair.

Osofsky, J. D., Osofsky, H. J., & Harris, W. W. (2007). Katrina's children: Social policy for children in disasters. *Social Policy Reports, Society for Research in Child Development, 21*(1), 1–20.

Palinkas, L. A. (2009). The Exxon-Valdez oil spill. In Y. Neria, S. Galea, & F. Norris (Eds.), *Mental health consequences of disasters* (pp. 454–472). New York: Cambridge University Press.

Palinkas, L. A., Petterson, J. S., Russell, J., & Downs, M. A. (1993). Community patterns of psychiatric disorder after the Exxon-Valdez oil spill. *The American Journal of Psychiatry, 150*, 1517–1523.

Pfefferbaum, B. (1997). Posttraumatic stress disorder in children: A review of the past 10 years. *Journal of the American Academy of Child and Adolescent Psychiatry, 36*, 1503–1511.

Picou, J. S., & Gill, D. A. (1996). The Exxon Valdez oil spill and chronic psychological stress. *American Fisheries Society Symposium, 18*, 879–893.

Picou, J. S., Marshall, B. K., & Gill, D. A. (2004). Disaster, litigation, and the corrosive community. *Social Forces, 82*, 1493–1522.

Piyasil, V., Ketuman, P., Plubrukarn, R., Jotipanut, V., Tanprasert, S., Aowjinda, S., et al. (2007). Post traumatic stress disorder in children after tsunami disaster in Thailand: 2 years follow-up. *Journal of the Medical Association of Thailand, 90*, 2370–2376.

Pynoos, R. (1993). Traumatic stress and developmental psychopathology in children and adolescents. In J. Oldham, M. Riba, & A. Tasman (Eds.), *American psychiatric press review of psychiatry* (Vol. 12, pp. 205–238). Washington, DC: American Psychiatric Press.

Pynoos, R., Goenjian, A., Tashjian, M., Karakashian, M., Manjikian, R., Manoukian, G., et al. (1993). Post-traumatic stress reactions in children after the 1988 Armenian earthquake. *The British Journal of Psychiatry, 163*, 239–247.

Pynoos, R. S., Steinberg, A. M., & Goenjian, A. (1996). Traumatic stress in childhood and adolescence: Recent developments and current controversies. In B. A. van der Kolk & A. C. McFarlane (Eds.), *Traumatic stress: The effects of overwhelming experience on mind, body, and society* (pp. 331–358). New York: Guilford Press.

Pynoos, R., Steinberg, A., & Piacentini, J. (1999). A developmental psychopathology model of childhood traumatic stress and intersection with anxiety disorders. *Biological Psychiatry, 46*, 1542–1554.

Roussos, A., Goenjian, A., Steinberg, A., Sotiropoulou, C., Kakaki, M., Kabakos, C., et al. (2005). Posttraumatic stress and depressive reactions among children and adolescents after the 1999 earthquake in Ano Liosia, Greece. *The American Journal of Psychiatry, 162*, 530–537.

Russoniello, C., Skalko, T., O'Brien, K., McGhee, S., Bingham-Alexander, D., & Beatley, J. (2007). Childhood posttraumatic stress disorder and efforts to cope after Hurricane Floyd. *Behavioral Medicine, 28*, 61–71.

Shaw, J. (2000). Children, adolescents and trauma. *Psychiatric Quarterly, 71*, 227–243.

Steinberg, A. M., Brymer, M. J., Decker, K. B., & Pynoos, R. S. (2004). The University of California at Los Angeles post-traumatic stress disorder reaction index. *Current Psychiatry Reports, 6*, 96–100.

Thienkrua, W., Cardozo, B. L., Chakkraband, M. L., Guadamuz, T. E., Pengjuntr, W., Tantipiwatanaskul, P., et al. (2006). Symptoms of posttraumatic stress disorder and depression among children in tsunami-affected areas in southern Thailand. *Journal of the American Medical Association, 296*, 549–559.

Vogel, J. M., & Vernberg, E. M. (1993). Psychological responses of children to natural and human-made disasters: I. Children's psychological responses to disasters. *Journal of Clinical Child Psychology, 22*, 464–484.

Watanabe, H. (2012). The manifold impact of radiation on children and families in Fukushima Paper presented at *The Great East Japan Earthquake and Disasters: One Year Later,* Sponsored by the UCSF Departments of Psychiatry and Pediatrics and Global Health Sciences, San Francisco.

Weems, C., Taylor, L., Cannon, M., Marino, R., Romano, D., Scott, B., et al. (2009). Post traumatic stress, context, and the lingering effects of the Hurricane Katrina disaster among ethnic minority youth. *Journal of Abnormal Child Psychology, 38*, 49–56.

Weems, C., Watts, S., Marsee, M., Taylor, L., Costa, N., Cannon, M., et al. (2007). The psychosocial impact of Hurricane Katrina: Contextual differences in psychological symptoms, social support, and discrimination. *Behaviour Research and Therapy, 45*, 2295–2306.

Chapter 8
Early Childhood Education and Care: Legislative and Advocacy Efforts

Helen Raikes, Lisa St. Clair, and Sandie Plata-Potter

Introduction

The focus of the current chapter is early childhood education and care, including a special examination of the role of research in relation to advocacy. Our focus encompasses the prenatal period through age 8. The topics of early childhood education and care have received intensive advocacy efforts over the past 20 years as investments and programs have grown extensively, due in part to these efforts.

These efforts have been spurred by increasing understanding of the importance of early development, particularly early brain development. Beginning before birth and continuing through the preschool years, the early childhood years characterize the most important and rapid growth period of any in the life span for proliferation of cells and synaptic connections within the human brain. Brain growth is influenced by health and nutrition but also by the types of relationships that children experience as well as by the quality and appropriateness of stimulation they receive. Moreover, these experiences affect the very architecture of the brain, forming the foundations of brain development that follow (Shonkoff & Phillips, 2000; National Scientific Council on the Developing Child, 2007). This underlying architecture is related to the many abilities that emerge during this period—language, reflective

H. Raikes, PhD (✉)
Department of Child, Youth and Family Studies, University of Nebraska,
257 Mabel Lee Hall, Lincoln, NE 68588-0236, USA
e-mail: hraikes2@unl.edu

L. St. Clair, PhD
Department of Education and Child Development, Munroe-Meyer Institute,
University of Nebraska Medical Center, Omaha, NE, USA

S. Plata-Potter, PhD
Department of Education, Mount Olive College, 634, Henderson,
Mount Olive, NC 28365, USA

A. McDonald Culp (ed.), *Child and Family Advocacy: Bridging the Gaps Between Research, Practice, and Policy*, Issues in Clinical Child Psychology,
DOI 10.1007/978-1-4614-7456-2_8, © Springer Science+Business Media New York 2013

thought, and gaining a sense that the world is a trustworthy and welcoming place to be, among others. While children's home environments and their relationships with parents form the bedrock for development during this period (Hart & Risley, 1995; Rodriguez & Tamis LeMonda, 2011), their early development is also influenced by experiences in child care and early childhood education settings, and this is particularly true for low-income children or children experiencing other adverse circumstances (Ludwig & Phillips, 2007; Reynolds, Temple, Robertson, & Mann, 2001). There is a well-documented achievement gap between low-income children and their more advantaged peers that is apparent at kindergarten entry (Hair, Halle, Terry-Humen, Lavelle, & Calkins, 2006; Lee & Burkham, 2002) and has been documented even earlier (Halle et al., 2009). This gap does not go away but often increases as children progress through school (Duncan et al., 2007). However, there is evidence that the gap at school entry can be reduced by high quality early education and care programs. Thus, influenced by developments and understanding of brain development and the general importance of early childhood education, there has been considerable activity in advocacy to promote early childhood education over the past 2 decades.

Work in advocacy and expansion in the early childhood education and care area has tended to focus on several issues, including a need to improve: (1) *access* to early care and education programs, (2) *quality* of education and care, and, (3) more recently, *continuities* for children between home and school and from infancy through school age. Many of the advocacy efforts focus on making changes that will improve children's developmental outcomes by leveling the playing field between less and more advantaged children. These efforts tend to target funding from federal or state sources, although funders may also be private, corporate, or business leaders.

We describe the state of the field and the issues around which advocacy efforts have been focused as well as where the efforts are focused today; we provide examples from one state—Nebraska—and we offer principles that have guided our work and may be helpful for scientists and practitioners as they consider their role in relation to advocacy.

Issues in Early Childhood Education and Care

Issues with Access

Access issues in early childhood are in two areas: (1) access for low-income children to programs that are either home-based (birth through 3, most typically, but not exclusively) or center-based (more typically for children ages 3–5 but also including some birth through 3 programs) and (2) access to child care so that parents can work. In the USA, typically, more advantaged children have had access to programs that supplement and support their development than has been true for low-income children.

For low-income children, access to early childhood education programs has been associated with improvements in children's school readiness and developmental outcomes (Love et al., 2005; Olds et al., 1997; Ramey & Campbell, 1991; Reynolds et al., 2001; Schweinharrt et al., 2005). While programs cited above have demonstrated gains for low-income children, in the past they were often limited to a few children in a concentrated program or to a single community. Despite growth in access to programs, there are still gaps for low-income children as we shall demonstrate.

Head Start, the nation's premier early childhood program for children whose parents live at or below the poverty line, began in 1965 with about half a million children and serves around a million children living at or below the poverty line today. State preschool programs—generally center-based programs for 3 and 4 year olds—serve approximately another million. Most, but not all of these programs are targeted towards children who live in low-income families, children with special developmental needs, or children whose families do not speak English. Despite extensive efforts to improve access to programs, particularly for low-income children, over the past 2 decades, access issues remain. For example, the *State of Preschool* reported that enrollment in pre-k (public and private) is about 65 % for the lowest 40 % of families by income and 90 % for the highest income quintile (Barnett, Carolan, Fitzgerald, & Squires, 2011). At age 3 years, enrollment is about 40 % for low-income and moderate-income families while it is 80 % for the top income quintile (Barnett et al., 2011). Moreover, programs may be part-day or part-year, which may be a problem for children in families who also have child care needs for full-day, full-year, requiring families to find multiple preschool and child care options for children in what is referred to as wrap-around care. While most Head Start and pre-k programs offer children meals and snacks and health screening, not all families have access to the supplemental services that these families may need to support preschool-age children's development, such as mental health or other health services.

Access to home visiting and other services for low-income prenatal/0- to 3-year olds has also increased over the past decade. Home visiting services provide child development and family support in individual visits to children's homes. Home visiting for children ages birth through 3 is currently in a ramping-up phase as states work to implement new home visiting programs, funded under the Affordable Health Care Act. This act will expand home visiting services for families with risk factors including poverty, being a single parent or low education. Approximately a half million to a million infants and toddlers are served in such programs, although there are large numbers of low-income parents today who do not receive prenatal care and mothers and fathers who do not receive parenting education or the kinds of supports that home visiting can provide. About 2 % of children under age 3, and with some level of risk (e.g., poverty, non-English speaking, single parents, low education, or mental health risks), are being served today (Astuto & Allen, 2009). The majority of these services are delivered to infants and toddlers and their parents or pregnant mothers in home visits.

The second area of focus of advocacy is access to *child care*. Access in regard to child care has improved over the past 4 decades as the market has expanded to meet demand of parental employment. Over half of the mothers of infants and toddlers are employed outside the home and in some states (e.g., Nebraska, South Dakota, Iowa), three-quarters of mothers of preschool-age children are employed outside the home, necessitating child care for a majority of children. Low-income children's child care is supplemented by federal and state child care subsidies that pay for some or all of the child care but states may or may not impose requirements for the quality of the care they pay for. Access to child care as purchased by public subsidies is a complicated issue as legislation and state efforts tend to concentrate on providing choices for families, use of local child care, and in spreading child care dollars over as many families as possible. These factors also raise issues about quality of the care that is being purchased (GAO, 2002; Raikes, 1998) and about the effects on children's development. Thus, while there may be areas and ages for which access to child care is lacking in the USA today, advocacy focus in regard to child care tends to be on quality, generally regarded to be an issue worthy of intensive focus.

Issues with Quality

Quality of early care and education has been consistently associated with children's developmental outcomes, a relationship even more pronounced for low-income children (Burchinal, Peisner-Feinberg, Bryant, & Clifford, 2000; Cost, Quality and Child Outcomes Study Team, 2005; NICHD Early Child Care Research Network, 2005; Peisner-Feinberg et al., 2001; Votruba-Drzal, Coley, & Chase-Lansdale, 2004). Moreover, the quality of much child care, whether center-based or family child care, in the USA has been found to be wanting (Cost, Quality and Child Outcomes Study Team, 2005; Kontos, Howes, Shinn, & Galinsky, 1995). Infant–toddler care has been found to be particularly questionable in regard to quality (Cost, Quality and Child Outcomes Study Team, 2005). Moreover, the quality of care purchased by public subsidies is either not well known (GAO, 2002) or, when it has been studied, it often has been found to be of lower quality than care more generally in states (Jones-Branch, Torquati, Raikes, & Edwards, 2004; Raikes, Raikes, & Wilcox, 2005; Whitebook, Kipnis, & Bellm, 2007). A sector of child care purchased by public subsidies, unlicensed but legally exempt child care offered in homes, has notably not been extensively investigated in regard to quality (Raikes et al., 2013).

Even public programs that have high standards of quality (e.g., the Head Start Program Performance Standards or state preschool programs that may have requirements aligned with those for public schools in the states, standards that are considerably higher than state licensing standards) have not *consistently* shown levels of quality that have been found to maximize children's developmental outcomes (Howes et al., 2008).

Thus, advocates have often focused efforts on quality improvement. For example, the recent federal Race to the Top competition (government-sponsored competition to encourage states to make major quality improvement steps) featured implementation of Quality Rating and Improvement Systems (QRIS; quality ranking systems) in states as a strategy for systematically improving child care and education programs and, thus states are implementing higher quality standards. Moreover, the National Institute for Early Education Research (NIEER), who rates states on five characteristics, demonstrates that states vary considerably in their ability to guarantee specific standards of quality (Barnett et al., 2011).

Issues with Continuities

Continuity is a broad umbrella for many problems related to fragmentation of the care and education for young children in the USA today. Young children, because of their immature emotional and cognitive development, develop best when their lives are most consistent and predictable, when they have predictable and loving relationships with a small number of consistent caregivers. It does not suit their development well when inconsistencies exist that make it difficult for them to feel at ease and make sense out of their world. Inconsistencies can be of many types— different language spoken at home and at child care; different cultural expectations; multiple child care environments over the course of a day or week; frequent changes in caregiving through the brief preschool years, to name a few. Inconsistencies are exacerbated by state and federal programs—however well intentioned—that have different rules for eligibility or rules that are not grounded in the wellbeing of young, vulnerable children (e.g., many states discontinue child care subsidies if parents are laid off work, causing children to lose consistency of child care due to lack of payment source). Moreover, there may be inconsistency between the early years and public schools (e.g., parents who have learned to be involved in early childhood programs may find their voice unwelcomed in elementary schools or children's preschool records may not be passed onto elementary schools so time is lost in addressing child problems).

Efforts in Addressing the Challenges in Early Childhood Education and Care

People seeking solutions in the area of early childhood education have been successful for several decades and these efforts are likely to accelerate and/or to provide a framework for the coming years.

Progress Toward Solutions Involving Access

There has been considerable progress as states have initiated programs for 4-year olds and to some extent for 3-year olds. Head Start is allowing programs to redesignate in order to serve infants and toddlers and 3-year olds where the schools and communities are otherwise now serving 4-year olds. Such work requires taking stock at the community level to determine how to spread resources so families' and children's experiences can be seamless. In the future, there will be considerable work to web together 0–3 home visiting and Early Head Start programs with pre-school programs for 3- and 4-year olds. Nationally, new programs initiated recently will greatly expand opportunities for children at greatest risk—expansion of Early Head Start (Head Start for pregnant women and children birth through age 3) and augmentation in child care subsidy funding through President Obama's economic stimulus in the American Recovery and Reinvestment Act (ARRA), funding of a number of states in the early childhood education Race to the Top competition, and inclusion of new 0–3 home visiting programs under the Affordable Care Act. Just how these three new programs are carried out varies from state to state. Early Head Start funding was doubled through ARRA, bringing opportunities to another 60,000 infants and toddlers at highest risk in the USA; in the first round of competition nine states received infusions of approximately $50 million each for improvements in early childhood education—improving access but also quality and continuities; states and jurisdictions, and Tribes are receiving grants in total of $224 million to improve health and development outcomes for at-risk children through evidence-based home visiting programs.

Research provides good support for advocacy relating to access to early child-hood education and care. As stated earlier, studies show that involvement in early childhood programs can help to reduce the achievement gap for low-income children. Children in the Perry Preschool project who received 2 years of quality early childhood education not only exceeded a control group at the end of the program but these children were more productive citizens 40 years later with an investment-to-benefit ratio of $17 reaped for every $1 invested in the program (Schweinharrt et al., 2005). Other programs such as the Abecedarian project showed a $4–1 ben-efit to cost, and the Chicago Parent-Child Program demonstrated benefits of over $10 to every $1 invested (Watt, Ayoub, Bradley, Puma, & Lebeouf, 2006). Moreover, the latter project demonstrated added value when out-of-school activi-ties were added during the elementary years. While these studies are some of the earliest to demonstrate the value of early childhood education programs, there have been countless other studies more recently demonstrating benefits, even in the cur-rent era when children in comparison groups also have access to early childhood services. For example, positive results have been found for state-sponsored pre-k programs affiliated with schools (Gormley, Gayer, Phillips, & Dawson, 2005), Head Start (U.S. Department of Health and Human Services, 2010) and Early Head Start (Love, Chazan-Cohen, Raikes, & Brooks-Gunn, 2013; Vogel et al., 2010) as well as for participation in home visiting programs (Sweet & Appelbaum, 2004). However, as noted, in child care programs, positive outcomes are dependent upon the child care being of good quality (Center on the Developing Child at Harvard University, 2007). Advocates can rely on a solid research base as well as on the principles from brain development research. In fact, Nobel Laureate James Heckman demonstrates through his econometric models that early investments in children's lives are better educational investments than investments that come later (Heckman & Masterov, 2004).

Advocates will encounter questions about "small effect sizes" (as some programs show significant effects but they are small compared to those of earlier programs). One counter argument is that many comparison group children also attend early childhood programs. They will hear questions about "fade out" (for programs with smaller effect sizes at end of project, longer term effects are not consistently seen), but can counter with findings showing that while cognitive impacts may not sustain into early elementary years, population studies show that children in Head Start and other early childhood programs have improved social capital outcomes into young adulthood (Deming, 2009; Garces, Thomas, & Currie, 2002; Johnson, 2011; Ludwig & Miller, 2007). Social capital outcomes include less crime, greater likelihood of completing high school, and adult employment.

Progress Toward Solutions for Improving Quality

There has been progress over the past several years with the implementation of QRIS (rating systems implemented in states giving parents information about the quality in child care programs) and other quality efforts (e.g., Barnett et al., 2011; National Institute for Early Education Research) but there is considerable work ahead. States will continue to try to monitor the quality of early education and child care; more work is needed in monitoring quality of care that the government purchases through subsidies. Moreover, as the recently released report from the Secretary's Advisory Committee on Head Start Research and Evaluation shows, Head Start and other early childhood education programs will benefit from systematic implementation of high quality, intensive, focused and targeted curricula (U.S. Department of Health and Human Services, 2012), augmented with a higher level and more focused training and technical assistance; and as higher education prepares for a more rigorous educational system for the next generation.

Research provides good support for advocacy efforts around quality. Recent efforts show larger effect sizes when all the working elements (high quality curriculum, high quality interactions, support and training for teachers in implementing the curriculum, child assessments, and parent involvement) are introduced simultaneously (Fantuzzo, 2012) and when children receive quality services over several years (Yazejian & Bryant, 2010). Advocates will find arguments that counter a push for quality. For example, they may hear that the effect sizes are small from quality increments; they may hear that some aspects of structural quality (features of quality somewhat more removed from the child's direct experience such as whether a program is licensed, staff education) do not consistently predict child outcomes (e.g., a college degree; Early et al., 2007). Research continues in an effort to identify the precise elements of quality that matter the most or in combination with one another (Raikes et al., 2006).

Progress Toward Solutions for Continuities Among Early Child Settings, Homes, and Public Schools

As we have noted, continuity can have multiple meanings. It may refer to consistencies between home and school; to high quality services that begin early and continue through the preschool years; to consistency throughout the child's day (e.g., not having a very young child in multiple caregiving environments), and in smooth transitions from early childhood to early elementary environments. There is increasing evidence that children who receive home environments and early childhood settings that are stimulating, safe, and healthy and are in sync with each other fare well in terms of developmental outcomes. Next, there is preliminary evidence that for low-income children, those whose high quality services begin early and continue to school entry, fare best. For example, the Early Head Start Research and Evaluation Project showed children who had received Early Head Start and preschool from ages 3 to 5 fared better than children who received one or the other or neither (Love et al., 2013). One example comes from a set of programs called "Educare." Educare programs are Early Head Start or Head Start programs that enhance what is typically offered to children. These enhancements are referred to as core features of these programs. To name just a few, Educare Staffs Master Teachers who provide reflective supervision to three or four classrooms. There are three teachers in every classroom, with a 3:8 ratio for infants and toddlers and a 3:17 ratio for preschool children. Children in Educare programs who enroll as infants and toddlers and stay enrolled until kindergarten score at national averages in language development compared to those who begin later who score around a half standard deviation lower (Yazejian & Bryant, 2010). Finally, federal government, states, and communities increasingly are interested in optimizing continuities from birth through early elementary school in multiple areas. Thus, a number of states have initiated departments of early childhood education to improve continuities at the policy level. In these states, a single department may combine programs in Health and Human Services, Education, and, possibly, other departments. Early childhood education programs have included outcomes from their programs in state longitudinal databases. For example, the recent Race to the Top competition emphasized integrating data and other systemic work in the area of early childhood education.

Promising Solutions for the Future

Thus, solutions for the future include still greater access to quality services particularly for children ages 0 through age 3, and particularly for children in low-income families or who are otherwise vulnerable. Solutions will also focus on improving quality across all types of programs, and, finally, solutions will increasingly be aimed at systemic efforts to create continuity within states and communities so children's experiences are continuous, consistent, and in keeping with the best developmental principles. Increasingly, efforts to advocate for these solutions can rely on existing and new research that pertains to the importance of early brain development and on evidence coming from an increasingly prolific and sophisticated early childhood education body of research literature.

Advocacy

There are many, many examples of effective advocacy in the area of early childhood education from the past several decades. In many ways, the advocacy is successful because of the solid research base that has been referred to above. The research base has been independently growing. That is, researchers completed rigorous research to answer critical questions about early childhood development, but increasingly the research results pointed to implications for increasing access, quality, and continuity in early childhood education. The purpose of the research was not advocacy but the research results have been immensely useful to the success of advocacy efforts.

First, we tell a story about advocacy in Nebraska and then in the final section of this chapter we discuss the relationship between the science and practice and advocacy as it pertains to early childhood education.

Advocacy Goal: Legislation to Increase Investment in Early Childhood in Nebraska

In the period from 2005 to 2008, Nebraska made huge strides in access/quality/continuity in two areas: (1) legislation to significantly increase the investment in early childhood education grants programs, including ongoing increases for funding for 4-year olds coming from the state school aide formula; and (2) legislation and a constitutional amendment to create a public–private endowed partnership for birth to 3 programs for children at risk. The efforts in Nebraska are examples and efforts of type have occurred throughout the USA in other states. Nationally, the works of First Five and the Pew Charitable Trusts, the Head Start Association, and others are examples of efforts that have garnered tremendous support and have demonstrated major success in effecting legislation that benefits young children.

Advocacy Action Steps

Invited Legislators, Initiated Pilot Program, and Testified

In 2001, Nebraska initiated an early childhood grants pilot program. This program had great "bones" in the sense the programs were administered through schools and education service units; they required local matches and collaboration with local early childhood providers; they could be administered by local early childhood providers; programs were required to meet high standards already stipulated in statute (e.g., Nebraska Rule 11 requiring teacher BS/A-level and encouraging National Association for the Education of Young Children certification). Also required were quality standards in classrooms that went considerably beyond licensing requirements, and the legislation allowed for alternative models for services birth through kindergarten. Eleven of Nebraska early childhood grants programs were in place in schools in 2005 when the advocacy-related phase of the story we will tell here begins.

Prior to introducing the legislation to increase the investment in these state-level programs, senators were invited by the Nebraska Children and Families Foundation to a reception at the Nebraska Governor's Mansion and Dr. Jack Shonkoff, Harvard University Center on the Developing Child, reviewed the science about the importance of early childhood and the opportunities for early childhood education. Even senators not engaged in early childhood education commented, "How can you argue with this?"

Legislation was introduced in 2005 that would add a cost of about $2.5 million a year to expand the program. The legislation also carried a clause whereby schools that successfully operated grants programs for 3 years could then roll the costs of serving 4-year olds into the state aid formula for matching funds, with needs and resources of the community determining the allocation from the state.

Many early childhood education researchers and practitioners testified to the Nebraska Unicameral Education Committee about the importance of early childhood education. Simultaneously, Nebraska Children and Families Foundation, a public–private partnership organization, provided support for the process—organizing the Shonkoff reception, providing weekly phone calls among advocates as constituents in senators' districts were identified for meeting with their senators. The Buffett Early Childhood fund provided support for the education of the general public and elected officials on the importance of investing early. The Nebraska children and families foundation successfully worked with both sides of the aisle providing senators information and rationale for the legislation. The legislation passed unanimously and last year the number of children served was over 3,000 in the grant programs and over 8,000 in district early childhood programs (Jackson, 2011). Each year the number served increases as expenses for 4-year olds are rolled into the state aid formula and more 3-year olds and new schools are added to the grants program.

Created a Public–Private Endowed Partnership for Birth to 3 Programs

In 2006, 1 year after the successful passage of the expanded early childhood grants program, the early childhood efforts (early childhood education leaders and stakeholders coordinated by the Nebraska Children and Families Foundation) to create more legislation to expand programs were renewed. This time, the emphasis was on programs for birth to 3-year olds. This early childhood education group proposed a private–public partnership whereby the private sector would raise $20 million matched to a state contribution of $40 million. The funds would endow a program for infants and toddlers at highest risk (e.g., risk due to poverty, being in families where English was not spoken, parental lack of high school education, single parent). The legislation was proposed and there was interest by senators but a question: where would the state $40 million come from? A senator proposed that school lands funds (funds available to every state through the Homestead Act of 1862) be made available for this purpose. There was a problem in that a constitutional amendment was required to allow preschool to be defined as eligible for school lands funds. First, the legislation passed—again with tremendous work on the part of the early childhood community to continue to make the case for the need for early childhood services and not to overlook the infant–toddler sector. The next summer the early childhood leaders who had been instrumental in passing the legislation remobilized to put the amendment on the ballot, campaign for the constitutional amendment. Of six amendments on the ballot in November of 2006, only this one and one other passed. The legislation called for establishment of a board of six members that would include two from the funding sector, two representing population centers of children at risk in the state (one urban and one rural), and one each from the NE Department of Education and the NE Department of Health and Human Services. This Board of Directors wrote requirements for the grants in keeping with the legislation and has provided oversight since. Approximately, 10 communities and 334 children and families are served by birth to 3 services that may be either center-based or home-visiting-based today (Jackson, Zweiback, & Alvarez, 2012).

Detailed Steps

We now turn to the principles that have been instrumental in the work from the examples provided in Nebraska. The efforts have a number of characteristics: (1) drawing on expertise and the latest science to augment the local stories; (2) engaging in big tent meetings across scientific and practitioner professionals in early childhood education to tell the story to policy makers; (3) organizing a central group of support from across the state; (4) building common sense strategies on working creatively with policy makers to find the way to fund the work; and (5) working with a supportive and creative funder.

Drawing on the science. Early childhood advocacy is able to be effective because the science so clearly points to the importance of access, quality, and continuities for children, especially for children with risk factors such as poverty. From our understandings about the developing brain, specific skill areas, and what early childhood programs are able to do (and not do), it is possible to truthfully inform policy makers about the opportunities afforded by early childhood education and child care access, quality, and continuity efforts. In many cases, thanks to organizations such as the Harvard Center on the Developing Child, explanations of complex scientific phenomena have been made interpretable to the lay person. Organizations such as that one were developed because there seemed to be a gap between what we knew and what we were doing. Fortunately, the gap is beginning to close but gaps still exist as we have discussed. The science continues to build as we refine understandings of preferred approaches, continuities needed for different groups, how to position programs when risks are greatest.

The relation between science and advocacy is a complex one and scientists may study questions of interest to advocates but science must always maintain its integrity for credibility and principle. Thus, advocates will not always like the findings that science brings forward but should be open to the discourse that robust science produces. We say more in the closing section about how scientists might think about advocacy in order to maintain the integrity of these two separate areas of emphasis. Today's advocate will need to know the science well and be able to faithfully report from it.

Organizing a "big tent." The efforts in Nebraska, in other states, and nationally have been as successful as they were because many people worked together to achieve aims. Often advocacy involves representatives in state systems, or even federal systems, to agree on what is needed to successfully pass legislation. A number of years ago (as recently as 20 years ago), the early childhood field was characterized by many voices and a lack of unanimity around goals. While there are still many healthy schools of thought about early childhood education issues, there is also more ability to rally around key changes, which has helped the field move forward. In addition, early childhood education and care cross many disciplines and fields from education to health and support services. There are different assumptions and definitions in these fields and there may also be differing technical requirements from legislation in different fields. Today's advocates will find it necessary to work in concert with many practitioners and scientists and policy makers and to be "multilingual" in being able to integrate across disciplines and fields.

Establishing a centralized group. Today in Nebraska, a new group called Nebraska First Five provides the centralized advocacy for the state. Many states have similar organizations. Other states have also organized early childhood efforts within the state into a centralized state governmental agency, as noted earlier. We have not done that in Nebraska, perhaps, in part, because we are a small state and traditionally have worked across agencies successfully. Because the programs for early childhood education are many and diverse, it is necessary to work centrally to achieve a common voice, to work through differences, and to achieve the most strategic approaches that make the most sense in the current climate. Thus, today's advocate will need to acquaint her/himself with persons in that unifying agency. The day of a single spokesperson making a big difference has probably passed as efforts become increasingly sophisticated, integrated, and part of a long-term strategy.

Building on strengths. There are no formulas for improving access, quality, and continuity for early childhood education. Thus, it is important to understand what others have done but to build on the strengths and possibilities that exist within a particular state or locality. In Nebraska, we built on an existing grants pilot program because it had all the quality elements in place and was aligned with schools. Other states have put their emphasis in other areas. Today's advocate will need to know the strengths to identify the opportunities that are unique and to recognize where a strategic leverage point exists for moving to the next level. In Nebraska, we found two unique funding mechanisms. A senator suggested the State Lands Fund, something no other state has initiated (though some may do so in the future) and we drew on the state funding formula for 4-year olds, which a few states have done. Further, advocacy efforts can sometimes be focused together to address even greater needs in an urban setting. This was the case in the development of two Educare of Omaha schools in North and South Omaha. The first opened its doors in 2002 and the other in 2009. Drawing from funding through Head Start and Early Head Start, along with school district and state funds, as well as private funding, this program served over 412 children and their families in 2011–2012. Long-term follow-up of their students in 2011–2012 demonstrated that former Educare students who participated 2 or more years in Educare earned an average score of 111 on the Nebraska state reading assessment (third to seventh grades), where "meeting standards" is set at 85 (St. Clair & Borer, 2012). Educare partners with others to move beyond the walls of a single program. Innovative programs such as Building Bright Futures-Early Childhood Services Network, a community-wide coaching quality enhancement project serving low-income community child care programs, systematically extract specific quality features and weave together community child care programs, experienced coaches (the staff providing the professional development "coaching" to community child care teachers), and comprehensive program evaluation in an effort to improve quality of early learning experiences for about 1,000 young children over the past 2 years.

At the end of 2 years, results showed significant improvements in external ratings of classroom quality using two tools: Environment Rating Scales overall with medium effect sizes ($d=0.66$) and the Classroom Organization domain of the Classroom Assessment and Scoring System-PreK ($d=0.69$). Children also showed significant improvements in auditory comprehension and expressive language on the Preschool Language Scale (fourth edition), with children approaching the goal of a 100 standard score (98.26) at exit, with modest change effect sizes ($d=0.26$) (Jackson, St. Clair, & Kumke, 2012).

Gaining support from a funder. We have been fortunate in Nebraska that a philanthropist, Susie Buffett, has a passion for early childhood education and for educating the public and others about its importance. Many funders are interested in making a difference in an area that matters and so early childhood education has been a popular area for funders. Moreover, there are a number of funders in states who have been supporting early childhood efforts. Alignment with philanthropy is helpful for the systems and long-term policy work needed in early childhood education and care.

Final Notes and Future Work

Advocacy in the realm of early childhood education and care is today an evolved and evolving effort. Contributors come from all sectors, yet, players are aware of the roles they can and cannot play in an advocacy world.

Researchers and scientists must be particularly careful to differentiate themselves from advocates in order to preserve the integrity of research. Thus, those entering the scientific professions who are drawn to help with the many compelling issues related to early education will want to give careful thought to their scientific responsibilities. Scientists and other professionals are helpful to those on the advocacy front by presenting and interpreting data in a way that is clear and solid. Preliminary findings or findings that are hard to interpret or ambiguous should not be shared as evidence of how programs work, no matter how tempting. Solid, well-vetted research with effect sizes should be reported. Negative findings as well as positive findings need to be reported and interpreted. Altogether, there is an art to reporting findings that the researcher thinks may be used in an advocacy world; it is best to report new findings in the context of extant findings to avoid overemphasizing any single finding. Scientists will need to synthesize the science, a role that the Center on the Developing Child has played well to date. There is also an art to synthesizing findings in such a way that provides sufficient information that the well-versed reader finds credible but not so much as to overwhelm policy makers with detail. Researchers who are interested in informing policy should always begin their work to discover the truth and be prepared to share findings that may not be pleasing.

Others—such as practitioners working for nonprofit or government agencies—may also have restrictions on their advocacy or political activity. It is always important to determine the ground rules in advance of advocacy-related efforts. Despite cautions, often they do not restrict all action. In many cases, one must separate what one can do as a private citizen from what one can do as representative of an agency or university.

There will always be a role for thoughtful and thorough reporting of knowledge about early childhood to help policy makers in decision making. Policy makers are appreciative of sources they can trust to tell them the truth.

In summary, we have addressed advocacy in early childhood education and care, an area that is richly informed by a growing knowledge base on brain development, other developmental areas, and the influence of early childhood education on early development. Many of the issues and current advocacy efforts focus on access, quality, and continuities in early education and care. Efforts tend to focus on leveling the playing field so that children from reduced socioeconomic circumstances or those who have not yet learned to speak English, as well as those with other risk factors, have experiences in early childhood education that are comparable to experiences of more advantaged children by the time they enter formal schooling. In Nebraska, as has been true in other states, advocacy has focused on expanding access, increasing quality, and developing continuity of early childhood education and care. Examples of these efforts were provided in this chapter. In Nebraska, the principles of the work have included building on the science of early development; having many diverse colleagues working together under a "big tent"; having a centralized organization leading the effort; working flexibly with state and community strengths and legislative predilections; and receiving support from a dedicated funder.

References

Astuto, J., & Allen, L. (2009). Home visitation and young children: An approach worth investing in? *Social Policy Report, 23*(4), 3–22.

Barnett, W. S., Carolan, M. E., Fitzgerald, J., & Squires, J. H. (2011). *The state of preschool 2011: State preschool yearbook.* New Brunswick, NJ: National Institute for Early Education Research.

Burchinal, M. R., Peisner-Feinberg, E., Bryant, D. M., & Clifford, R. (2000). Children's social and cognitive development and child-care quality: Testing for differential associations related to poverty, gender, or ethnicity. *Applied Developmental Science, 4*(3), 149–165.

Center on the Developing Child at Harvard University. (2007). *A science-based framework for early childhood policy: using evidence to improve outcomes in learning, behavior, and health for vulnerable children.* Retrieved from http://www.developingchild.harvard.edu, September, 2012

Cost Quality and Outcomes Study Team. (2005). Cost, Quality and child outcomes in child care centors: key finding and recommendation. *Young Children, 50*(40), 40–44.

Deming, D. (2009). Early childhood intervention and life-cycle skill development: Evidence from Head Start. *American Economic Journal: Applied Economics, 1*(3), 111–134.

Duncan, G. J., Dowsett, C. J., Claessens, A., Magnuson, K., Huston, A. C., Klebanov, P., et al. (2007). School readiness and later achievement. *Developmental Psychology, 43*(6), 1428–1446.

Early, D., Maxwell, K. L., Burchinal, M., Bender, R., Ebanks, C., & Zill, N. (2007). Teachers' Education, classroom quality, and young children's academic skills: Results from seven studies of preschool programs. *Child Development, 78*(2), 558–580.

Fantuzzo, J. (2012). *A model of generating across domain learning experiences through intentional, systematic and "intense enough" integrated curricula.* In Presentation at the 2012 Head Start research conference, Washington, DC, June 18–20.

Garces, E., Thomas, D., & Currie, J. (2002). Longer-term effects of Head Start. *American Economic Association, 92*(4), 999–1012.

Gormley, W., Gayer, T., Phillips, D., & Dawson, B. (2005). The effects of universal pre-K on cognitive development. *Developmental Psychology, 41*, 872–884.

Government Accounting Office. (2002). *States have undertaken a variety of quality improvements, but more evaluations of effectiveness are needed.* GAO-02-897.

Hair, E., Halle, T., Terry-Humen, E., Lavelle, B., & Calkins, J. (2006). Children's school readiness in the ECLS-K: Predictions to academic, health, and social outcomes in first grade. *Early Childhood Research Quarterly, 21*(4), 431–454.

Halle, T., Forry, N., Hair, E., Perper, K., Wandner, L., Wessel, J., et al. (2009). *Disparities in early learning and development: Lessons from the Early Childhood Longitudinal Study-Birth Cohort (ECLS-B).* Washington, DC: Child Trends.

Hart, B., & Risley, T. (1995). *Meaningful differences in the everyday experiences of young American children.* Baltimore, MD: Paul H. Brookes.

Heckman, J. J., & Masterov, D. V. (2004). *The productivity argument for investing in young children.* Working Paper No. 5. Washington, DC: Invest in Kids Working Group.

Howes, C., Burchinal, M., Early, D., Pianta, R., Bryant, D., Clifford, R., et al. (2008). Ready to learn? Children's pre-academic achievement in pre-kindergarten programs. *Early Childhood Research Quarterly, 23*, 27–50.

Jackson, B. (2011). *Early childhood education in Nebraska school districts and educational service units, 2010–2011 state report.* Retrieved from http://www.education.ne.gov/oec/index.html, September, 2012

Jackson, B., St. Clair, L., & Kumke, J. (2012). *Evaluation findings: Early childhood services network of excellence coaching model.* Omaha, NE: University of Nebraska Medical Center.

Jackson, B., Zweiback, R., & Alvarez, L. (2012). *Sixpence annual evaluation report 2011–12.* Retrieved from www.nebraskachildren.org, September, 2012

Johnson, R. C. (2011). *School-quality and the long-run effects of Head Start.* Unpublished paper.

Jones-Branch, J. A., Torquati, J., Raikes, H., & Edwards, C. P. (2004). Child care subsidy and quality. *Early Education and Development, 15*(3), 329–341.

Kontos, S., Howes, C., Shinn, M., & Galinsky, E. (1995). *Quality in family child care and relative care.* New York, NY: Teachers College Press.

Lee, V. E., & Burkham, D. T. (2002). *Inequality at the starting gate: Social background differences in achievement as children begin school.* Washington, DC: Economic Policy Institute.

Love, J. M., Chazan-Cohen, R., Raikes, H., & Brooks-Gunn, J. (Eds.). (2013). What makes a difference: Early Head Start evaluation findings in a developmental context. *Monographs of the Society for Research in Child Development 78*(1), vii–viii, 1–173.

Love, J. M., Kisker, E. E., Ross, C., Raikes, H., Constantine, J., Boller, K., et al. (2005). The effectiveness of Early Head Start for 3-year-old children and their parents: Lessons for policy and programs. *Developmental Psychology, 41*(6), 885–901.

Ludwig, J., & Miller, D. L. (2007). Does Head Start improve children's life changes: Evidence from a regression discontinuity design. *The Quarterly Journal of Economics, 122*(1), 159–208.

Ludwig, J., & Phillips, D. (2007). *The benefits and costs of Head Start* (Vol. 21, No. 3, pp. 3–11). Social Policy Report. Cambridge, MA: National Bureau of Economic Research, Society for Research on Child Development.

National Scientific Council on the Developing Child (2007). The science of early childhood development. Retrieved from http://developingchild.harvard.edu/resources/reports.

NICHD Early Child Care Research Network. (2005). *Child care and child development: Results from the NICHD Study of Early Child Care and Youth Development.* New York, NY: Guilford.

Olds, D. L., Eckenrode, J., Henderson, C. R., Jr., Kitzman, H., Powers, J., Cole, R., et al. (1997). Long-term effects of home visitation on material life-course and child abuse and neglect: Fifteen year follow up of a randomized trial. *Journal of the American Medical Association, 278*(8), 637–643.

Peisner-Feinberg, E. S., Burchinal, M. R., Clifford, R. M., Culkin, M. L., Howes, C., Kagan, S. L., et al. (2001). The relation of preschool child-care quality to children's cognitive and social developmental trajectories through second grade. *Child Development, 72*, 1534–1553.

Raikes, H. H. (1998). What are we buying? The need for research on child care subsidy. *Society for Research in Child Development Social Policy Reports, 12*(2), 1–18.

Raikes, H. A., Raikes, H. H., & Wilcox, B. (2005). Regulation, subsidy receipt and provider characteristics: What predicts quality in child care homes? *Early Childhood Research Quarterly, 20*, 164–184.

Raikes, H. H., Torquati, J., Hegland, S., Raikes, H. A., Scott, J., Messner, L., et al. (2006). Studying the culture of quality early education and care: A cumulative approach to measuring characteristics of the workforce and relations to quality in four Midwestern states. In M. Zaslow & I. Martinez-Beck (Eds.), *Critical issues in early childhood professional development* (pp. 111–136). Baltimore, MD: Paul Brookes.

Raikes, H. H., Torquati, J. C., Jung, E., Peterson, C., Atwater, J., Messner, L., (2013). Family child care in four Midwestern states: Multiple measures of quality and relations to outcomes by licensed status and subsidy program participation, *Early Childhood Research Quarterly*

Ramey, C. T., & Campbell, F. A. (1991). Poverty, early childhood education, and academic competence: The Abecedarian experiment. In A. C. Houston (Ed.), *Children in poverty: Child development and public policy* (pp. 190–221). Cambridge: Cambridge University Press.

Reynolds, A. J., Temple, J. A., Robertson, D. L., & Mann, E. A. (2001). Long-term effects of an early childhood intervention on educational achievement and juvenile arrest: A 15-year follow-up of low-income children in public schools. *JAMA: The Journal of the American Medical Association, 285*(18), 2339–2346.

Rodriguez, E., & Tamis LeMonda, C. (2011). Trajectories of the home learning environment across the first 5 years: Associations with children's vocabulary and literacy skills at prekindergarten. *Child Development, 82*(4), 1058–1075.

Schweinharrt, L. J., Montie, J., Xiang, Z., Barnett, W. S., Belfield, C. R., & Nores, M. (2005). *Lifetime effects: The HighScope Perry Preschool study through age 40.* Ypsilanti, MI: HighScope Press.

Shonkoff, J., & Phillips, D. (Eds.). (2000). *From neurons to neighborhoods: The science of early childhood development.* Washington, DC: National Academy Press.

St. Clair, L., & Borer, M. (2012). *Annual evaluation report for Educare of Omaha 2011-12.* Retrieved from www.Educareomaha.org, September, 2012.

Sweet, M., & Appelbaum, M. (2004). Is home visiting an effective strategy? A meta-analysis of home visiting programs for families with young children. *Child Development, 74,* 1435–1456.

U.S. Department of Health and Human Services, Administration for Children and Families (USDHHS). (2010). *Head Start impact study. Final report.* Report #2011-7. Washington, DC: Office of Planning, Research and Evaluation, Administration for Children and Families, U.S. Department of Health and Human Services.

U.S. Department of Health and Human Services, Administration for Children and Families (USDHHS) (2012). *Advisory committee on head start research and evaluation: Final Report.* Retrieved on May, 2013 from http://www.act.hhs.gov/programs/opre/resource/advisory committee_on-head-start-research-and-evaluation-final-report.

Vogel, C. A., Xue, Y., Moiduddin, E. M., Kisker, E. E., & Carlson, B. L. (2010). *Early Head Start children in grade 5: Long-term follow-up of the early head start research and evaluation study sample.* OPRE Report # 2011-8. Washington, DC: Office of Planning, Research and Evaluation, Administration for Children and Families, U.S. Department of Health and Human Services.

Votruba-Drzal, E., Coley, R. L., & Chase-Lansdale, P. L. (2004). Child care and low-income children's development: Direct and moderated effects. *Child Development, 75,* 296–312.

Watt, N., Ayoub, C. C., Bradley, R. H., Puma, J. E., & Lebeouf, W. A. (2006). *The crisis in youth mental health: Critical issues and effective programs. Early intervention programs and policies* (Vol. 4). Westport: Praeger Press.

Whitebook, M., Kipnis, F., & Bellm, D. (2007). *Disparities in California's child care subsidy system: A look at teacher education, stability and diversity.* Berkeley: Center for the Study of Child Care Employment, University of California. Retrieved from http://search.ebscohost.com/login.aspx?direct=true&db=eric&AN=ED499065&site=ehost-live

Yazejian, N., & Bryant, D. M. (2010). *Promising early returns: Educare implementation study data, January 2010.* Chapel Hill, NC: FPG Child Development Institute, UNC-CH.

Chapter 9
Education Reform Strategies for Student Self-Regulation and Community Engagement

Lauren M. Littlefield and Robert A. Siudzinski

How well does the US public school system fare in student achievement when wcompared to educational systems in other countries? How satisfied is the American public with the effectiveness of US schools? The answers to these questions speak to whether or not education reform is needed.

- Graduation trends recorded in 2009 revealed that the average high school graduation rate of the Organization for Economic Cooperation and Development's (OECD) 34-member countries was 82 %, compared with the US rate of 76 % (OECD, 2011). Upwards of three million eligibly aged US young adults in 2009 were without a high school diploma or GED (Chapman, Laird, Ifill, & Kewal Ramani, 2011).
- US student scores revealed a decline in reading ability from year 2000 to year 2009, with the decline being particularly notable in female students and in the number of students in the top proficiency range (OECD, 2012).
- The math literacy of US 15-year-olds was deemed below average when rank ordered among participating OECD countries (Aud et al., 2011).

The USA is either behind, or losing ground, in critical educational areas. Given how the USA compares, it is surprising that the USA spends about $3,000 more per student annually on educational expenditures than the OECD average (OECD, 2011).

A second way to gauge effectiveness of, and satisfaction with, the current educational system is to examine how people view it. While public schooling continues to be the most popular choice among available US educational options, there is some evidence that faith in traditional public education is declining.

L.M. Littlefield, Ph.D. (✉)
Department of Psychology, Washington College, Chestertown, MD, USA
e-mail: llittlefield2@washcoll.edu

R.A. Siudzinski, Ph.D.
Department of Education, Washington College, Chestertown, MD, USA

A. McDonald Culp (ed.), *Child and Family Advocacy: Bridging the Gaps Between Research, Practice, and Policy*, Issues in Clinical Child Psychology,
DOI 10.1007/978-1-4614-7456-2_9, © Springer Science+Business Media New York 2013

- With a general population growth in school-aged children from 2007 to 2010 being approximately 2.11 %, Ray (2011) found that there was at least a 7 % increase during the same time period in homeschooled students as compared to only 0.59 % growth in the non-homeschooled group.
- The most recent Gallup poll conducted by Phi Delta Kappa, the professional association for educators in the U.S., revealed that at least 70 % of random US adults surveyed endorsed the charter school concept (Bushaw & Lopez, 2011). Charter schools are non-tuition-based alternatives to traditional public schools. While they still rely on public funding, they are typically designed to meet a perceived community need, to allow innovations in teaching practices, and to provide a smaller learning community. Charter schools are not fully constrained by state educational regulations. Three times the number of US charter schools existed in 2008/2009 than in 1999/2000 (Aud et al., 2011).

Collectively, the statistics indicate discontent and unrest within the US public educational system. Shrinking budgets, bullying behavior, and the pressure of teacher accountability for student achievement are concerns that weigh heavily on politicians, school administrators, teachers, and parents alike. However, these constituencies do not share a common vision for how to positively impact American school reform. Many potentially positive efforts have been abandoned due to limited funds or terminated due to inconsistent follow through. It is time for a common vision that will drive systematic change.

Approaches to School Reform

International education expert Vivien Stewart (n.d.) has authoritatively delineated essential factors for effective school reform; these include modernization of the curriculum and student engagement, among others. This chapter argues that the best way to teach children is to engage them in the learning process. Increased student involvement occurs when students become active participants, rather than observers, in their own learning. Engaging students helps them to learn in the short term and provides the foundation for them to become responsible, self-motivated critical thinkers in the long term (Dweck, 2006). Through hands-on lessons, children develop self-confidence during the learning process. Further, children learn best by discovering the value of their lessons (Brophy, 2008). Students who realize the real-world context and meaningfulness of a concept are likely to be motivated to learn more about it.

Public school students need opportunities to develop their self-regulation skills in support of the learning process. They also need access to the physical spaces and teaching techniques that create an atmosphere of meaningful, active learning. Teaching self-regulation skills and using the community as the expanded classroom are both associated with improvements in student behavior and with increases in academic achievement.

Fig. 9.1 Academic learning in the schools begins with building character, reinforcing good behavior, and gaining command of one's cognitive processing

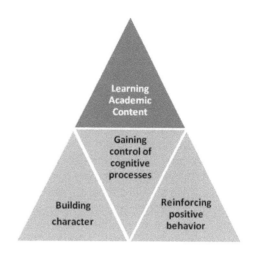

Teaching Self-Regulation Skills

Definitions and Background

It sometimes takes significant internal motivation to persevere in the school environment. Especially when boring or difficult topics are being taught, many students have difficulty inhibiting prepotent responses like doodling, daydreaming, or chatting with friends. Off-task and rule-breaking behavior detract from learning engagement, while order in the late elementary school classroom is directly related to student gains in literacy and mathematics (Gaskins, Herres, & Kobak, 2012). Similarly, positive student social skills are predictive of higher standardized test scores in reading and mathematics (DiPerna & Elliott, 1999; Ray & Elliott, 2006). Welsh and colleagues report a reciprocal statistical model, showing that stronger report card grades positively impact student behavior and that, in turn, level of social competence demonstrated by students directly influences academic achievement (Welsh, Parke, Widaman, & O'Neil, 2001). It is clear that well-behaved students are poised to absorb the academic curriculum. Therefore, we contend that good character, positive behavior, and control of cognitive processes are basic building blocks for self-regulated learning. Figure 9.1 depicts the multifaceted, tripartite base that supports successful academic learning. The three different lines of research that correspond to Fig. 9.1's building blocks are described in this section.

Building character. Character development, or teaching an appreciation of right from wrong, is inherent to academic learning (Elias, 2009; Howard, Berkowitz, & Schaeffer, 2004). Character-building programs carry a noble mission of fostering personal strengths so that sound judgments can be made, both in and out of the school environment. The many faces of character education are reviewed by Howard et al. (2004); with a main goal of preventing unhealthy behaviors, character education includes: (1) teachings in religion, values, and moral philosophy; (2) service-learning approaches; and (3) specific training in practical life skills and methods. While some programs have been criticized for consisting of highly structured lessons followed by repetition and drills until students recite what are deemed to be the correct answers (Kohn, 1997), aspects of character education exist in many American schools.

Reinforcing positive behavior. Personal growth occurs through experiences when children learn that certain actions are encouraged and others are discouraged. Programs involving positive behavior support (PBS) have slightly different names (e.g., PBIS or positive behavioral interventions and supports, and SWPBS or school-wide positive behavior support), but regardless of name, the united goal is to foster prosocial student behaviors. Perhaps most cited for his work on PBS, Edward G. Carr describes it as a flexible, research-based movement that views students as able to be competent (Carr et al., 2002). Children are taught what is expected of them. The expectations are consistent and pervasive. Students are acknowledged for good behaviors through an established reward system. Some are recognized for being exceptionally good role models. When rules are broken, consequences for misbehavior are consistent and intervention is targeted. Many PBS programs incorporate aspects of character education by using keywords for guiding behavior, such as responsibility, respect, fairness, safety, and achievement. At least 10 % of public schools incorporate content that focuses on decreasing asocial behaviors and interpersonal conflicts (Arndt, 2010).

Gaining control of cognitive processes. Supported by positive character traits and well-developed emotions and behaviors, cognitive strategies for self-regulation can be taught to maximize learning potential. In other words, children can be taught to monitor their own learning through the incorporation of specific study skills techniques, such as calendaring, organizing, and mnemonic systems. Executive functioning skills include a wide array of intentional behaviors such as maintaining focus of attention, planning before acting, and learning by effectively updating one's memories. At the core of cognitive control for students is the ability to target their attention on lessons and incorporate new information into their long-term store of knowledge. This is precisely what working memory allows students to do. Working memory is a temporary attention system with limited capacity for information storage and manipulation (Baddeley & Hitch, 1974). It involves the information that a person chooses to pay attention to and process at any given moment. The convenience and adaptability of working memory is that a person can hold concepts, words, pictures, or ideas within memory and integrate the ideas simultaneously (Baddeley, 1983; Fockert, Rees, Frith, & Lavie, 2001; Hitch et al., 1983).

How to Teach Basic Learning Skills

Today's strength-based approaches emphasize student competencies, rather than focusing on weaknesses. Most children can learn to modulate their own impulses and adjust them to environmental demands. Programs can be woven into existing academic curricula and/or direct skills instruction can be implemented to teach character, positive behavior, and cognitive processing strategies.

How to build character. Advocates of character education declare that "it is not a question of whether to do character education but rather questions of how consciously and by what methods" (Howard et al., 2004, p. 210). Effective practices for implementation of character education are outlined by Berkowitz (2011). These include, but are not limited to, student service work in the school and community, parental involvement, role modeling (i.e., school role models and vicarious learning about heroes and historical figures), character-based school mission statements, and time and money apportioned for professional development of teachers, administrators, and guidance counselors. Character-building strategies are diverse and can be applied quite differently across schools, depending on the age of students being served, the problems unique to certain communities, and the philosophy of school administrators.

How to reinforce positive behavior. Long ago, it was discovered that teachers' responses toward students can have a direct impact on the number of disruptive vs. prosocial behaviors displayed by students (Thomas, Becker, & Armstrong, 1968). Rules in and of themselves cause little effect on behavior in the classroom, whereas showing clear approval for expected behaviors makes a strong, positive effect on gaining control of the classroom (Madsen, Becker, & Thomas, 1968). When school personnel are committed to PBS, behaviors are consistently reinforced and modeled, allowing students the motivation to change their behavior (Safran & Oswald, 2003). As is the case with good decision-making, students benefit from mechanisms to apply what they have learned in real-world contexts. Teaching children to think critically about situations can assist them in mediating their own disputes.

How to teach students to gain control of their cognitive processes. Cleary and Zimmerman (2004) explain case study techniques that have been used for developing empowered, self-regulated learners: showing them how they can set goals and how to monitor their own progress; teaching them study strategies (e.g., such as use of graphic organizers and tables); and instructing them about how to adjust their study plans. Teaching writing as a process as early as the elementary school years is helpful so that the steps become routinized as writing assignments increase in length and complexity. Coaching students to set their own realistic goals toward task completion or discussing how they will study for a future test at the beginning of a new unit can assist them in goal-setting and follow through, particularly when faced with long-term projects. Using school calendars or planners can make the planning process more visual and concrete. Similarly, specific task processing can be facilitated by using number lines, wall charts, and memory note cards. Rehearsal strategies can be taught and time can be apportioned during class time so that there is less repetition offered by the teacher and more retrieval practice performed by the student. While research examining the efficacy of attention and memory training is a relatively new pursuit, recent findings are promising. Preliminary work shows that executive functioning skills are moldable and trainable (Bryck & Fisher, 2012; Flook et al., 2010; Mackey, Hill, Stone, & Bunge, 2011).

How to incorporate all three basic learning skills. Integrated school programs that develop character, reinforce good behavior, and teach explicit cognitive strategies provide a solid foundation for academic learning. A model School Development Program (SDP) began in 1968 when James Comer started directing a Yale Child Study Center project in two schools (Panjwani, 2011). The collaboration for SDPs is between a researcher, a child development center, and a school or school district. A school management team made up of the principal, a mental health worker, elected teachers, and elected parents creates school policy, making decisions about academic, extracurricular, and social programs. Students are expected to demonstrate character and are taught social skills and problem-solving strategies. Parents are offered classes about how their children learn and are invited to be on the team that discusses any academic or behavioral problems. Teachers are provided with equal access to resources and regularly communicate with one another. The SDP model focuses on all aspects of the student—social, emotional, behavioral, and academic. Since 1968, the model has expanded to positively impact students in schools across 20 different states, showing dramatic improvements in test scores, student behavior, attendance, confidence in abilities, and feelings of safety and belongingness in the school environment (Panjwani, 2011).

Research Findings

What not long ago was anecdotal evidence is now a growing body of literature evidencing the impact of positive behavior programs and cognitive skill training programs in the schools.

Research on character building. There is a paucity of peer-reviewed literature that assesses the impact of character education. Available studies that isolate character education use vastly different teaching materials and yield mixed findings, so they are not reported in detail here. However, it is worth noting than none of the character education studies reported adverse effects and that many positive behavior programs incorporate some aspect of character education.

Research on reinforcing positive behavior. Reviews of the available literature present evidence that children low in social–emotional or cognitive control tend to be disruptive and less engaged in classroom activities; ultimately, they achieve lower levels of academic competence (Eisenberg, Sadovsky, & Spinrad, 2005; Eisenberg, Valiente, & Eggum, 2010). Moreover, reinforcing prosocial student behavior consistently leads to positive outcomes.

- When properly implemented, SWPBS leads to gains in student academic achievement (Sailor, Stowe, Turnbull, & Kleinhammer-Tramill, 2007). SWPBS implemented in a North Texas elementary school resulted in higher scores on the statewide standardized achievement test as well as reductions in rule violations and office referrals (Menendez, Payne, & Mayton, 2008).
- PBS has been shown to be successful in urban high schools. Bohanon et al. (2006) found decreases in office disciplinary referrals and the number of stu-

dents needing individual intervention. As a result of program implementation, Lassen, Steele, and Sailor (2006) revealed improved student behavior and significant increases in reading and mathematics scores.

- White and Warfa (2011) examined the effectiveness of a prosocial development program which included whole-class character education lessons in an elementary school in England. As a result of the intervention, they found that content delivery from teachers and on-task behavior of students increased while the need for behavior management in the classroom decreased. The number of disruptive incidents and office referrals decreased significantly from pre- to post-program implementation.
- A meta-analysis of 213 social and emotional learning programs for school-aged children showed clear, positive gains on a number of indices, such as more developed social skills, better controlled behavior, and higher academic achievement as a result of intervention (Durlak, Weissberg, Dymnicki, Taylor, & Schellinger, 2011).

Research on gaining control of cognitive processes. Children with well-developed executive functioning skills consistently and predictably obtain higher scores on standardized academic tests of reading, writing, and mathematics (Best, Miller, & Naglieri, 2011; Neuenschwander, Röthlisberger, Cimeli, & Roebers, 2012; Roebers, Cimeli, Röthlisberger, & Neuenschwander, 2012). One type of executive functioning, working memory capability, is said to be in place by the time children start school, between 4 and 6 years old (Alloway, Gathercole, Willis, & Adams, 2004). Working memory skills are directly related to important academic indicators. Strong working memory skills measured in children attending Head Start programs predicted better development of literacy and numeracy skills through kindergarten (Welsh, Nix, Blair, Bierman, & Nelson, 2010). Furthermore, working memory measured at school entry has been deemed an excellent predictor of student success on national assessment measures of reading, math, and language comprehension in third grade (Gathercole, Brown, & Pickering, 2003).

Preschool is not too early to begin programs to promote development of executive functioning skills, and working memory skills in particular. Early work (reviewed by Bryck & Fisher, 2012) indicates that working memory training can even influence brain development. Working memory task performance is associated with increased activity in the prefrontal cortex (Olsen, Westerberg, & Klingberg, 2004), the part of the brain known to be associated with goal-directed behaviors like planning, decision-making, and impulse control. Research performed by Diamond and colleagues boasts an effective, inexpensive curriculum designed for preschoolers that resulted in decreased negative student behaviors (such as impulsivity and conduct-related problems) as well as better ability to inhibit and appropriately respond to changing task demands on a complex computerized task (Diamond, Barnett, Thomas, & Munro, 2007). The training curriculum is intensive, requiring teachers to spend approximately 80 % of each school day focusing on preschool-level executive functioning activities like talking out loud as a mechanism for monitoring one's behavior, various mnemonic devices, and dramatic play. Simple, inexpensive, and less time-intensive interventions can also assist students in honing their cognitive skills. Mackey et al. (2011) used commercially available games (i.e., computer, hand-held video, and board games) twice weekly during 8 weeks of after-school programming with a sample of early elementary students drawn from lower socioeconomic backgrounds. The games were chosen for the reasoning, attention, and memory skills they required. Students improved considerably from pre- to post-testing on visual working memory and speed of information processing. Children with the lowest scores at pretesting showed the greatest gains as a result of intervention, which is a finding replicated by other researchers. Executive training appears to work when using an array of executive function training techniques (i.e., mindfulness, martial arts, games, and guided speech strategies), but those with the poorest functioning at the onset tend to demonstrate the greatest gains (Diamond & Lee, 2011; Wang, Chen, & Zhong, 2009).

Using the Community as the Classroom

Definition and Background

Philosophers and learning theorists have long discussed and attempted to articulate the processes of experiential education through models and theoretical abstractions (Dewey, 1938; Joplin, 1981; Kolb, 1984). Young American learners are missing out on formative cultural and natural experiences that are crucial in their development as sophisticated thinkers and societal contributors. As Louv (2005, 2011) points out, students are suffering from nature deficit disorder, and the cultural shift indoors has caused children to spend more time watching television, playing video games, and surfing the Internet. Long ago, John Dewey viewed students "as being engaged in community life that reflects the larger society" (Totten & Pedersen, 2012, p. 43). Instead of the modern-day emphasis on passive information absorption, students are better served when encouraged to "make connections, find new patterns, [and] imagine new possibilities" (Kozol, 2005, pp. 131–132). Ideas about learning environments have dramatically changed over the last decade, with learning sites increasing in communities and informal learning environments such as gardens, woodlands, and watersheds, as well as museums, aquaria, and state and national parks.

Adventure learning, field trips, and experiential learning are all student-centered programs that engage learners by making use of natural spaces that are relevant to the teaching of multiple disciplines. Through service-learning, students learn and develop by active participation in a thoughtfully organized service that is conducted in the community, and meets the needs of students' educational objectives. Place-based education (PBE) expands the classroom into both the community and outdoor environment. PBE occurs when children, teachers, and adults in the community use the natural environment in which they live as an inquiry-based learning laboratory for students to gain knowledge and skills across the curriculum (Sobel, 2004).

A commonly accepted definition of PBE was articulated by the Rural School and Community Trust in 2005 and endorsed by Smith and Sobel (2010):

> Place-based education is learning that is rooted in what is local—the unique history, environment, culture, economy, literature, and art of a particular place. The community provides the context for learning, student work focuses on community needs and interests, and community members serve as resources and partners in every aspect of teaching and learning. This local focus has the power to engage students academically, pairing real-world relevance with intellectual rigor, while promoting genuine citizenship and preparing people to respect and live well in any community they choose. (p. 23)

PBE is a multisensory educational approach that uses all aspects of the local environment, including its culture, history, and socio-politics, natural and built environments, as the integrating context for interdisciplinary learning. This values-driven approach, designed to advance educational goals together with locally identified objectives, allows for resource sharing and team teaching with community partners. It is a hands-on, learner-centered approach focused on problem-solving projects that adapts to students' individual skills and abilities (Duffin, Chawla, Sobel, & PEER Associates, 2005). Alliances formed between schools and external organizations can be mutually beneficial, with the organization supporting the school and the students performing service for the organization. Progressive social change can be influenced by efforts in the schools.

Learners who are engaged, be they young or old, show sustained behavioral involvement in learning activities accompanied by a positive emotional tone. They select tasks that challenge their competencies, initiate action when given the opportunity, and exert intense effort and concentration in the implementation of learning tasks. They show generally positive emotions during ongoing action, including enthusiasm, optimism, curiosity, and interest (Reyes, Brackett, Rivers, White, & Salovey, 2012). Making community the larger classroom enhances the learning environment and provides unique opportunities for engaging with inquiry-based and interdisciplinary projects, including work in science, math, language arts, fine arts, and social studies (Rural School and Community Trust, 2011; Sobel, 2004).

PBE provides students with opportunities to connect with their communities and public lands through hands-on, real-world learning experiences with community-based projects (PEEC, 2008). Place-based educational practices can often parallel or overlap methods with experiential, adventure, service-learning, discovery, and environmental pedagogies. Varying in definition, purpose, and relationship to the regular school curriculum, educators stress the importance of direct, contextual experiences often found in communities (McInerney, Smyth, & Down, 2011; Smith & Knapp, 2011). Learners involved in community-based experiential learning are given the opportunity to engage in reflective observation, to form abstract conceptualizations, and to pursue active experimentation and practical application of what they're learning (Hirsch & Lloyd, 2005; McClellan & Hyle, 2012). Characteristics consistent with PBE include:

- Situated in the socio-cultural, natural, and built environments in which students live

- Multidisciplinary and interdisciplinary in process and product
- Partners learners, educators, advocates, and organizations with community
- Promotes academic rigor, investigation, and applied action
- Encourages active and responsible citizenship via community/environment stewardship

A growing number of schools across the USA and abroad have initiated this approach, which is distinguished by its focus on community (Gruenewald & Smith, 2008; Smith & Sobel, 2010), with a deepening connection of students to their homes, neighborhoods, and regions with the goal of empowering youth with the capacity to contribute solutions to local challenges. At its very core, PBE involves tapping all the local community has to offer for the sake of learning. "Solutions-based" education presents youth with a convincing model of how they as citizens have the capacity to address the challenging dilemmas facing humanity by thinking through issues and taking action within the context of their own community (Smith, 2011). By cultivating a sense of care (Noddings, 2005), participants in such programs begin to recognize their agency in bringing care and attention to issues in their immediate environment as a skill that can be transferred to broader world issues.

How to Use the Community as a Classroom

The nature of PBE means it can take on many forms, depending upon the particulars of each project. Below are examples of this approach.

- Kindergarteners work with a local artist to develop an ABC coloring book about the creatures found at a local nature center and the book is sold to raise funds for nature education.
- Concord Carlisle High School in Massachusetts is taking students of varied academic achievement into the community for 2-week learning expeditions led by teams of six teachers. By exploring interdisciplinary topics, through the lenses of literature, math, science, and history, faculty engage their students through student-driven discussions that guide the formation of connections within and across disciplines (Wu, 2010).
- Ambitious projects for citizen-scientists recording salamander populations in Manhattan (Foderaro, 2011) teach young students to examine local ecology through the lenses of community, systems, and sustainability.
- Fifth-grade students develop and publish an illustrated walking tour booklet of a historic neighborhood, including a map, commentary, and photographs of each building.
- Several effective models (Schultz, 2008; Wade, 2007; Westheimer & Kahne, 2004) illustrate how content areas such as math, science, or English language skills can be simultaneously developed through sustainable teaching practices emphasizing social action and civic engagement.
- Eighth-grade students collect data on ground-level ozone damage to plants growing in their schoolyard, as part of a national study.

- Eleventh-grade students collaborate to write a weekly newspaper column about the special cultural and natural places of their community, including interviews, photo-documentation, and other primary research.
- Geographic Information Systems and other science-based tools can help target important land and resources for conservation, while illuminating powerful, context-specific sites for student learning.

The role of mobile learning devices in PBE holds tremendous potential. With the ubiquitous presence of smartphones in our pockets, GPS units in our backpacks, and laptops on our fieldtrips, technology enables information access by students and teachers practically anyplace and anytime. Blurring the traditional boundaries surrounding physical and virtual teaching spaces suggests a need for reflective consideration of, and research into, what are the new "ecologies" of learning (Barron, 2006; Borgman et al., 2008; Israel, 2012; Veletsianos, Doering, & Henrickson, 2012).

Research Findings

Recognition of the value of informal learning and PBE can be noted in the tremendous rise in National Science Foundation funded research and increasing occurrence in academic journals (Ucko, 2010). Research supports that active learning tends to be more efficient than passive or highly directed learning (Beard & Wilson, 2009; Herbert, 1995; Jernstedt, 1980). When students are disengaged with school learning, negative consequences emerge such as lower grades, more classroom disruptions, and a lower likelihood of aspiring to higher educational goals (Reyes et al., 2012; Skinner & Belmont, 1993).

Place-based learning can translate into higher self-efficacy, for as students gain experience, they gain confidence. Authentic learning activities provide experience operating in settings much like those in which they will eventually find themselves as employees and adult citizens. Children benefit by being challenged to manage and prioritize activities, engage in formal teamwork, and learn to work effectively with those different from themselves (Lareau, 2003). Outcomes yield a long list of additional advantages including: improved academic attainment, school attendance, sense of direction and self-esteem; reductions in disruptive and/or violent behaviors, expulsions, suspensions and referrals; increased student motivation; enhanced health awareness; and better ability to develop and sustain relationships, communicate and cope with authority (Gutherson, Davies, & Daszkiewicz, 2011). Emphasizing hands-on, real-world learning experiences, the place-based approach to education increases academic achievement, helps students develop stronger ties to the community, enhances student appreciation for the natural world, and creates a heightened commitment to serving as active, contributive citizens.

The National Park Service (NPS) and the Appalachian Trail Conservancy (ATC) have piloted an alternative educational program called the Trail to Every Classroom (TTEC) exploring the potential for heritage and natural resource sites as classrooms for multidisciplinary education. TTEC seeks to provide educators with the tools and resources to create programs for students using experiential learning and sense-of-place development. Recent evaluations of the program found that participating students were engaged through many subject areas and partners, with positive impacts on students including "appreciation of nature, academic engagement, and volunteering on the AT (Appalachian Trail)" (PEER Associates, Inc., 2009) and "higher levels of civic responsibility, volunteerism, and environmental stewardship" (PEER Associates, Inc., 2010). To date, over 300 teachers have been trained in 14 states, with an approximate 25,000 students engaged in place-based instruction between 2006 and 2012 (Hennessy, 2012).

Two decades of research completed by the Place-based Education Evaluation Collaborative suggest that such programs offer effective opportunities for improving academic achievement and environmental literacy (Duffin et al., 2005; SEER, 2000), citizenship and stewardship development (PEEC, 2008; Powers, 2004a), while providing young people opportunities to do valuable, local work with immediate impact (Comber, Nixon, Ashmore, Loo, & Cook, 2006; Harrison, 2010; Sobel, 2004). Studies examining the use of community and the local environment as an integrating context for learning suggest its use in increasing student motivation toward achievement, agency, and dispositions towards critical thinking (Athman & Monroe, 2004; Rodriguez, 2008) and mitigating the achievement gap (Emekauwa, 2004; Lieberman & Hoody, 1998; SEER, 2000). In fact, schools that have adopted place-based or environment-based educational approaches demonstrate statistically significant academic benefits when compared to traditional classroom-based programs (Duffin, Powers, Tremblay, & PEER Associates, 2004; Lieberman & Hoody, 1998; SEER, 2005; Smith, 2011; Von Secker, 2004). For instance, researchers in California analyzed over 12,700 sets of student data collected at eight study schools over a 5-year period, and found that students in the environment-based schools outperformed their peers in the control schools on standardized test scores in reading, math, language, and spelling (California Student Assessment Project, 2005). Lieberman and Hoody (1998) investigated 40 schools using PBE as a context for teaching history/social studies, English/language arts, math and science to discover higher scores on standardized academic achievement tests, reduced discipline problems, increased student engagement in learning, and greater ownership/pride in students' accomplishments.

Advocacy Goal: Engaging Students in Their Learning

Through experiential education programs that also teach student self-regulation, deep roots can form in students' habits of critical thinking and responsible action. In light of the fact that the USA is falling behind peer countries in achievement indices and statistical indications that the US public is growing in dissatisfaction with the current status of the public educational system, it is time for a change. The overarching advocacy goal for school reform is to engage our students in their learning and thereby increase the pace in US education, rather than stagnate and continue to fall behind.

Advocacy Steps

There are four steps to take in order to make a change in school reform so that students take an active role in their learning. The four steps we propose are: (1) cultivate partnerships and make community connections; (2) revamp teacher education programs; (3) engage in high-quality research and program evaluation; and (4) revise the state and national educational budgets.

Cultivate Partnerships and Make Community Connections

Administrative understanding and support, at the school and district level, is critical to the integration of place-based learning practices in schools and the development of learning partnerships in the community (Coyle, 2010; Ernst, 2012; Hennessy, 2012; PEER Associates, Inc., 2007). Partnering with local community education/service organizations and school reform organizations across the country (e.g., the Orion Society, the Foxfire Fund, the Coalition of Community Schools, the Rural School and Community Trust, and the National Park Service National Leadership Council) will bolster public and alternative school educators' efforts to push back against the current educational system that is failing our children due to its overprescribed system now controlled through external accountability processes and pressures generated by a centralized curriculum and high-stakes testing. "Going local" (Smith, 2002) through PBE represents the refreshing future in national educational practice starting at the grassroots level of students, teachers and families, communities and schools, districts and states.

The list of potential local school sponsors is endless, and can include businesses, community-based nonprofit organizations, neighborhood associations, universities, teacher unions, Rotary Clubs, 4-H, YMCA, Boy/Girl Scouts, churches, Junior Achievers, Kiwanis Clubs, international school partnerships/exchanges, and more. National organizations also offer support for launching such projects. An arm of the Corporation for National and Community Service (called Learn and Serve America) provides learning resources for educators to begin service-learning initiatives (see http://www.learnandserve.gov/ for details).

As applied to any new initiative, it will not be sustainable without a system of support, including technical assistance and staff development. Collaborative partnerships can be achieved with low overall financial demands. For the sake of consistency, school-wide changes need to be accompanied by an investment in training and sustained professional development. Relationships with community stakeholders need to be formed early in the planning process and then continually cultivated.

In the end, the curriculum needs to be directly aligned with state assessment goals and standards, thereby having the power to enhance participating schools' improvement goals and student performance expectations.

Revamp Teacher Education Programs

The proposed reform efforts cannot be effectively accomplished without changes to teacher education programs. Teacher preparation programs need innovative transformation for the twenty-first century, yet this cannot be accomplished without new strategic partnerships to share in the responsibility of preparing teachers in radically different ways. The National Research Council (2010) recently identified "field experience" as one of the three "aspects of teacher preparation that are likely to have the highest potential for effects on outcomes for students," along with content knowledge and the quality of teacher candidates (p. 180). Elliot (2012) suggests that any reform or reconstruction of teacher education should primarily involve the development of teachers' situational understandings, so that they can make wise and better decisions in complex, ambiguous, and dynamic learning contexts. Now, more than ever, in-service and pre-service teachers require appropriate professional development for new pedagogies, curricular models, and learning environments.

One method for front-loading the successful launch of place-based pedagogies is to train pre-service educators in the theory, philosophy, and methodology before they graduate from schools of education. Required in many states as a high school graduation requirement, service-learning in K-12 classrooms has historical roots and numerous examples reported in research (Burns, 1998; Parsons, 1996; Wade, 1997). Only recently, though, have teacher education programs begun to enhance the personal learning and professional growth of their pre-service teachers through the connection of academic study with a program of service (Gallego, 2001; Spencer, Cox-Peterson, & Crawford, 2005; Zeller, Griffith, Zhang, & Klenke, 2010). Service-learning assignments that provide community service outside the formal classroom encourage meaningful connections of learning theory to practice, while applying service directly to community needs. Enhancing pre-service teachers' comfort with relating subject matter through place-based learning practices increases the likelihood of those teachers incorporating place-based pedagogy during their early teaching careers (Israel, 2012; PEER Associates, Inc., 2006; Powers, 2004b; Stern, Wright, & Powell, 2012). Backed by theoretical studies and knowledge of experiential learning, graduates become the informed, experienced, and motivated individuals who can lead curricular change in their schools as early-service teachers. Novice teachers can bring innovative practices and engaging energy to their new schools. In fact, insights drawn from comparative studies of educational approaches and the conclusions of the 1999 Third International Mathematics Science Study (TIMSS) prompted Stigler and Hiebert (2009) to assert that educational reform must begin with dramatic changes in the cultures of teaching, followed by changes to the curriculum.

Similarly, an articulated and infused approach to child development needs to be included in teacher education programs. This includes more focused training in the development of emotional and behavioral control as well as teaching teachers about memory skills and cognitive functioning, a pursuit strongly advocated for by Moely et al. (1986). Being able to set the stage for student learning through implementation of validated social–emotional and cognitive programs, new teachers should be more marketable. Once they obtain positions, new teachers should be better prepared to manage student behavior and to encourage positive learning experiences. Various teaching techniques and reinforcement tactics can be employed to address student motivation, thus encouraging a "growth mindset" in learners (Dweck, 2006). Pre-service teachers who have learned aspects of character-building exercises and memory strategy training can share their experiences with veteran teachers. Some states, such as Maryland, e.g., have statewide character/positive behavior initiatives and have mandated an environmental literacy requirement for all their graduating high school students, thereby requiring public schools to incorporate lessons about conservation, sustainable growth, and studies about the natural world into a variety of subjects.

Engage in High-Quality Research and Program Evaluation

Research is essential to purposeful school improvements. When research findings reveal evidence that new programs are worthwhile, these findings should be widely disseminated and readily accessible in a format that is usable to teachers, school leaders, and caregivers. Research deepens understanding of which programs work and under what conditions.

We make several recommendations for research that is needed. PBS is widely used, but more research is required to better understand its true impact. While more than 9,000 schools nationwide have implemented some form of PBS system, Bradshaw, Mitchell, and Leaf (2010) call for research that evaluates school contexts, teacher efficacy, and quality of implementation to determine how and when PBS can be most effective and sustainable. Further, Diamond and Lee (2011) advocate for curricula that incorporate aspects of social–emotional development and executive function training; well-designed research is necessary to explore if an integrative approach yields more achievement and behavioral gains than either one alone. More place-based educational research is needed to examine the efficacy of hybrid learning environments mediated by technology (Veletsianos et al., 2012), to investigate the learning gains achieved by involving students in community-based action research (Malone, 2012), and to measure the long-term impact of place-based learning on stewardship beliefs and behaviors (Meyer, 2012).

Unfortunately, much educational research is based on small samples or self-report methods with low statistical control of variables of interest. There is a general lack of solid educational research. When quantifiable measures are used, they sometimes fail to meet standards for adequate reliability or validity. This causes bias and makes it difficult to generalize findings to new situations. For instance, schools often use different training models so it is difficult to conduct cross-school comparisons. Conflicting results exist for studies with similar goals or methods.

Evidence-based research can mold educational practices and play a powerful role in influencing policies. Yet, research in the education field has been variously referred to by political constituencies as "awful," "mediocre," "irrelevant," and "useless" (Kaestle, 1993). While it is true that research projects always have limitations, rigorous and high-quality research can help isolate the aspects of programs that are most efficient and effective (Baker & Welner, 2012). Questions can be effectively answered with either controlled, randomized between-subjects designs (i.e., matched control and intervention groups), or within-subjects designs where baseline measures are taken before implementation and post-testing is completed with the same measurement tools. Demographic characteristics such as age, sex, race, and socioeconomic status of participants, as well as multiple outcome variables (i.e., school grades, school attendance record, standardized achievement test scores, number of office referrals, behavior rating scales, objective observations performed by trained researchers) are useful in determining the true impact of a given intervention. Integrative research, wherein teams of researchers explain multiple facets of the same program, likely provides the most complete picture of any educational phenomena. There is much to learn, but much to gain, through cross-disciplinary discovery. Neuro-education, for instance, is a new area of interdisciplinary study that seeks to blend established disciplines, like cognitive psychology, neuroscience, and education, for the purposes of impacting curriculum and educational policy (Carew & Magsamen, 2010).

Revise the State and National Education Budgets

When faced with decreasing budgets, it is a reality that operating expenses are cut and educational research funds become scarce. Unfortunately, such cost-saving measures inevitably impact school children. Class sizes grow. New textbooks aren't purchased. After-school programming is eliminated. Field trip funding is reduced. Programs for gifted students are terminated. Teacher and teacher's aide positions are eliminated. Instead of funding having a rate-limiting factor on education, the needs of American schools should determine the funding streams. We recommend redirection of funds to programs that engage students.

The budgets of district, state, and national offices need to be studied. Are educational administrative costs growing, and is there a measureable payoff to allotting high salaries to bureaucrats to oversee all of the regulation? A subject of great debate is whether bureaucracy plays a facilitative or a negative role in public school performance. In other words, do administrators contribute toward valuable performance indicators, or do administrators impose controls that limit teaching innovations? A 2001 regression analysis of district-level indicators in the Texas public schools revealed that the more administrators, the more negative impact there was on student reading, writing, and arithmetic test performance, and this relationship was especially present at the elementary and middle school levels (Bohte, 2001). Further, the percentage of teachers within a given district was positively related to student academic performance. While Smith and Larimer's (2004) study of Texas school districts concurs with Bohte's discovery of the negative relationship between number of school administrators and academic outcomes, Smith and Larimer point out that other indicators show a positive relationship with the number of administrators, namely dropout rates and attendance. While it may very well be true that reducing bureaucracy too much will impair teachers' ability to perform (Smith & Meier, 1994), there is a delicate balance between having too many administrators and expecting teachers to perform multiple administrative tasks. Noninstructional and clerical tasks can be doled out to trusted support staff. In the end, budgets need to be examined and revised so that programs that support student learning are the funding priority.

Next Steps: A Call to Action

We believe that US public school teachers should teach self-regulation skills to students and make use of local communities as extensions of traditional classrooms. Despite the apparent benefits of the suggested educational models, it would be naïve to believe that wide scale reform will be readily welcomed. Locked in the behavioral and programmatic regularities of school (Sarason, 1996) and concerned about potential controversy, there is a tendency for most public school administrators to question whether any new model matches the common vision of what "real school" should be (Metz, 1989; Stevenson, 1987). However, today's alternative educators are laying the foundation for a pedagogical revolution that will demand a redefinition of "real school," and require deep changes in the thinking of teachers, policymakers, and the public about the purposes of education.

Individuals can impact, and help lead, the pedagogical revolution of engaged learning.

- Parent leaders can play a role as the agents of community change. For instance, parents, guardians, and caregivers can assert their desire for engaged approaches to learning in local schools. They can advocate for the use of sound educational programs that encourage cognitive, social, emotional, and behavioral development in children.
- Community members can assist in forming partnerships between schools and their own property or places of work.
- Teachers and administrators can seek grant support and join with community partners.
- Researchers can adopt a school and assist with well-designed outcomes research.
- All interested parties can become active in parent–teacher associations/councils and demand engaged learning initiatives, which can be implemented both during the school day and during after-school programming.

How can the general public have a broad and lasting impact? Political pressures can support or stymie implementation of any program. People can contact local school boards with letters and petitions to ask for a change. At the state level, Senators and members of the House of Representatives receive calls, emails, and personal letters that may impact the formation of bills, the wording of the bills, and how those legislators choose to vote on bills. This is why bringing research evidence to the attention of educational policy makers is essential. In addition to informing the public officials about the success of promising programs, demands should be made for regularized grant support that is accessible to schools. State education associations and teachers unions can form special interest groups that serve as a collective voice that influences votes of various legislators. School boards can become advocates for students in the reform movement. Project Smart Vote, a non-partisan organization that records statements made by politicians, as well as their voting records on various issues, can be accessed online at votesmart.org. Political Action Committees are organizations that raise money in efforts to campaign for specific candidates. When contemplating who to vote for to begin with, find out their position on education, share this information with others, and vote for the person who aligns with meaningful educational reform.

By fostering community commitment while providing students practical life lessons in self-control, the US could continue to compete in the ever-changing global marketplace. Transformative policies, plans, and practices can turn the tide in the US from educational mediocrity to educational excellence. The broader the community segment influenced by the reform process, the more public confidence will grow in its initiatives. Bodilly, Karam, and Orr (2011) recommend developing best practices in feeder schools and then scaling these up to the district to eventually impact local and state education policies. Exemplar schools can affect teaching practices in other district schools thereby demonstrating the power to both reshape learning experiences that improve academic performance and enhance the wellbeing of local social, cultural, and natural environments (Smith, 2011).

Positive changes in education will occur by relying on solid research findings, by solidifying community partnerships, by redirecting educational budgets from buildings and administrators to front-line teachers and student learning initiatives, and by revamping the way teachers are trained.

References

Alloway, T. P., Gathercole, S. E., Willis, C., & Adams, A.-M. (2004). A structural analysis of working memory and related cognitive skills in young children. *Journal of Experimental Child Psychology, 87*, 85–106.

Arndt, K. J. (2010). Conflict management. In T. C. Hunt & T. J. Lasley II (Eds.), *Encyclopedia of educational reform and dissent, 1*. Thousand Oaks, CA: Sage.

Athman, J., & Monroe, M. (2004). The effects of environment-based education on students' achievement motivation. *Journal of Interpretation Research, 9*, 9–25.

Aud, S., Hussar, W., Kena, G., Bianco, K., Frohlich, L., Kemp, J., et al. (2011). *The condition of education 2011* (NCES 2011-033). U.S. Department of Education, National Center for Education Statistics. Washington, DC: U.S. Government Printing Office.

Baddeley, A. D. (1983). Working memory. *Philosophical Transactions of the Royal Society of London. Series B, Biological Sciences, 302*, 311–324.

Baddeley, A., & Hitch, G. J. (1974). Working memory. In G. A. Bower (Ed.), *Recent advances in learning and motivation* (8th ed., pp. 47–89). New York, NY: Academic.

Baker, B., & Welner, K. G. (2012). Evidence and rigor: Scrutinizing the rhetorical embrace of evidence-based decision making. *Educational Researcher, 41*, 98–101. doi:10.3102/0013189X12440306.

Barron, B. (2006). Interest and self-sustained learning as catalysts of development: A learning ecology perspective. *Human Development, 49*, 193–224.

Beard, C., & Wilson, J. P. (2009). *Experiential learning: A best practice handbook for educators and trainers* (2nd ed.). London: Kogan Page.

Berkowitz, M. W. (2011). What works in values education. *International Journal of Educational Research, 50*, 153–158.

Best, J. R., Miller, P. H., & Naglieri, J. A. (2011). Relations between executive function and academic achievement from ages 5 to 17 in a large, representative national sample. *Learning and Individual Differences, 21*(4), 327–336. doi:10.1016/j.lindif.2011.01.007.

Bodilly, S. J., Karam, R., & Orr, N. (2011). *Continuing challenges and potential collaborative approaches to education reform*. Santa Monica, CA: Rand Corporation.

Bohanon, H., Fenning, P., Carney, K. L., Minnus-Kim, M. I., Anderson-Harriss, S., Moroz, K. B., et al. (2006). Schoolwide application of positive behavior support in an urban high school: A case study. *Journal of Positive Behavior Interventions, 8*, 131–145. doi:10.1177/10983007060080030201.

Bohte, J. (2001). Bureaucracy and student performance at the local level. *Administration Review, 61*, 92–99.

Borgman, C. L., Abelson, H., Dirks, L., Johnson, R., Koedinger, K. R., Linn, M. C., et al. (2008). *Fostering learning in the networked world: The cyberlearning opportunity and challenge*. Report of the NSF Task Force on cyberlearning.

Bradshaw, C. P., Mitchell, M. M., & Leaf, P. J. (2010). Examining the effects of schoolwide positive behavioral interventions and supports on student outcomes: Results from a randomized controlled effectiveness trial in elementary schools. *Journal of Positive Behavior Interventions, 12*, 133–148. doi:10.1177/1098300709334798.

Brophy, J. (2008). Developing students' appreciation for what is taught in school. *Educational Psychologist, 43*, 132–141. doi:10.1080/00461520701756511.

Bryck, R. L., & Fisher, P. A. (2012). Training the brain: Practical applications of neural plasticity from the intersection of cognitive neuroscience, developmental psychology, and prevention science. *The American Psychologist, 67*, 87–100. doi:10.1037/a0024657.

Burns, L. T. (1998). Make sure it's service-learning, not just community service. *Education Digest, 62*, 38–41.

Bushaw, W. J., & Lopez, S. J. (2011). Betting on teachers: The 43rd annual Phi Delta Kappa/Gallup poll of the public's attitudes toward the public schools. *Phi Delta Kappan, 93*, 9–26.

Carew, T. J., & Magsamen, S. H. (2010). Neuroscience and education: An ideal partnership for producing evidence-based solutions to guide 21st century learning. *Neuron, 67*, 685–688. doi:10.1016/j.neuron.2010.08.028.

Carr, E. G., Dunlap, G., Horner, R. H., Koegel, R. L., Turnbull, A. P., Sailor, W., et al. (2002). Positive behavior support: Evolution of an applied science. *Journal of Positive Behavior Interventions, 4*, 4–16. doi:10.1177/109830070200400102.

Chapman, C., Laird, J., Ifill, N., & Kewal Ramani, A. (2011). *Trends in high school dropout and completion rates in the United States: 1972–2009* (NCES 2012-006). U.S. Department of Education. Washington, DC: National Center for Education Statistics. Retrieved from http://nces.ed.gov/pubsearch

Cleary, T. J., & Zimmerman, B. J. (2004). Self-regulation empowerment program: A school-based program to enhance self-regulated and self-motivated cycles of student learning. *Psychology in the Schools, 41*, 537–550. doi:10.1002/pits.10177.

Comber, B., Nixon, H., Ashmore, L., Loo, S., & Cook, J. (2006). Urban renewal from the inside out: Spatial and critical literacies in a low socioeconomic community. *Mind, Culture, and Activity, 13*, 228–246. doi:10.1207/s15327884mca1303_5.

Coyle, K. (2010). *Back to school: Back outside.* National Wildlife Federation. Retrieved from http://www.nwf.org/News-and-Magazines/Media-Center/News-by-Topic/Get-Outside/2010/~/media/PDFs/Be%20Out%20There/Back%20to%20School%20full%20report.ashx

Dewey, J. (1938). *Experience and education.* New York, NY: Macmillan.

Diamond, A., Barnett, W. S., Thomas, J., & Munro, S. (2007). Preschool program improves cognitive control. *Science, 318*, 1387–1388. doi:10.1126/science.1151148.

Diamond, A., & Lee, K. (2011). Interventions shown to aid executive function development in children 4 to 12 years old. *Science, 333*(6045), 959–964. doi:10.1126/science.1204529.

DiPerna, J. C., & Elliott, S. N. (1999). Development and validation of the academic competence evaluation scales. *Journal of Psychoeducational Assessment, 17*, 207–225. doi:10.1177/073428299901700302.

Duffin, M., Chawla, L., Sobel, D., & PEER Associates. (2005). *Place-based education and academic achievement.* Retrieved from http://www.peecworks.org/PEEC/FV4-0001B456/01795C0D-001D0211.19/PBE.

Duffin, M., Powers, A., Tremblay, G., & PEER Associates. (2004). *Place-based Education Evaluation Collaborative: Report on cross-program research and other program evaluation activities, 2003-2004.*

Durlak, J. A., Weissberg, R. P., Dymnicki, A. B., Taylor, R. D., & Schellinger, K. B. (2011). The impact of enhancing students' social and emotional learning: A meta-analysis of school-based universal interventions. *Child Development, 82*, 405–432. doi:10.1111/j.1467-8624.2010.01564.x.

Dweck, C. S. (2006). Boosting achievement with messages that motivate. *Education Canada, 47*, 6–10.

Eisenberg, N., Sadovsky, A., & Spinrad, T. L. (2005). Associations of emotion-related regulation with language skills, emotion knowledge, and academic outcomes. *New Directions for Child and Adolescent Development, 109*, 109–118.

Eisenberg, N., Valiente, C., & Eggum, N. D. (2010). Self-regulation and school readiness. *Early Education and Development, 21*, 681–698. doi:10.1080/10409289.2010.497451.

Elias, M. J. (2009). Social-emotional and character development and academics as a dual focus of educational policy. *Educational Policy, 23*, 831–846. doi:10.1177/0895904808330167.

Elliot, J. (2012). *Reconstructing teacher education:* Teacher development (2nd ed.). New York, NY: Routledge.

Emekauwa, E. (2004). *They remember what they touch: The impact of place-based learning in East Feliciana parish.* Rural School and Community Trust. Retrieved from http://www.seer.org/pages/research/Emekauwa2004.pdf.

Ernst, J. (2012). Influences on and obstacles to K-12 administrators' support for environment-based education. *The Journal of Environmental Education, 43*, 73–92.

Flook, L., Smalley, S. L., Kitil, M. J., Galla, B. M., Kaiser-Greenland, S., Locke, J., et al. (2010). Effects of mindful awareness practices on executive functions in elementary school children. *Journal of Applied School Psychology, 26*, 70–95. doi:10.1080/15377900903379125.

Fockert, J. W., Rees, G., Frith, C. D., & Lavie, N. (2001). The role of working memory in visual selective attention. *Science, 291*, 1803–1806.

Foderaro, L. (2011, October 7). Unleashing the scientist in the student. *New York Times.* Retrieved from http://www.nytimes.com/2011/10/08/nyregion/salamander-study-enlists-new-york-city-seventh-graders.html?pagewanted=all&_r=0

Gallego, M. (2001). Is experience the best teacher? The potential of coupling classroom and community-based field experiences. *Journal of Teacher Education, 52*, 312–325.

Gaskins, C. S., Herres, J., & Kobak, R. (2012). Classroom order and student learning in late elementary school: A multilevel transactional model of achievement trajectories. *Journal of Applied Developmental Psychology, 33*(5), 227–235. doi:10.1016/j.appdev.2012.06.002.

Gathercole, S. E., Brown, L., & Pickering, S. J. (2003). Working memory assessments at school entry as longitudinal predictors of National Curriculum attainment levels. *Educational and Child Psychology, 20*, 109–122.

Gruenewald, D., & Smith, G. (2008). *Place-based education in the global age: Local diversity.* New York, NY: Routledge.

Gutherson, P., Davies, H., & Daszkiewicz, T. (2011). *Achieving successful outcomes through alternative education provision: An international literature review.* CfBT Education Trust. Retrieved from http://www.cfbt.com/evidenceforeducation/pdf/5671_AEP(Report)_v3.pdf

Harrison, S. (2010). "Why are we here?" taking "place" into account in UK outdoor environmental education. *Journal of Adventure Education and Outdoor Learning, 10*, 3–18.

Hennessy, R. (2012, October). Reconnecting in 2012. *Trail to Every Classroom Fall Newsletter, 3*, 1–2

Herbert, T. (1995). Experiential learning: A teacher's perspective. In R. J. Kraft & J. C. Kielsmeier (Eds.), *Experiential learning in schools and higher education* (pp. 201–211). Boulder, CO: AEE.

Hirsch, P., & Lloyd, K. (2005). Real and virtual experiential learning on the Mekong: Field schools, e-Simms and cultural challenge. *Journal of Geography in Higher Education, 29*, 321–337.

Hitch, G. J., Halliday, M. S., Hulme, C., Le Voi, M. E., Routh, D. A., & Conway, A. (1983). Working memory in children. *Philosophical Transactions of the Royal Society of London. Series B, Biological Sciences, 302*, 325–340.

Howard, R. W., Berkowitz, M. W., & Schaeffer, E. F. (2004). Politics of character education. *Educational Policy, 18*, 188–215. doi:10.1177/0895904803260031.

Israel, A. L. (2012). Putting geography education into place: What geography educators can learn from place-based education, and vice versa. *Journal of Geography, 111*, 76–81.

Jernstedt, G. C. (1980). Experiential components in academic courses. *Journal of Experiential Education, 3*, 11–19.

Joplin, L. (1981). On defining experiential education. *Journal of Experiential Education, 4*, 155–158.

Kaestle, C. F. (1993). The awful reputation of education research. *Educational Researcher, 22*, 23–31.

Kohn, A. (1997). How not to teach values: A critical look at character education. *Phi Delta Kappan, 78*, 428–439.

Kolb, D. A. (1984). *Experiential learning: Experience as the source of learning and development.* New Jersey: Prentice-Hall.

Kozol, J. (2005). *The shame of the nation: The restoration of apartheid schooling in America.* New York, NY: Crown.

Lareau, A. (2003). *Unequal childhoods: Class, race, and family life.* Berkeley: University of California Press.

Lassen, S. R., Steele, M. M., & Sailor, W. (2006). The relationship of school-wide positive behavior support to academic achievement in an urban middle school. *Psychology in the Schools, 43*(6), 701–712. doi:10.1002/pits.20177.

Lieberman, G. A., & Hoody, L. (1998). *Closing the achievement gap: Using the environment as an integrating context for learning.* San Diego, CA: State Education and Environment Roundtable.

Louv, R. (2005). *Last child in the woods: Saving our children from nature-deficit disorder.* Chapel Hill, NC: Algonquin Books.

Louv, R. (2011). *The nature principle: Human restoration and the end of nature-deficit disorder.* Chapel Hill, NC: Algonquin Books.

Mackey, A. P., Hill, S. S., Stone, S. I., & Bunge, S. A. (2011). Differential effects of reasoning and speed training in children. *Developmental Science, 14*, 582–590. doi:10.1111/j.1467-7687.2010.01005.x.

Madsen, C. H., Jr., Becker, W. C., & Thomas, D. R. (1968). Rules of praise and ignoring: Elements of elementary classroom control. *Journal of Applied Behavior Analysis, 1*, 139–150.

Malone, K. A (2012). "The future lies in our hands": Children as researchers and environmental change agents in designing a child-friendly neighbourhood. *Local Environment: The International Journal of Justice and Sustainability*, 1–24. doi:10.1080/13549839.2012.719020.

McClellan, R., & Hyle, A. (2012). Experiential learning: Dissolving classroom and research borders. *The Journal of Experiential Education, 35*, 238–252.

McInerney, P., Smyth, J., & Down, B. (2011). Coming to a place near you? The politics and possibilities of a critical pedagogy of place-based education. *Asia-Pacific Journal of Teacher Education, 39*, 3–16.

Menendez, A. L., Payne, L., & Mayton, M. R. (2008). The implementation of positive behavioral support in an elementary school: Processes, procedures, and outcomes. *Alberta Journal of Educational Research, 54*, 448–462.

Metz, M. (1989). Real school: A universal drama amid disparate experience. *Politics of Education Association Yearbook*, 75–91.

Meyer, S. R. (2012). *Center for research on sustainable forests: 2012 annual report*. Orono, ME: University of Maine.

Moely, B. E., Hart, S. S., Santulli, K., Leal, L., Johnson, T., Rao, N., et al. (1986). How do teachers teach memory skills? *Educational Psychologist, 21*, 55–71.

National Research Council. (2010). *Preparing teachers: Building evidence for sound policy* (Committee on the Study of Teacher Preparation Programs in the United States, Division of Behavioral and Social Sciences and Education). Washington, DC: National Academy Press.

Neuenschwander, R., Röthlisberger, M., Cimeli, P., & Roebers, C. M. (2012). How do different aspects of self-regulation predict successful adaptation to school? *Journal of Experimental Child Psychology, 113*(3), 353–371. doi:10.1016/j.jecp.2012.07.004.

Noddings, N. (2005). *The challenge to care in schools: An alternative approach to education* (2nd ed.). New York, NY: Teachers College Press.

Olsen, P. J., Westerberg, H., & Klingberg, T. (2004). Increased prefrontal and parietal activity after training of working memory. *Nature Neuroscience, 7*, 75–79.

Organization for Economic Cooperation and Development (OECD). (2011). *Education at a glance 2011: OECD indicators*. OECD: Author. http://dx.doi.org/10.1787/eag-2011-en

Organization for Economic Cooperation and Development (OECD). (2012). *OECD factbook 2011-2012: Economic, environmental and social statistics*. OECD: Author. doi: 10.1787/factbook-2011-en

Panjwani, N. (2011). Saving our future: James Comer and the school development program. *The Yale Journal of Biology and Medicine, 84*, 139–143.

Parsons, C. (1996). *Serving to learn, learning to serve: Civics and service from A to Z*. Thousand Oaks, CA: Corwin Press.

PEER Associates, Inc. (2006). *An evaluation of a trail to every classroom summer institute*. Appalachian Trail Conservancy Appalachian Trail Park Office of the National Park Service.

PEER Associates, Inc. (2007). *Building a foundation for change: Place-based education at an Urban Middle School*. An evaluation of project CO-SEED at the Henry Dearborn Middle School in partnership with the Appalachian Mountain Club, 2003–2006. Antioch New England Institute.

PEER Associates, Inc. (2009). *An evaluation of a trail to every classroom summer institute*. Appalachian Trail Conservancy Appalachian Trail Park Office of the National Park Service.

PEER Associates, Inc. (2010). *An evaluation of a trail to every classroom summer institute*. Appalachian Trail Conservancy Appalachian Trail Park Office of the National Park Service.

Place-Based Education Evaluation Collaborative (PEEC). (2008). *The benefits of place-based education*. Richmond, VT: Author.

Powers, A. L. (2004a). An evaluation of four place-based education programs. *The Journal of Environmental Education, 35*, 17–32.

Powers, A. L. (2004b). Teacher preparation for environmental education: Faculty perspectives on the infusion of environmental education into pre-service methods courses. *The Journal of Environmental Education, 35*, 3–11.

Ray, B. D. (2011). *2.04 million home school students in the United States in 2010*. National Home Education Research Institute. Retrieved from nheri.org

Ray, C. E., & Elliott, S. N. (2006). Social adjustment and academic achievement: A predictive model for students with diverse academic and behavior competencies. *School Psychology Review, 35*, 493–501.

Reyes, M., Brackett, M., Rivers, S., White, M., & Salovey, P. (2012). Classroom emotional climate, student engagement, and academic achievement. *Journal of Educational Psychology, 104*, 700–712.

Rodriguez, A. (Ed.). (2008). *The multiple faces of agency: Innovative strategies for effecting change in urban school contexts*. Rotterdam: Sense Publishers.

Roebers, C. M., Cimeli, P., Röthlisberger, M., & Neuenschwander, R. (2012). Executive functioning, metacognition, and self-perceived competence in elementary school children: An explorative study on their interrelations and their role for school achievement. *Metacognition and Learning, 7*(3), 151–173. doi:10.1007/s11409-012-9089-9.

Rural School and Community Trust. (2011). Rural students channel hundreds of thousands of dollars to their communities. *Rural Policy Matters, 13*.

Safran, S. P., & Oswald, K. (2003). Positive behavior supports: Can schools reshape disciplinary practices? *Exceptional Children, 69*, 361–373.

Sailor, W., Stowe, M. J., Turnbull, H. R., & Kleinhammer-Tramill, J. (2007). A case for adding a social-behavioral standard to standards-based education with schoolwide positive behavior support as its basis. *Remedial and Special Education, 28*, 366–376.

Sarason, S. (1996). *The culture of the school and the problem of change* (2nd ed.). New York, NY: Teachers College Press.

Schultz, B. D. (2008). *Spectacular things happened along the way*. New York, NY: Teachers College Press.

Skinner, E. A., & Belmont, M. J. (1993). Motivation in the classroom: Reciprocal effects of teacher behavior and student engagement across the school year. *Journal of Educational Psychology, 85*, 571–581.

Smith, G. (2002). Going local. *Educational Leadership, 60*, 30.

Smith, G. A. (2011). Linking place-based and sustainability education at Al Kennedy High School. *Children, Youth and Environments, 21*, 58–78.

Smith, T. E., & Knapp, C. (2011). *Sourcebook of experiential education: Key thinkers and their contributions*. New York, NY: Routledge.

Smith, K. B., & Larimer, C. W. (2004). A mixed relationship: Bureaucracy and school performance. *Public Administration Review, 64*, 728–736.

Smith, K. B., & Meier, K. J. (1994). Politics, bureaucrats, and schools. *Public Administration Review, 54*, 551–558.

Smith, G., & Sobel, D. (2010). *Place- and community-based education in schools*. New York, NY: Routledge.

Sobel, D. (2004). *Place-based education*. Great Barrington, MA: Orion Society Press.

Spencer, B. H., Cox-Peterson, A. M., & Crawford, T. (2005, Fall). Assessing the impact of service-learning on pre-service teachers in an after-school program. *Teacher Education Quarterly*.

State Education and Environment Roundtable (SEER). (2000). *California student assessment Project: The effects of environment-based education on student achievement*. Retrieved from http://www.seer.org/pages/csap.pdf

State Education and Environment Roundtable (SEER). (2005). *California student assessment project—Phase two: The effects of environment-based education on student achievement*. Poway, CA: SEER.

Stern, M. J., Wright, E. M., & Powell, R. B. (2012). Motivating participation in national park service curriculum-based education programs. *Journal of Visitor Studies, 15*, 28–47.

Stevenson, R. (1987). Schooling and environmental education: Contradictions in purpose and practice. In I. Robottom (Ed.), *Environmental education: Practice and possibility* (pp. 69–82). Geelong, VIC: Deakin University Press.

Stewart, V. (n.d.). *Top 10 ways to reform schools.* Retrieved from http://asiasociety.org/initiativel-wtw/top-10-ways-reform-schools

Stigler, J. W., & Hiebert, J. (2009). *The teaching gap: Best ideas from the world's teachers for improving education in the classroom.* New York, NY: Free Press.

Thomas, D. R., Becker, W. C., & Armstrong, M. (1968). Production and elimination of disruptive classroom behavior by systematically varying teacher's behavior. *Journal of Applied Behavior Analysis, 1,* 35–45.

Totten, S., & Pedersen, J. E. (2012). John Dewey and teaching and learning about social issues. In S. Totten & J. E. Pedersen (Eds.), *Educating about social issues in the 20th and 21st centuries: A critical annotated bibliography* (Vol. 1). Charlotte, NC: Information Age.

Ucko, D. (2010). The learning science in informal environments study in context. *Curator: The Museum Journal, 53,* 129–136.

Veletsianos, G., Doering, A., & Henrickson, J. (2012). Field-based professional development of teachers engaged in distance education: Experiences from the Arctic. *Distance Education, 33,* 45–59.

Von Secker, C. (2004). *Bay schools project: Year three summative evaluation.* Annapolis, MD: Chesapeake Bay Foundation.

Wade, R. (Ed.). (1997). *Community service-learning: A guide to including service in the public school curriculum.* Albany, NY: State University of New York Press.

Wade, R. (2007). *Social studies for social justice: Teaching strategies for the elementary classroom.* New York, NY: Teachers College Press.

Wang, J., Chen, Y., & Zhong, N. (2009). Training on low executive function in primary school students. *Chinese Journal of Clinical Psychology, 17,* 777–779.

Welsh, J. A., Nix, R. L., Blair, C., Bierman, K. L., & Nelson, K. E. (2010). The development of cognitive skills and gains in academic school readiness for children from low-income families. *Journal of Educational Psychology, 102,* 43–53. doi:10.1037/a0016738.

Welsh, M., Parke, R. D., Widaman, K., & O'Neil, R. (2001). Linkages between children's social and academic competence: A longitudinal analysis. *Journal of School Psychology, 39,* 463–481.

Westheimer, J., & Kahne, J. (2004). What kind of citizen?: The politics of educating for democracy. *American Educational Research Journal, 41,* 237–269.

White, R., & Warfa, N. (2011). Building schools of character: A case-study investigation of character education's impact on school climate, pupil behavior, and curriculum delivery. *Journal of Applied Social Psychology, 41,* 45–60.

Wu, J.Q. (2010). Teaching outside the box: Interdisciplinary program offers alternative to classroom education. *Boston Globe.* August 18, 2010.

Zeller, N., Griffith, R., Zhang, G., & Klenke, J. (2010). From stranger to friend: The effect of service-learning on pre-service teachers' attitudes towards diverse populations. *Journal of Languages and Literacy Education, 6*(2), 34–50.

Chapter 10
Media Violence and Children: Applying Research to Advocacy

John P. Murray

Research and advocacy concerning children and media violence has a long and conflicted history. In recent times, the focus of discussion has been on video games. However, the history of concern began in the early 1900s with questions about the effects of comics and comic books, and their stories of crime and violence. The same concern continued with questions about the effects of radio programs of crime and mystery and the influence of violence in films. By the late 1940s, however, a new medium bursts on the scene in America: television!

Although television was demonstrated as a novelty at the 1939 World's Fair in New York, further development of the medium was forestalled by the advent of World War II. In the postwar years, of the late 1940s, television development and production boomed and television sets started humming in American homes in 1948–1949. In 1949, only 2 % of American homes had a TV set, but by 1950, the ownership rose to 10 % of all homes (Condry, 1989). Over the next decade, the diffusion of TV set ownership increased rapidly so that by the 1960s, almost 90 % of American households had at least one TV set (Condry, 1989). Within the next decade TV ownership in America reached full saturation levels of 98–99 % (there were always a few holdouts for reasons of personal values or geography that prevented receiving a television signal).

Along with the rapid diffusion of television (faster diffusion than indoor plumbing or radios or electric toasters) came an equally fast diffusion of criticism and concern about the content of TV programs. The particular focus was the amount of violence in cartoons—deemed to be children's programming—and the frequency of shooting and fighting in Westerns and Crime dramas (Barnouw, 1982; Cole, 1981).

J.P. Murray, Ph.D. (✉)
Department of Psychology, Washington College, Chestertown, MD, USA

Center on Media and Child Health, Children's Hospital, Boston, MA, USA
e-mail: jmurray2@washcoll.edu

A. McDonald Culp (ed.), *Child and Family Advocacy: Bridging the Gaps Between Research, Practice, and Policy*, Issues in Clinical Child Psychology, DOI 10.1007/978-1-4614-7456-2_10, © Springer Science+Business Media New York 2013

Research on Media Violence

The questions about TV violence were first raised by teachers and parents and were echoed by various organizations in the fields of health and education. By the early-to-mid-1950s these concerns began to stimulate the interest of social scientists and even members of Congress. Indeed, the first Congressional hearings on the topic of TV violence were held in 1952 (United States Congress, House of Representatives Committee on Interstate and Foreign Commerce) and 1955 (United States Congress, Senate Committee of the Judiciary, Subcommittee to Investigate Juvenile Delinquency). Two of the social scientists who testified at these Congressional hearings were Lazarsfeld (1955), a sociologist at Columbia University, and Maccoby (1954), a developmental psychologist at Stanford University (Murray, 1980).

Following these early Congressional hearings, there was a steady increase in research interest in the impact of television and film violence. Foremost among the early researchers were Wilbur Schramm and his colleagues (Schramm, Lyle, & Parker, 1961) at Stanford and Hilde Himmelweit and her colleagues (Himmelweit, Oppenheim, & Vince, 1958) at the London School of Economics, who conducted surveys in the United States/Canada and England, respectively. Also central to this early research were the experimental studies of psychologists Albert Bandura (Bandura, Ross, & Ross, 1961) at Stanford and Berkowitz (1962) at the University of Wisconsin who studied the impact of viewing violence on children and adolescents, respectively.

By the mid-1960s, the concern about violence and media had greatly increased. Some of the stimulus events were the series of assassinations of President John F. Kennedy, followed by Dr. Martin Luther King, Jr., and Robert Kennedy. At this point, President Lyndon Johnson established the National Commission on the Causes and Prevention of Violence. This Commission released a seven-volume report in 1969 in which one of the volumes was devoted to the impact of media violence (Baker & Ball, 1969). Following on this report, which suggested that media violence was one part of the cause of increases in violence in American society, Congress held new hearings on the impact of TV violence on children. As a result of this hearing, Congress authorized the establishment of special research program, under the direction of the United States Surgeon General, to investigate the effects of TV violence on children and adolescents. The 12-member panel of experts in psychology, psychiatry, communications, and political science, known as the Surgeon General's Scientific Advisory Committee on Television and Social Behavior, was established to award research contracts from the National Institute of Mental Health to over 60 researchers throughout the country, and to write a summary report of the findings from these special studies. The Surgeon General's Committee (United States Department of Health, Education and Welfare, 1972) released its report entitled *Television and Growing Up: The Impact of Televised Violence* in 1972 and this report is summarized by Murray (1973). The Committee report concluded that viewing violence on television did lead to increases in aggressive behavior among those children and adolescents who regularly viewed such programs.

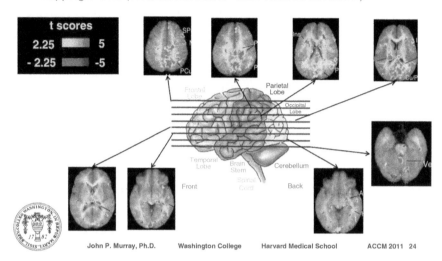

Fig. 10.1 Location of significant brain scans in slices of composite brains of 8–13 years old boys and girls

In the years following the Surgeon General's report, there were several reviews and reports that affirmed and extended the initial findings. Foremost among these reports was the review published by the National Institute of Mental Health (1982), which concluded that the majority of social scientists who have studied the issue of the impact of televised violence agree that viewing violence is one cause of increases in aggression in children and teens. In addition to the NIMH report, there were reviews and reports from the American Psychological Association (APA) (Huston et al., 1992), the American Academy of Pediatrics (AAP, 1990), and the Group for the Advancement of Psychiatry (1982). All of these reports confirm that viewing violence can lead to increases in aggressive behavior, changes in attitudes and values favoring the use of aggression to solve conflicts, and desensitization to the harm caused by violence.

By the beginning of the twenty-first century, researchers added a focus on the neurological correlates of violence viewing (Mathews et al., 2005; Murray, 2001; Weber, Ritterfeld, & Mathiak, 2006). For example, I and my colleagues (Murray et al., 2006) have conducted research showing the unique brain activation patterns of children viewing video violence (in this case, clips of boxing scenes from Sylvester Stallone's Rocky IV) in which children activate the threat arousal systems involving the amygdala and limbic system and seem to be storing the violence in the posterior cingulate in a manner that allows for instantaneous recall of the violence to serve as a schematic for planning aggressive behavior (see Fig. 10.1). The results of these studies, using functional Magnetic Resonance Imaging (fMRI) to assess brain activation patterns in children and adolescents viewing video violence, confirm that viewing violence is associated with activation of areas of the brain involved in arousal and perception of threat (e.g., the amygdala and thalamus) and memory storage of the violent actions in areas reserved for long-term memory of traumatic and frightening events (e.g., the posterior cingulate).

Taken together, the studies undertaken over the past 50 years demonstrate that exposure to violence in television, movies, and video games can be harmful to the social development of children and teens (Pecora, Murray, & Wartella, 2007). This then leads to questions about the ways in which developmental scientists can advocate for policies and programs that mitigate and reduce the impact of media violence.

The Roots of Advocacy

The late 1960s saw the beginnings of advocacy for enhancing children's television. The Surgeon General's report provided a sweeping study of the impact of televised violence and the advent of an advocacy group, Action for Children's Television (ACT) provided a focused group of advocates for change in the nature of children's television. ACT was particularly focused on demanding more educational television opportunities for children (Action for Children's Television, 1971). Also, in the 1960s, the newly appointed Chairman of the Federal Communications Commission, Newton Minow, addressed the annual convention of the National Association of Broadcasters and expressed his shock and displeasure with commercial television programming and declared that "television is a vast wasteland" in terms of programming available to the American public, and especially for children. Indeed, in the 1990s he reaffirmed that conclusion in his book *Abandoned in the Wasteland: Children, Television and the First Amendment* (Minow & LaMay, 1995). The scorching speech by Newton Minow expedited the establishment of the Corporation for Public Broadcasting and the launch of the Public Broadcasting System (PBS). Furthermore, continuing pressure from advocacy organizations like ACT encouraged philanthropic foundations and government agencies to provide funding to the Children's Television Workshop (CTW) and the launch of Sesame Street in 1969.

This ferment in the 1960s and 1970s ultimately led Congress to pass the Children's Television Act of 1990 which provided, among other things, the requirement that all new television sets must have a pre-installed "V-Chip" (Violence Chip) to allow parents to block certain violent programs on their sets (Kunkel, 1991).

Nevertheless, the struggle continues with the development of very violent video games marketed to children and teens. The most recent example was a regulation passed by the California Legislature and signed into law by the then Governor of California, Arnold Schwarzenegger. Indeed, this issue found its way to the Supreme Court of the United States (SCOTUS) in 2011. Its rocky journey and difficult resolution is summarized in two articles in the APA's Division 37 newsletter, *The Advocate*, entitled "The Terminator Meets SCOTUS" (Murray, 2010) and "Pulling

Their Punches: The Supreme Court and Video Game Violence" (Murray, 2011) and in a *Mayo Clinic Proceedings* article (Murray et al., 2011). In brief, the Court ultimately ruled that the State of California did not have the right to ban the sale or rental of violent video games to minors under the age of 18—thereby, holding the California law to be unconstitutional in its current form (Brown, 2011).

What Developmental Scientists Can Do: Advocacy Steps

So what role can developmental scientists play in advocating for policy and practices that improve children's access to useful experiences with television and video games? At the outset, it is important to have clear goals for one's advocacy and the ways in which research and professional expertise can be applied to the issues. In the case of media violence, the goal is to reduce the frequency and severity of such violence in children's lives. We know from various studies conducted over the years that the pathway of effect of media violence on viewers includes changes in the viewer that lead to a belief that the world is a mean and dangerous place and that violence is seen as a normal and acceptable response to perceived feelings of injustice. This desensitization of the viewer allows for the increased likelihood of aggression and violent outbursts. The task for developmental scientists is to find ways to reduce exposure to violent media and mitigate its effects on youngsters.

For those with an interest in advocacy, it is important to start with the basic research findings on the given topic. Any policy that is not based on sound research is a flawed policy. Therefore, if you wish to advocate in any particular area you should begin with a review of the research literature. A quick search of the databases provided by the APA or the National Library of Medicine, for example, would result in a fairly useful listing of journal articles or review papers. And, as in all things, you need to take a careful view of the nature of the publication and the background of the author (including this present author, of course). Yes, there are differing opinions—not only on television and children but virtually any topic you care to choose. Sometimes, the differences of opinion reflect differing interpretations of research, but sometimes there are subtle biases based upon the author's employment or experiences. When in doubt, ask colleagues about their opinions and their thoughts about the authors of various papers.

Once you have satisfied yourself that the topic has a satisfactory research base and that the positions that you favor are within the framework of justified conclusions, you are ready to advocate for your position and policy. You can pursue this activity in many different ways:

- Joining a national or regional organization that is concerned about your issues.
- Inquiring about the policy statements or issue papers available from your professional organization, such as the APA, Society for Research in Child Development (SRCD), AAP, National Education Association (NEA), National Association for the Education of Young Children (NAEYC), or other similar groups. For example, various Divisions of APA have special interest groups who

hold online discussions of relevant topics. Also, SRCD publishes **quarterly Social Policy Reports** and the associated **Social Policy Report Briefs** (which are two-page summaries of the full report). These reports and briefs are sent to any relevant member of Congress, along with wide distribution to other interested parties. Examples of recent reports, such as an article on Uses of Research in Policy and Practice by Vivian Tseng, Vice President of the William T. Grant Foundation (Tseng, 2012) are available on the SRCD website (www.srcd.org).

- Writing an opinion article for a professional newsletter or writing an OpEd article for a newspaper.
- Giving presentations to local groups who are interested in these topics.
- Writing a policy brief for government agencies and regulatory bodies, or even better, join other like-minded professionals to write an Amicus Curia brief for the Supreme Court (a difficult task that requires the assistance of an appropriate law firm and some sort of "legal standing" in the court's deliberations about the issue). An excellent example of an Amicus Curia Brief is the so-called Gruel Brief filed by Steven F. Gruel as Counsel of Record for the Amicus Brief of Senator Leland Y. Yee and the California Chapter of the AAP and the California Psychological Association (Gruel Brief, 2010).
- Testifying before Congress on issues related to your professional experience and research evidence. You could testify on your own behalf or in behalf of a professional association or advocacy group. Often, the opportunity to testify is the result of a direct invitation from a member of Congress or a staff member who serves on the Committee that is conducting the hearing, but you can volunteer your testimony by contacting the relevant member of Congress. In some cases, you will be invited to testify in person or, in other cases, you may be asked to provide comments in a written submission.

Each of these activities entail a different level of commitment. However, if you are very interested in the issue you will find the time and the appropriate entry point for your involvement.

Outcomes and Next Steps

Of course, the trajectory of my own advocacy experiences leads to a final caveat: **One does not always win in advocacy efforts**. Sad, but true, and one must be prepared for any outcome. Even when solid research evidence exists and as an advocate you believe that your policy views are on the correct side, there are other factors that may intervene. The other factors may be cultural preferences, conflicting laws and statutes, extremely organized opposition, or just simply entrenched vested interests that will collide with the proposed policy recommendations. For example, one dedicated opponent of the harmful effects of media violence on children and youth is a psychologist at Texas A & M International, Christopher Ferguson, who believes that the case is "not proven." In one article, Ferguson and his colleague (Ferguson & Kilburn, 2009) conducted a meta-analysis of a selection of research papers and decided that the results of research findings were not sufficiently robust to serve as a basis for policy proposals. In part, his conclusion rests on a very carefully selected group of studies that were not representative of the full range of research available at that point. One would have thought that the comprehensive reviews of research by the National Institute of Mental Health (1982), the AAP (1990), and the APA (Huston et al., 1992) would be sufficient to dispel the faulty conclusions by Ferguson. Therefore, if one is dedicated to the value of one's proposals, one should continue to refine them by taking into account the criticism of one's opponents, as well as additional research findings on the topic.

In my own case, I began this journey on the effects of television on children and youth in 1969, when I was hired to serve as "scientist-administrator" at the National Institute of Mental Health to help coordinate studies in the Surgeon General's Scientific Advisory Committee on Television and Social Behavior. The Surgeon General's investigation of the impact of TV violence on children was requested and funded by Congress and was thought to take about 1 year although extended into 3 years. The outcome of this research program was very successful in demonstrating the harmful effects of TV violence on children and launched my interests in the field (when I was a *very young* developmental psychologist). Despite the challenges, one can remain convinced that policy and research move forward in a slow incremental pattern and advocates should keep adding their voice to the discussions. So, my final advice to readers is "simply become engaged" in the process—it will lead to better policies for society.

References

Action for Children's Television. (1971). *The first national symposium on the effect of television programming and advertising on children*. New York, NY: Avon Books.

American Academy of Pediatrics. (1990). Children, adolescents, and television. *Pediatrics, 85*, 1119–1120.

Baker, R. K., & Ball, S. J. (1969). *Mass media and violence: A staff report to the national commission on the causes and prevention of violence*. Washington, DC: U.S. Government Printing Office.

Bandura, A., Ross, D., & Ross, S. (1961). Transmission of aggression through imitation of aggressive models. *Journal of Abnormal and Social Psychology, 63*, 575–582.

Barnouw, E. (1982). *Tube of plenty: The evolution of American television* (Rev. ed.). New York, NY: Oxford University Press.

Berkkowitz, L. (1962). *Aggression: A social psychological analysis*. New York, NY: McGraw-Hill.

Brown, Governor of California, et al v Entertainment Merchants Association, et al., No. 08-1448. Argued November 2, 2010. Decided June 27, 2011. Retrieved from http://www.supremecourt. gov/opinions/10pdf/08-1448.pdf.

Cole, B. (1981). *Television today: Readings from TV guide*. New York, NY: Oxford University Press.

Condry, J. (1989). *The psychology of television*. Hillsdale, NJ: Erlbaum.

Ferguson, C. J., & Kilburn, J. (2009). The public health risks of media violence: A meta-analytic review. *Journal of Pediatrics, 154*(5), 759–763.

Group for the Advancement of Psychiatry. (1982). *The child and television drama: The psychosocial impact of cumulative viewing.* New York, NY: Mental Health Materials Center.

Gruel Brief. (2010). *Brief of Amicus Curia of California State Senator Leland Y. Yee, Ph.D., The California chapter of the American Academy of Pediatrics and the California Psychological Association in Support of the Petitioners, Arnold Schwarzenegger, Governor of California, et al, v Entertainment Merchants Association, et al.* No. 08-1448 (2010). (U.S. July, 19, 2010) 2010 WL 2937557.

Himmelweit, H. T., Oppenheim, A. N., & Vince, P. (1958). *Television and the child: An empirical study of the effects of television on the young.* London: Oxford University Press.

Huston, A. C., Donnerstein, E., Fairchild, H., Feshbach, N. D., Katz, P. A., Murray, J. P., et al. (1992). *Big world, small screen: The role of television in American society.* Lincoln, NE: University of Nebraska Press.

Kunkel, D. (1991). Crafting media policy: The genesis and implications of the Children's Television Act of 1990. *American Behavioral Science, 35,* 181–202.

Lazarsfeld, P. F. (1955). Why is so little known about the effects of television and what can be done? *Public Opinion Quarterly, 19,* 243–251.

Maccoby, E. E. (1954). Why do children watch television? *Public Opinion Quarterly, 18,* 239–244.

Mathews, V. P., Kronenberger, W. G., Wang, Y., Lurito, J. T., Lowe, M. J., & Dunn, D. W. (2005). Media violence exposure and frontal lobe activation measured by functional magnetic resonance imaging in aggressive and nonaggressive adolescents. *Journal of Computer Assisted Tomography, 29,* 287–292.

Minow, N. N., & LaMay, C. L. (1995). *Abandoned in the wasteland: Children, television, and the first amendment.* New York, NY: Hill & Wang.

Murray, J. P. (1973). Television and violence: Implications of the Surgeon General's research program. *American Psychologist, 28*(6), 472–478.

Murray, J. P. (1980). *Television & youth: 25 Years of research & controversy.* Boys Town, NE: The Boys Town Center for the Study of Youth Development.

Murray, J. P. (2010). Advocacy—The terminator meets SCOTUS. *The Advocate, 33*(2), 16–18.

Murray, J. P. (2011). Pulling their punches: The supreme court and video game violence. *The Advocate, 34*(3), 24–28.

Murray, J. P., Biggins, B., Donnerstein, E., Kunkel, D., Menninger, R. W., Rich, M., et al. (2011). A plea for concern regarding violent video games. *Mayo Clinic Proceedings, 86*(8), 818–820.

Murray, J. P. (October, 2001). TV violence and brainmapping in children. *Psychiatric Times,* 70–71

Murray, J. P., Liotti, M., Ingmundson, P., Mayberg, H. S., Pu, Y., Zamarripa, F., et al. (2006). Children's brain response to TV violence: Functional Magnetic Resonance Imaging (fMRI) of video viewing in 8-13 year-old boys and girls. *Media Psychology, 8,* 25–37.

National Institute of Mental Health. (1982). *Television and behavior: Ten years of scientific progress and implications for the eighties: Vol. 1. Summary Report.* Washington, DC: United States Government Printing Office. Retrieved from http://www.eric.ed.gov/PDFS/ED222186.pdf

Pecora, N., Murray, J. P., & Wartella, E. A. (2007). *Children and television: Fifty years of research.* Mahwah, NJ: Erlbaum.

Schramm, W., Lyle, J., & Parker, E. B. (1961). *Television in the lives of our children.* Palo Alto, CA: Stanford University Press.

Tseng, V. (2012). The uses of research in policy and practice. *Social Policy Report, 26*(2). www.srcd.org

United States Congress, House Committee on Interstate and Foreign Commerce. (1952). *Investigation of radio and television programs, hearings and report, 82nd Congress, 2nd session, June 3–December 5, 1952.* Washington, DC: United States Government Printing Office.

United States Congress, Senate Committee of the Judiciary, Subcommittee to Investigate Juvenile Delinquency. (1955). *Juvenile delinquency (television programs), hearings, 83rd Congress, 2nd Session, June 5–October 20, 1954.* Washington, DC: United States Government Printing Office.

United States Department of Health, Education, and Welfare; Surgeon General's Scientific Advisory Committee on Television and Social Behavior. (1972). *Television and growing up: The impact of televised violence*. Washington, DC: United States Government Printing Office. Retrieved from http://profiles.nlm.nih.gov/ps/access/NNBCGX.pdf

Weber, R., Ritterfeld, U., & Mathiak, K. (2006). Does playing violent video games induce aggression? Empirical evidence of a functional magnetic resonance imaging study. *Media Psychology, 8*(1), 39–60.

Chapter 11
Changing Juvenile Justice Policy and Practice: Implementing Evidence-Based Practices in Louisiana

Joseph J. Cocozza, Debra K. DePrato, Stephen Phillippi Jr., and Karli J. Keator

Overview

This chapter will describe how the gap between existing juvenile justice policies and programs, and research-based practices was closed in Louisiana as a result of advocacy efforts at the state and local level with support from a national foundation.

Youth in the Juvenile Justice System

Large numbers of youth come in contact with the juvenile justice system each year. In 2009, the most recent year for which data are available, 1.9 million youth under the age of 18 were arrested (Puzzanchera & Adams, 2011). Estimates indicate that up to 600,000 youth cycle through detention centers annually, with more than 70,000 youth in a juvenile correctional setting or other residential placement on any given day (Sickmund, Sladky, Kang, & Puzzanchera, 2010).

J.J. Cocozza, Ph.D. (✉) • K.J. Keator, M.P.H.
National Center for Mental Health and Juvenile Justice, Policy Research Associates, Inc., 345 Delaware Avenue, Delmar, NY 12054, USA
e-mail: jcocozza@prainc.com

D.K. DePrato, M.D.
Institute for Public Health and Justice, Louisiana State University Health Sciences Center, New Orleans, LA, USA

S. Phillippi Jr., Ph.D., L.C.S.W.
School of Public Health, Louisiana State University Health Sciences Center, New Orleans, LA, USA

A. McDonald Culp (ed.), *Child and Family Advocacy: Bridging the Gaps Between Research, Practice, and Policy*, Issues in Clinical Child Psychology, DOI 10.1007/978-1-4614-7456-2_11, © Springer Science+Business Media New York 2013

Over the years, states and local jurisdictions have developed a variety of programs and practices for responding to justice-involved youth. Unfortunately, until recently the effectiveness of these practices was not supported by research. Findings from a review of over 200 studies in the late 1980s found that rehabilitative efforts had no appreciable effect on recidivism (Gendreau & Ross, 1987). The resulting concern in the field was that "nothing works." This conclusion has changed dramatically over the last 15–20 years as a result of the growth and demonstrated effectiveness of evidence-based practices (EBPs).

EBPs are defined as standardized and manualized interventions with demonstrated positive outcomes based on repeated rigorous evaluation studies. EBPs were developed as a method to use research to improve decision-making and practice within the context of the medical field. This method has expanded to other fields, including juvenile justice. Within the juvenile justice context, EBPs utilize research and knowledge of processes and tools that can improve outcomes for youth, families, and communities. EBPs used with justice-involved youth have demonstrated reduced rates of rearrest, improved family functioning, improved school performance, decreased drug use and decreased psychiatric symptoms, and reduced out-of-home placements (Halliday-Boykins, Schoenwald, & Letournea, 2005; Lipsey, 2009; Robbins & Szapocznik, 2000; Substance Abuse and Mental Health Services Administration 2009a, 2009b). Further research has shown that EBPs commonly used within the juvenile justice context have an economic benefit (Lee et al., 2012). For example, Functional Family Therapy (FFT) is estimated to save $21.57 in future costs to the juvenile justice and related systems for every $1 spent on treatment.

A few examples of EBPs commonly used with justice-involved youth that have a significant research base showing effectiveness and have a demonstrated economic benefit include FFT, Multi-Systemic Therapy (MST), and Multidimensional Treatment of Foster Care (MTFC). FFT is an intervention with demonstrated success for reducing recidivism and violent behavior, and for having a positive effect on family relations (Alexander et al., 1998). It can be delivered in a variety of service settings within the community to meet the needs of the justice-involved youth and their families. MST is focused on treating factors that contribute to delinquency and violence risk within the youth's social network and changing the behavior of the youth in order to achieve decreased recidivism and improved social and mental health outcomes (Henggeler, Melton, Brondino, Scherer, & Hanley, 1997). MST is a community-based intervention and can be utilized in the home, school, or other community setting. MTFC is used primarily with youth who have been removed from their home (Chamberlain & Reid, 1991). This intervention treats the youth in a skilled foster home setting while the youth's parent/guardian receives simultaneous treatment in the community. The goal of MTFC is to help youth live successfully within their community with their biological family, relatives, or adoptive parents when foster care placement ends.

Challenges of Adopting and Implementing EBPs

Despite the transformation from "nothing works" to solid research support for the effectiveness of certain interventions, the implementation and spread of EBPs has been slow. At least one researcher estimated that access to these effective practices was as low as 5 % among juvenile offender populations (Greenwood, 2008). In addition, the adoption of these services has not been systematic and service availability is too often fragmented. There are a number of issues that have significantly impeded the widespread adoption and implementation of EBPs. Many of these can be viewed as challenges related to collaboration, funding, and training.

Addressing the challenge of collaboration, the first step towards implementing any EBP is the development of community-wide support for the adoption and use of EBPs. This includes obtaining buy-in from policy makers, service system administrators and providers, advocates, and family members. This process may be assisted by educating stakeholders through personal discussion, public workshops, factsheets and information papers, and targeted use of media venues. Any of these educational efforts should be followed by targeted consensus building meetings. Collaboration among stakeholders is essential to successfully adopt and implement EBPs, and there must be ongoing support for these efforts to address changing leadership and personnel.

Another challenge for the adoption and implementation of EBPs is the lack of dedicated funding to support these efforts. Implementing EBPs requires funding to purchase manuals and other materials for the particular treatment, funding to train clinicians and service providers in how to deliver the EBP, and funding to support the delivery or reimbursement of the EBP. Too often funding for EBPs, in particular for the delivery or reimbursement of the EBP, is grant-funded and sustainability of the practice is jeopardized when the grant period ends. Although grants can be an effective resource to cover initial start-up costs, to increase the likelihood that these services become institutionalized and are sustained, dedicated funding and reimbursement mechanisms must support the delivery of services.

Finally, EBPs require ongoing training for staff and supervision of these staff. In order to realize positive outcomes and for the intervention to be most effective, EBPs must be implemented with fidelity to the standardized and tested model. This means that there are not only initial training costs but also ongoing continuing education to discourage drift, or deviation from the model. Additional costs are incurred both in terms of the direct cost for providing the training and staff time to attend the training. There is a loss of staff time for providing reimbursable services that must be considered. Finally, turnover should be anticipated and new staff, including administration, must be trained in the EBP when hired.

Lawsuit in Louisiana

In November of 1998, the U.S. Department of Justice filed a lawsuit against the State of Louisiana for failure to provide adequate education, medical and mental health care to youth in detention and correctional facilities, and for failure to provide safe conditions for these youth (Butterfield, 1998). This suit followed 2 years of investigations into the conditions of the juvenile justice system in Louisiana and a failure by the Louisiana Department of Public Safety and Corrections to address the Justice Department's findings. Juvenile correctional settings—filthy, violent, and chronically understaffed—earned one Louisiana facility the title of the worst in the nation (Butterfield, 1998).

In response to Justice Department's findings and the lawsuit, advocates in Louisiana sought to redefine the juvenile justice system from one based heavily on punishment and incarceration to one reliant on community-based alternatives and diversion. The State partnered with the Louisiana State Health Sciences Center to develop and implement best practice medical, dental, and mental health care in all the facilities. This partnership was a major step in the reform process, and where stakeholders were first exposed to evidence-based assessments and treatment. In 2001, the Louisiana legislature created a Juvenile Justice Commission (JJC) purposed to "study the Louisiana juvenile justice system and make recommendations for system improvement" (Juvenile Justice Implementation Commission, 2012). Two years later, the JJC delivered recommendations to overhaul the juvenile justice system, key pieces of which were used in the Juvenile Justice Reform Act of 2003. This piece of legislation set the tone for the juvenile justice reform, making it possible for Louisiana to embark on radical systems change.

The federal lawsuit and actions taken by state leaders and advocates in Louisiana resulted in a major reform of the state's juvenile justice system. The focus was now on reducing the number of youth placed in long-term juvenile correctional systems and providing better care to those youth who remained within the facilities in partnership with higher education. In fact, the achievements of this effort were impressive. Over a period of less than a decade, the number of youth housed in secure facilities in Louisiana dropped from 2,000 to below 500 (Louisiana Office of Juvenile Justice, 2012). While a tremendous accomplishment, the Louisiana juvenile justice system was confronted with a major challenge. Many youth who previously would have been incarcerated were now remaining in the community and required a range of community-based services that were often nonexistent or, at best, inadequate. While the juvenile justice system and local communities in Louisiana were struggling with this issue, an opportunity developed that provided a chance to couple the need for community-based services with the trend toward providing services that work and produce effective outcomes.

The Models for Change Initiative

The John D. and Catherine T. MacArthur Foundation is a large private foundation that supports creative people and effective institutions committed to building a more just, verdant, and peaceful world. Beginning in 1996, the MacArthur Foundation funded a Research Network on Adolescent Development and Juvenile Justice. This Research Network focused on adolescent development research and the implications of the research for juvenile justice policy and practice.

As a follow-up to the Research Network, and reflective of emerging trends, the MacArthur Foundation established the Models for Change initiative (Hurst, 2012). The goal of this initiative was to accelerate the reform of juvenile justice systems across the country to systems that would hold young people accountable for their actions, provide for their rehabilitation, protect them from harm, increase their life chances, and manage the risk they pose to themselves and to public safety. The aim of the Models for Change effort was to use the experiences of a select number of states and communities to help create sustainable, effective, and research-based reform models.

Four states were initially selected to participate in this effort—Pennsylvania in 2004, Illinois in 2005, Louisiana in 2006, and Washington in 2007. These states were strategically chosen using criteria such as leadership, commitment to change, geography, and needs and opportunities for change (John D. and Catherine T. MacArthur Foundation, States for Change, 2012b). Additional states joined the effort later through the development of Action Networks, or multistate groups focused on sharing and disseminating best practices for addressing common issues. In addition to the support given directly to the states, the MacArthur Foundation also made grants to expert organizations forming a National Resource Bank (NRB). The NRB was available to guide efforts, provide technical assistance to the states and jurisdictions participating in Models for Change, and disseminate the knowledge and shared experiences of this effort with other states and jurisdictions through the development of resources and various publications (John D. and Catherine T. MacArthur Foundation, National Resource Bank, 2012a). In each of the four core states, stakeholders from the state and local jurisdictions, in conjunction with a designated lead entity, worked with the Foundation and the NRB to identify targeted areas for improvement, develop a strategic plan, and implement and subsequently diffuse models for reforming the juvenile justice system.

While there are several states across the nation working on similar goals under the umbrella of Models for Change, the information that follows highlights the reform efforts in Louisiana in order to delineate the specific goals and action steps with a state model.

Programmatic and Advocacy Goal for Louisiana: Develop Focus on EBPs

As described above, Louisiana's participation in Models for Change came at a time when the State was in the process of reforming juvenile justice practices—moving towards a system of increased community-based services and a reduced reliance on deep-end juvenile justice system penetration. Through its participation in Models for Change, Louisiana identified as one of its primary focus areas "increasing access to evidence-based services" (John D. and Catherine T. MacArthur Foundation, 2007). Specifically, the aim was to implement empirically supported community-based interventions using existing research. The overarching goal was to foster the development of a system in which justice-involved youth could be quickly screened and assessed using research-based tools, leading to the efficient and appropriate diversion to a community-based system offering a range of EBPs designed to address their specific needs. This system would lead to better outcomes for communities, and youth and their families. The new services needed to be community-based and sustainable at the local level, taking into account funding, training, and other forms of support.

In response, the Louisiana Models for Change team developed a plan for the adoption and implementation of sustainable and replicable strategies for the incorporation of EBPs for justice-involved youth. Grants from the MacArthur Foundation supported efforts by the Louisiana team to design the framework, develop an education and adoption strategy, and allowed for the implementation of the adopted EBPs within selected pilot jurisdictions and statewide. In tandem, the Louisiana team focused on the adoption and implementation of research-based screening and assessment practices across the spectrum of the juvenile justice system in order to identify youth to divert to the community-based interventions. The MacArthur Foundation provided grants to support these efforts as well.

Advocacy Steps in Louisiana: Education, Research, and Implementation

The Louisiana Models for Change team introduced and supported the adoption of EBPs in community-based settings through a three-pronged approach. This approach encompassed educating stakeholders, utilizing sound research, and strategically implementing EBPs using a phased approach. Each of these advocacy steps are described below:

Educate Stakeholders

The first prong of this approach was education. This included, "conducting statewide meetings, workshops, and other educational activities to raise awareness of the benefits of evidence-based practices" (John D. and Catherine T. Louisiana models for, 2007). Understanding that adoption and implementation requires the full support of policy makers, agency administrators, providers, and the communities, the Louisiana team focused early reform efforts on the development of awareness and increased knowledge of the various stakeholders regarding the empirical support for EBPs and standardized screening and assessment procedures. Any efforts to increase availability of and access to EBPs would require the complete support from the various stakeholders including providers and policy makers.

Several large workshops and conferences, such as the "Evidence-Based Practice Summit for Louisiana Leadership," were convened to support the education and awareness campaign undertaken through the Louisiana Models for Change project. This particular event, and other similar smaller events, included state administrators, legislatures, judges, district attorneys, and public defenders. Other events were attended by juvenile justice professionals, service providers, and advocates. In audience-tailored and often practice-specific settings, training was provided to front-line staff. For example, clinicians were provided training on EBPs and juvenile justice professionals, such as probation officers, received training on standardized screening. Wrap around technical assistance was also provided to support the implementation efforts with the local jurisdictions and support the continued efforts to educate and raise awareness of the need for increased availability and access to EBPs. In summary, these educational efforts entailed:

- A general training on the benefits of EBPs for state policy makers and agency leadership
- Stakeholder awareness of the benefits and rationale for EBP adoption and utilization
- Technical assistance to review current EBPs, workforce demands to adopt such practices, and evaluation of the readiness of the local area to implement the practice
- Practice-specific education regarding EBPs that fit local needs
- Practice skills related to specific EBPs and screening and assessment tools chosen to meet the needs of local communities and state organizations

These efforts helped establish an infrastructure of key stakeholders in local communities and at the state level. It was understood that obtaining buy-in from local leaders was a necessary and critical first step in the planning and implementation process. Local pilot sites with community leaders ready and able to develop models for collaboration between the juvenile justice and community service provider systems were identified for select projects. Ongoing stakeholder education strengthened the process and built a foundation for ensuring long-term success and sustainability as judges, prosecutors, and other justice personnel developed an understanding of the value of EBPs and began to refer youth only to EBPs within their community. Finally, the Louisiana team engaged with professional organizations to provide ongoing education to support the systematic adoption and implementation of EBPs. Grants were made to support these activities and to encourage dialogue about EBPs in a peer-to-peer setting. These organizations engaged constituents and peers in ongoing dialogue which reinforced why EBPs are important for achieving positive outcomes for youth, their families, and communities.

Utilize Research

At the core of the Louisiana Models for Change efforts was the desire that all reforms should be data-driven, and that informed and calculated decisions should be based on data in order to identify the areas of most need, use limited resources efficiently, and monitor outcomes of these efforts. To lay the groundwork for efforts and monitoring outcomes, the National Center for Mental Health and Juvenile Justice (NCMHJJ) and the Louisiana State University Health Sciences Center (LSUHSC) jointly developed a "Juvenile Justice System Screening, Assessment and Treatment Services Inventory." The *Inventory* is a web-based tool used to assess and track the types of services available to justice-involved youth. The data from the *Inventory* were used to aid strategic planning by the local stakeholder groups around the implementation of EBPs. The *Inventory* was initially used by several parishes (i.e., counties) that were awarded grants by the MacArthur Foundation to support efforts to identify the availability of EBPs within the community and to identify the baseline knowledge of community stakeholders—it has now been used statewide. Specifically, this inventory:

- Surveyed screening and assessment practices
- Surveyed juvenile justice service provider programs and practices
- Gathered self-report information regarding whether those practices were evidence-based
- Identified points where EBPs were utilized and where there were gaps

The use of pilot projects to develop research-based screening and assessment policies and procedures created mechanisms which allowed for data collection and analysis of the initial screening and follow-up assessment results. These data were then used by the local Children and Youth Planning Boards to guide the decision-making on which EBPs could best meet the needs of the community. This data-driven approach to the selection and implementation of EBPs increased the likelihood that the services provided would meet the needs of the target populations.

Implement EPBs

The third strategy included strategic implementation of EBPs and support for the consistent use of screening and assessment tools across the juvenile justice system. Activities included the following:

- *Joint position statement*: NCMHJJ, LSUHSC, and the Technical Assistance Collaborative, Inc. collaborated with the child serving agencies in Louisiana to develop a joint position statement supporting the development, implementation, and sustainability of EBPs at the local level, completed a survey of current and projected EBPs, and planned regional meetings to develop broad support for the planned development of community-based EBPs.

- *Readiness evaluation*: LSUHSU and NCMHJJ developed a readiness survey to identify a community's readiness to adopt EBPs. This tool helped the local group to identify priorities and key areas of concern for local stakeholders, and guided the identification of EBPs that fit the local context and need. The results of this survey were used to guide the next steps of the effort; in particular, to help assess and discuss areas such as target population, level of collaboration, workforce requirements, and organizational readiness.
- *Adoption of screening and assessment*: The parishes within the state worked with the National Youth Screening Assistance Project to facilitate the adoption of research-based screening and assessment instruments, to develop policies and procedures to ensure the proper and continued administration of these tools, and to establish a referral process to link youth and families with appropriate services based on the results of the screening and assessment.
- *Revision of contracting*: The State's Office of Juvenile Justice (OJJ) adopted new procedures for their request for proposals and contracting processes to support adoption and expansion of EBPs. Local jurisdictions with local tax-based funds also worked to revise contracting procedures. These efforts emphasized preference given to providers who delivered EBPs in contract awards.
- *Implementation of EBPs*: The state and local parishes worked to increase access to EBPs. Initial efforts focused, in particular, on increasing the availability of FFT which was identified as an EBP that would fit an identified service gap within the State. Other efforts centered on giving priority to utilizing EBPs that matched the assessed needs of youth on probation as determined by a statewide implemented research-based risk and needs screening tool.

The Louisiana team was able to successfully implement EBPs in large part by recognizing and addressing barriers as they occurred. One of the first challenges encountered was the fact that many agencies were "wedded" to their home-grown screening and assessment tools and treatment programs that seemed to work, conclusions which were based on personal experience rather than on evaluation data. To overcome this challenge, the team encouraged a change in philosophy among all key stakeholders in the juvenile justice and community service provider systems. Another challenge was in deciding which EBPs could be developed that were affordable and necessary for the target population, which requires time and funds to support these efforts. There was a lack of availability of EBPs in the community and providers needed to be engaged in the process. Developing EBPs can be a difficult process, requiring start-up funds, support for monitoring outcomes, and access to reimbursement dollars. Therefore, providers often needed supplemental funding to support these start-up activities. Finally, a knowledge base had to be developed which would guide stakeholders in making referrals to appropriate EBPs. With all implementation comes barriers—if these barriers are recognized and addressed as they arise, successful outcomes are more likely to occur.

Advocacy Outcomes

The comprehensive and coordinated effort undertaken by Louisiana appears to be having a significant impact in a number of ways at both the state and local level. Among some of the key accomplishments are:

- *Increase in availability of EBPs*: The initial survey in 2006 found that, in the communities surveyed, only 11 % of programs and services were evidence-based (Cocozza, Shufelt, & Phillippi, 2007a, 2007b) whereas by 2009 this had grown to 54 % (Phillippi & Cuffie, 2009), and by 2011 58 % of juvenile justice serving programs reported the use of EBPs in spite of significant economic barriers (Phillippi & Arteaga, 2011). In one local jurisdiction of Louisiana, an approach was piloted where the contracting process for services encouraged the use of EBPs. Data from that large metropolitan jurisdiction show that the number of contracts awarded to support EBPs rose from approximately 20 % of contracts in 2007 to 90 % in 2010.
- *Increase in the number of youth referred to EBPs*: At the state level, in 2006, less than one in every five youth receiving services from juvenile justice providers were reported to be accessing an EBP (Cocozza et al., 2007a, 2007b). By 2011, almost half were reported to be accessing EBPs (Phillippi, Cocozza, & DePrato, 2012). At a local level, one metropolitan parish demonstrated trends showing the proportion of youth referred to an EBP rose more than 400 % between 2007 and 2010. Another way to look at this increase is that in 2007 only 19 % of youth on probation in the parish were referred to an EBP. By 2010 this percentage had increased to 95 %. This sharp increase is attributed to both a change in local contracting practices favoring EBPs and policy changes in regard to probation officer referral practices.
- *Development and expansion of EBPs*: The Louisiana OJJ, with state funding, supported the implementation of FFT. OJJ provided a full year of start-up and licensing costs and 3 years of funding for FFT teams in select jurisdictions that were being supported by the technical assistance available under the Models for Change initiative. By 2007, the OJJ financial support had backed the implementation of the state's first five FFT teams, resulting in 31 clinicians providing services in six parishes to over 300 families on any given day. The success of these pilot teams led the Louisiana legislature in 2009 to pass legislation establishing a statewide FFT pilot program (15 LA Rev. Statutes § 971 et. seq.). The aim of this legislation was to increase the access to effective treatment for youth in contact with the juvenile justice system. As of 2012, the state has eight functioning FFT teams spread throughout the state in both rural and urban districts.
- *Increase in use of research-based screening and assessment*: Research-based screening and assessment tools and procedures have been adopted in a number of Louisiana parishes and dissemination of this model throughout the state is ongoing. A survey of Louisiana juvenile drug courts found an increase in the use of research-supported screening and assessment tools (Cocozza et al., 2007a, 2007b). Furthermore, a survey of juvenile justice providers statewide demonstrated

a 16 % increase in the utilization of research-based, standardized screening and assessment instruments between 2007 (51 %) and 2011 (67 %). Most importantly this equates to just over 16,000 youth now being evaluated annually using a research-driven standardized screening instrument as of 2011 (Phillippi et al., 2012).

- *Adoption and implementation of the SAVRY*: Another accomplishment of this effort has been the statewide planning and systematic adoption of the SAVRY, an empirically based instrument for assessing risk of juvenile offenders. The SAVRY was initially implemented in pilot communities and evaluated for effectiveness and efficiency. The result from the evaluation studies of the SAVRY implementation demonstrated success with increased public safety and improved youth outcomes, and has now been expanded statewide. This practice alone has been credited as one of the more significant reforms resulting in the transformation of case processing and service planning efforts by both courts and probation officers. The data from this tool are now also being utilized to examine risk and need trends throughout the state in order to better plan for services.

Conclusion and the Next Steps in Our Advocacy Efforts

Can a state bridge the gaps among research, policy, and practice? While not easy, the answer does seem to be yes. The State of Louisiana started at a point where they were criticized for overreliance on long-term institutional care for their juvenile justice population and had little understanding or availability of research-based interventions. Despite this, in a relatively short time Louisiana was able to:

- Decrease long-term care
- Increase awareness of EBPs
- Increase use of research-based screening and assessment
- Increase availability of EBPs
- Develop support by state

These were all achieved with no apparent threat to public safety as arrest rates and detention rates have also continued to decline in Louisiana. The extent of their success is reflected in the recent statement by Greenwood, Welsh, Rosica, Barber, and Mederano (2012) that Louisiana is "among the top four states in the country to show growth in evidence-based community programs." The state was able to make this remarkable progress as a result of the confluence of a number of factors:

- Federal lawsuit with ensuing development of institutional best practices
- Partnership between higher education and the juvenile justice system
- Funding from the MacArthur Foundation
- Involvement of national and state experts
- Support by the State and Local Governments
- Leadership by key stakeholders

While the coming together of so many critical factors may be unusual, what this demonstrates is that it is possible to bring about significant system-wide reform under difficult conditions and in a relatively short period of time. What has happened in Louisiana is not just the development of a single program in one part of the state, nor tinkering with a minor component of the process, nor educating one portion of the relevant stakeholders. Rather, it succeeded in reorienting the state's juvenile justice system in a way that brought together the latest and best research of what interventions actually work for these youth with developing state and local policies and practices. The body of research on EBPs would suggest that this integration will result in significantly better outcomes for the youth and the communities in Louisiana.

The challenge remains, of course, as to how to maintain this reform as Foundation support, access to technical assistance through the NRB, and other aspects fade away. To their credit, a number of concrete steps have already been taken with the state to build the infrastructure necessary to ensure the likelihood that these reforms will be sustained and expanded.

- New state policies for reimbursing community providers for the delivery of evidence-based services has been enacted.
- Contracting processes tied to funding streams have been revised in order to support EBPs.
- An Institute for Public Health & Justice at the LSUHSC has been established to provide ongoing support for EBPs and to inform the public and policy making process.

Clearly these and other ongoing actions are needed to document the impact of these changes and to ensure the ongoing expansion and fidelity to the new models. Whether these actions are enough to sustain the reform in the long run is uncertain and dependant on a number of fiscal, political, and programmatic factors. What is clear is that as a result of these efforts the gaps among research, policy, and practice for youth in contact with the justice system in Louisiana have been bridged.

References

Alexander, J., Barton, C., Gordon, D., Grotpeter, J., Hansson, K., Harrison, R., et al. (1998). Functional family therapy: Blueprints for violence prevention, book three. In D. Elliott (Ed.), *Blueprints for violence prevention series*. Boulder, CO: Center for the Study and Prevention of Violence, Institute of Behavioral Science, University of Colorado.

Butterfield, F. (1998, November 6). U.S. suing Louisiana on prison ills. *The New York Times*.

Chamberlain, P., & Reid, J. B. (1991). Using a specialized foster care community treatment model for children and adolescents leaving the state mental hospital. *Journal of Community Psychology, 19*, 266–276.

Cocozza, J. J., Shufelt, J. L., & Phillippi, S. W. (2007a). *Louisiana juvenile justice system service provider survey: A report of findings*. Delmar, NY: National Center for Mental Health and Juvenile Justice.

Cocozza, J. J., Shufelt, J. L., & Phillippi, S. W. (2007b). *Report to the Louisiana supreme court drug court office on the Louisiana juvenile drug court survey*. Delmar, NY: National Center for Mental Health and Juvenile Justice.

Gendreau, P., & Ross, R. (1987). Revivification of rehabilitation: Evidence from the 1980s. *Justice Quarterly*.

Greenwood, P. (2008). Prevention and intervention programs for juvenile offenders: The benefits of evidence-based practices. *The Future of Children, 18*, 11–36.

Greenwood, P., Welsh, B., Rosica, B. A., Barber, E., & Mederano, M. (2012). Making it happen: States that lead in providing top-rated evidence-based programs. *Blueprints for violence prevention conference*, San Antonio, TX.

Halliday-Boykins, C., Schoenwald, S., & Letournea, E. (2005). Caregiver-therapist ethnic similarity predicts youth outcomes from an empirically based treatment. *Journal of Consulting and Clinical Psychology, 73*(5), 808–818.

Henggeler, S., Melton, G., Brondino, M., Scherer, D., & Hanley, J. (1997). Multisystemic therapy with violent and chronic juvenile offenders and their families: The role of treatment fidelity in successful dissemination. *Journal of Consulting and Clinical Psychology, 65*(5), 821–833.

Hurst, H. (2012). *Models for Change Update 2012: Headlines*. Pittsburg, PA: National Center for Juvenile Justice.

John, D., & Catherine T. MacArthur Foundation. (2007). *Louisiana models for change work plan*.

John, D., & Catherine T. MacArthur Foundation. (2012a). National Resource Bank. Retrieved September 24, 2012, from Models for Change: Systems Reform in Juvenile Justice: http://www.modelsforchange.net/about/National-Resource-Bank.html

John, D., & Catherine T. MacArthur Foundation (2012b). States for Change. Retrieved September 24, 2012, from Models for Change: Systems Reform in Juvenile Justice: http://www.modelsforchange.net/about/States-for-change.html?tab=states

Juvenile Justice Implementation Commission. (2012). Retrieved September 24, 2012, from Juvenile Justice Initiative: State of Louisiana: http://www.louisianajuvenilejustice.la.gov/index.cfm?md=misc&tmp=aboutCommiss

Lee, S., Aos, S., Drake, E., Pennucci, A., Miller, M., & Anderson, L. (2012). *Return on investment: Evidence-based options to improve statewide outcomes*. Olympia, WA: Washington State Institute for Public Policy.

Lipsey, M. W. (2009). The primary factors that characterize effective interventions with juvenile offenders: A meta-analytic overview. *Victims and Offenders, 4*, 124–147.

Louisiana Office of Juvenile Justice. (2012, March 12). Retrieved September 24, 2012, from http://ojj.la.gov/ojj/files/Demographic_Profiles_for_Secure(3).pdf

Phillippi, S. W., & Arteaga, P. (2011). *Louisiana juvenile justice system service provider survey: A report of findings*. New Orleans, LA: Louisiana State University Health Sciences Center.

Phillippi, S. W., Cocozza, J. J., & DePrato, D. K. (2013). Improving community services for youth: Implementation strategies and outcomes from advancing evidence-based practices for juvenile justice reform (in press).

Phillippi, S. W., & Cuffie, D. (2009). *Louisiana juvenile justice system service provider survey: A report of findings*. New Orleans, LA: Louisiana State University Health Sciences Center.

Puzzanchera, C., & Adams, B. (2011). *Juvenile arrests 2009*. Washington, DC: U.S. Department of Justice, Office of Justice Programs, Office of Juvenile Justice and Delinquency Prevention.

Robbins, M., & Szapocznik, J. (2000). *Brief strategic family therapy. Office of justice programs*. Washington, DC: U.S. Department of Justice.

Sickmund, M., Sladky, T. J., Kang, W., & Puzzanchera, C. (2010). Easy access to the census of juveniles in residential placement. Retrieved September 24, 2012, from Office of Juvenile Justice and Delinquency Prevention Statistical Briefing Book: http://www.ojjdp.gov/ojstatbb/ezacjrp/asp/display.asp

Substance Abuse and Mental Health Services Administration. (2009a). *SAMHSA model programs: Brief strategic family therapy*. Rockville, MD: Substance Abuse and Mental Health Services Administration.

Substance Abuse and Mental Health Services Administration. (2009b). *SAMHSA model programs: Multisystemic therapy*. Rockville, MD: Substance Abuse and Mental Health Services Administration.

Chapter 12
Advocacy for Child Welfare Reform

Mary I. Armstrong, Svetlana Yampolskaya, Neil Jordan, and Rene Anderson

Defining the Issue

Child welfare system (CWS) in the United States commonly refers to services and institutions concerned with the physical, social, and psychological well-being of children (Child Welfare, 2012). The main goals of the CWS are to protect children who have been abused and/or neglected or who are at risk of being maltreated; to provide a stable, safe, and caring environment for them; and to support families that are under stress. The system is designed to provide an array of prevention and intervention services and oriented toward ameliorating conditions that put these families at risk (National Association of Social Workers, 2005). These services include screening and responding to reports of child abuse and neglect, maintaining children in out-of-home (foster) care, supporting families who experienced maltreatment, and preparing for and supporting adoption of children whose parents have lost their parental rights.

In the United States, child welfare is largely the responsibility of state, county, and local agencies, with considerable financial support and oversight from the federal government. The federal government also plays an important role in ensuring that provided programs and services lead to improved outcomes for children. Although all child protection systems are monitored by the federal government, the organization of child welfare agencies varies significantly across states. Whereas in some states the CWS is administered at the state level, in others it is administered at

M.I. Armstrong, Ph.D. (✉) • S. Yampolskaya, Ph.D. • R. Anderson
Department of Child and Family Studies, University of South Florida,
13301 Bruce B. Downs Boulevard, Tampa, FL 33612, USA
e-mail: miarmstr@usf.edu

N. Jordan, Ph.D.
Department of Psychiatry & Behavioral Sciences, Northwestern University Feinberg
School of Medicine, 420 East Superior Street, Chicago, IL 60611, USA

A. McDonald Culp (ed.), *Child and Family Advocacy: Bridging the Gaps Between Research, Practice, and Policy*, Issues in Clinical Child Psychology,
DOI 10.1007/978-1-4614-7456-2_12, © Springer Science+Business Media New York 2013

the county level (Bass, Shields, & Behrman, 2004). In addition, state laws, policies, and practices substantially vary.

In 2010 the CWS received approximately 3.3 million reports of alleged child abuse and neglect across the United States (U.S. DHHS, 2010). Nearly 1.8 million of these reports were accepted by state and local child protective services agencies for investigation or assessment, and about one-quarter (24.3 %) of investigations or assessments resulted in a disposition of substantiated abuse or neglect. In addition, 408,425 children were in foster care in 2010 with a median length of stay of 14 months, and 254,375 children entered out-of-home care. Between 2 and 12 % of children experience maltreatment recurrence every year and approximately 1,500 children die annually due to maltreatment. The CWS faces numerous challenges that increase the complexity of the tasks related to child protection and improving outcomes for children.

Efforts to Reform the Child Welfare System

The need for CWS reform has been long recognized by legislators and policy makers. This need for reform can be attributed to both growing numbers of children entering CWS as well as a substantial increase in the foster care population. In 1996, approximately 900,000 American children were victims of abuse or neglect, 520,000 children were in foster care, and 11 % of these youth had been in foster care for 3–4 years (U.S. DHHS, 1998). The passage of the Child Abuse Prevention and Treatment Act (CAPTA) of 1974, the Adoption Assistance and Child Welfare Act of 1980, the Family Preservation and Support Act of 1993, and the Adoption and Safe Families Act (ASFA) of 1997 were the most important federal legislative efforts directed at improving child welfare outcomes.

CAPTA was the first federal legislation concerning child maltreatment. It focused on child protection and authorized financial assistance for programs aimed at prevention, identification, and treatment of child abuse and neglect. In addition, CAPTA required states to establish child abuse reporting procedures and investigation systems. CAPTA has been reauthorized several times with amendments that expanded the scope of the law. For more information on CAPTA and the prevention of child maltreatment, please read Chapter 5 of this volume.

To address concerns about the unnecessary removal of children from home and the adverse consequences associated with unnecessary removal, Congress enacted the Adoption Assistance and Child Welfare Act of 1980 (Public Law 96-272), which emphasized the importance of establishing permanency plans, such as reunification with biological families or placement with adoptive families. This act required states to make "reasonable efforts" to prevent the placement of children in out-of-home care. In addition, this legislation provided a separate title of the Social Security Act (Title IV-E) and transferred Aid to Families with Dependent Children (AFDC)-Foster Care to the new title. These funds could then be used for states' costs related to the placement of poor children in out-of-home care and for adoption assistance for poor children leaving care.

In 1993, the federal government passed the Family Preservation and Support Services Act (Public Law 103-66). This act provided approximately $1 billion over 5 years to states to establish prevention and family preservation services. This legislation was an attempt to make state CWSs more responsive to the needs of families and better equipped to provide intervention before families go into crisis (Ahsan, 1996). It also emphasized the importance of prevention and encouraged states to switch from treatment-oriented to more integrated, preventive CWSs.

Another key piece of child welfare legislation was the ASFA enacted in 1997. ASFA prioritized child safety over reunification or placement and focused on reducing the time children are in out-of-home care settings. ASFA was the first federal law to address kinship care as a potential permanent placement. ASFA marked a fundamental change in the CWS by not only stressing the importance of achieving timely permanency but also underscoring two other critical outcomes for children: safety and well-being.

In response to the demands of ASFA requirements, the federal government created the Child and Family Services Review (CFSR) to evaluate each state's ability to achieve safety, permanency, and well-being for children (U.S. DHHS, 2001). CFSR pressed states to establish legal, administrative, and practice structures that ensure higher quality services for children, and develop systems that promote better outcomes. States that do not meet federal standards are required to submit performance improvement plans. After 2 years, states that have not demonstrated improvement may face financial penalties.

Title IV-E Waivers

Although states made considerable progress toward addressing the needs of children and families entering the CWS, a critical limitation remained in the financing structure of the CWS. Fiscal restrictions imposed by the federal government required states to use a larger portion of federal funds for children who were removed from their families. Available on an unlimited entitlement basis, Title IV-E reimburses states for a portion of foster care maintenance expenses paid on behalf of eligible children and related administrative costs. Among the requirements for eligibility was that children must be removed from a family that would have qualified for the former AFDC (welfare, poor children).

Restricting the use of funds to foster care hindered the ability of states to develop innovative and effective alternative service delivery models to keep families together and discouraged investment in prevention, intervention, and treatment services. Also, considering that most children and their families served by the CWS have multiple problems (Marsh, Ryan, Choi, & Testa, 2006), states needed greater flexibility in the use of available child welfare funds in order to provide a diverse array of services.

In 1994, in response to concerns about the federal child welfare financing structure, Congress authorized child welfare demonstration waivers (as part of the Social Security Amendments of 1994, Public Law 103-432). The program, known as Title

IV-E waiver, was designed to enable states to test innovative approaches to delivering and financing child welfare services, with the goal of producing better outcomes for children. Title IV-E waivers granted states greater financial flexibility and allowed them to directly access Title IV-E funds for investments in a broad continuum of services for children and families, including prevention, early intervention, treatment, family preservation, and post-permanency services. Since 1996, 32 states have participated in the waiver program, with several states having multiple waivers approved (Wulczyn, 2010). The majority of waivers have aimed at reducing a child's length of stay in out-of-home care, but waiver projects have also included assisted guardianship/kinship permanency, services to substance-abusing caretakers, adoption services, intensive service options, and tribal administration of Title IV-E funds (Houshyar, 2011). Most recently, the Child and Family Services Improvement and Innovation Act of 2011 (Public Law 112-34) restored waiver authority to extend programs funded under Title IV-B and Title IV-E through federal fiscal year 2016 and authorized new demonstration projects through federal fiscal year 2014.

Reform at the State Level

While the federal government continued to make efforts in reforming the CWS, some states responded to the pressure of attending to the needs of a rapidly growing foster care population by forming public–private partnerships and moving toward the privatization of services. In general, privatization is a process where functions and responsibilities in whole or in part are shifted from government agencies to the private sector. The contracting models for privatization vary widely across states, from statewide reforms to a range of smaller reforms covering specific geographic regions of a state or to specific service populations. Privatization efforts also include different purchase-of-service arrangements and community-based partnerships for child protection, as well as various types of outsourcing (Craig, Kulik, James, & Nielsen, 1998; Freundlich & Gerstenzang, 2003; Petr & Johnson, 1999). Typically, "contracting out" (or subcontracting) can be described as a process where the government seeks competition among private agencies or organizations to perform services previously provided by government agencies. With subcontracting, the government remains the financier and is responsible for managing and setting policies regarding the services to be provided (U.S. GAO, 1997).

Types of contracting: outsourcing services. There are different models of privatization, and they vary by geography, financial arrangements, type of services privatized, and child welfare provider type. For example, a state may contract with a specific region or county as was done in Florida during the first stage of privatization (Yampolskaya, Paulson, Armstrong, Jordan, & Vargo, 2004), or have a single, statewide contract similar to Pennsylvania's arrangement (Jones, 1999). States may also contract with a single provider to be responsible for various types of services, such as case management, adoption, or foster care. Alternatively, these contracts can be arranged with multiple providers, with each provider responsible for one type of service. The most important aspect of privatization, however, is the financial arrangement itself. Contractors can be paid in one of three ways: (1) on a fee-for-service basis, receiving payments for specific services, or (2) based on a case rate, when they receive a fixed amount of money per client served, or (3) with a global amount that is based on the number of eligible clients, regardless of how many clients actually receive services. Recently, many state child welfare agencies have shifted their contracting process to increase the emphasis on outcomes and their link with explicit fiscal incentives (McCullough & Associates, Inc., 2005).

Privatization has been viewed as a mechanism to improve performance of the CWS, delivering services more efficiently and reducing costs. At least 14 states currently have some level of privatization (Alliance for Children & Families, 2011). Some states began to privatize their CWS in response to legislative mandates (e.g., Florida and Colorado), whereas others were prompted by positive feedback from the Kansas and Florida initiatives. Many states relocated services into local communities in the hope of improved outcomes (Geen & Tumlin, 1999). Although states were motivated to outsource or contract out child welfare services for many different reasons, including a need to respond to ASFA requirements and to reduce costs (Westat & Chapin Hall Center for Children, 2002), the assumption was that private agencies have the potential to provide higher quality and greater efficiency in services at lower cost and the flexibility to use innovative ways to improve child welfare (Gibelman & Demone, 1998).

However, critics of privatization have expressed a number of concerns. These concerns include decreased public accountability and control; difficulty in establishing and monitoring performance standards; unrealized cost savings (partially caused by greater monitoring and contracting costs); unreliable and ineffective contractors; and the subjection of private agencies to public policy shifts and budget cuts that threaten the viability and stability of the agency (Gibelman & Demone, 1998). The Center for Public Policy Priorities (2005) points out that states with privatized services struggle with the same issues that challenge public agencies, including obtaining adequate services, reducing caseloads, and reducing staff turnover. Others have argued that the very nature of social services makes them inappropriate for privatization and expressed particular concerns about the use of for-profit providers (Quality Improvement Center, 2006). To further complicate tradeoffs between the benefits and shortcomings of privatization, evaluation studies have yielded mixed results as to whether privatization results in better outcomes for children.

What We Know Based on State Data

Improving outcomes for youth in the CWS is both essential and extremely challenging. As with most social service systems, system reform requires an advocacy base that is organized and empowered. Advocates also need solutions that are evidence-based to strengthen their arguments. In this section, we describe the evidence base for CWS reform efforts at the state level.

Findings from IV-E Flexible Funding Waiver Demonstration Projects

Although the impact of flexible funding due to IV-E waivers has not been consistently positive across all waiver states, many positive findings have been reported (Lehman, Liang, & O'Dell, 2005; U.S. DHHS, 2011a, 2011b). Several states have shown significant improvements in prevention of out of-home placements, exits to permanency, placement duration, and foster care reentry. Demonstration project data show that maltreatment recurrence has been no higher overall among child welfare populations assigned to experimental counties/groups or over time, which implies that children with access to waiver-funded services are at least as safe as those without access. However, of the six states that have received flexible funding waivers, only Florida and Indiana have demonstrated consistently positive and statistically significant findings across most major outcome areas (U.S. DHHS, 2011a, 2011b).

Privatization Findings

Kansas. Kansas has privatized all components of child welfare with the exception of child protective investigations, which is the initial investigation of allegations of abuse and neglect reports. Kansas adopted a lead agency model, in which a public agency is responsible for service provision within a designated region. During the first 4 years of this model (1996–2000), Kansas used a case rate arrangement, where contracted service providers were paid a fixed amount per client (rather than per client per day), which exposed them to substantial financial risk for youth who needed high cost services or a lengthy stay in out-of-home care. In response to underestimation of unit costs and financial problems private providers faced, Kansas abandoned the case rate system and reverted to a fee-for-service system. This transition appeared to be the state's acknowledgement that the implemented system was not successful.

Despite a lack of success with reforming the financing model, the Kansas CWS experienced some positive outcomes. In particular, the number of adoptions dramatically increased, and the proportion of adoptions finalized within 180 days rose from 18 % before privatization to 30 % after privatization (Unruh & Hodgkin, 2004). Also, child welfare service providers met and exceeded outcome goals related to child safety, minimizing placement moves, maintaining siblings together in placement, and placing the children in or close to the child's home community.

Florida. In 1996, the Florida Legislature mandated the outsourcing of child welfare services via a reform known as community-based care (CBC). Florida's CBC is based on a lead agency model where a not-for-profit agency is contracted to provide (or subcontract for) all foster care-related services for a specified geographic region. A lead agency is given a fixed budget and becomes responsible for coordinating and providing all services needed to all children who enter the CWS in the lead agency's geographic area of responsibility. All child protection-related services are outsourced with the exception of child protective investigations and child welfare legal services. The intent of the original statute was to strengthen the support and commitment of local communities to the "reunification of families and care of children and their families" and increase the efficiency and accountability of services.

Florida's reform effort was associated with some positive outcomes for youth. During state fiscal years (SFYs) 2002, 2003, and 2004, as implementation of CBC expanded throughout the state, the proportion of children exiting care within 12 months increased while the average length of stay in foster care decreased. During the same timeframe, the maltreatment recurrence rate remained stable, and the rate of out-of-home care reentry increased only slightly (Vargo et al., 2006).

Illinois. Illinois' child welfare reform effort shows another example of outsourcing. In 1997, anticipating the impact of the upcoming federal ASFA, the state sought a new way to deliver services that directly rewarded performance on key permanency outcomes. The Illinois Department of Children and Family Services implemented a performance-based contracting (PBC) model. First piloted in Cook County (Greater Chicago), foster care agencies under this model were required to accept a certain percentage of their caseload in new referrals, and transition a certain percentage of their caseload to permanency each year. By exceeding the permanency expectations, an agency could secure future caseload reductions without a loss in revenue. The Illinois PBC reform also involved an additional state investment in services to support permanency, including reunification/after care and therapeutic services (O'Brien, 2005). In conjunction with the new contracting model, the state implemented a new risk assessment protocol, redefined relative placements, and implemented an extended family support program.

Permanency outcomes improved substantially after implementation of the PBC model. During SFY 1999, more children were adopted than in the 7-year period of 1987 through 1994 combined. The number of children placed permanently with relatives also doubled in SFY 1999 compared to the previous year. By 2006, Illinois' foster care caseload had fallen by 65 %. There is evidence that the state used agency performance data to retain better performing agencies and eliminate ineffective ones (Blackstone, Buck, & Hakim, 2004).

In sum, privatized models vary across states, and although states continue to struggle with multiple challenges, there has been an overall positive trend towards improved performance in child safety and permanency outcomes (Missouri Department of Social Services Children's Division, 2010; Shaver, 2006; Watt, Porter, Renner, & Parker, 2007). Furthermore, there is modest evidence that financial models linking reimbursement or payment amounts to improved performance are having the desired impact, and such models offer the potential to further improve child outcomes and quality of services (O'Brien & Watson, 2002). A major barrier to child welfare financing reform has been the restrictions placed on the use of federal child welfare funds, but IV-E flexible funding waivers have enabled many states to implement successful reforms.

Other Factors Affecting Solutions

While privatization and IV-E waivers represent key structural opportunities for reforming CWS, there are several other key ingredients needed to support such system reforms. As shown in the IV-E waiver demonstrations, reliable data and adequate data systems are required to measure and assess changes in child welfare outcomes over time. Consistent with privatization models and the role of both public funders and private providers of child protection services, CWSs should be based on a public/private partnership. This partnership should feature leadership from both sectors as well as a governance structure with clear delineation of authority, roles and responsibilities, and a jointly implemented quality assurance system.

The other distinctive feature of CWSs is their local nature. Although primarily funded by federal and state funds, child welfare services are almost entirely provided locally, and require local direction through a community-driven process. While advocacy at the federal and state levels is essential for promoting child welfare reform, there is also tremendous need for a local advocacy base that is organized and empowered to promote the needs of youth and families in the CWS. The data from the state sources have revealed many issues, two of which are concerning to us and upon which we will focus in this chapter: kinship caregivers and gay and lesbian youth.

Goals of the Advocacy Effort for Child Welfare System Reform

Among the numerous advocacy needs in the CWS, we have chosen to focus on two issues highlighted in the state studies. First, kinship caregivers receive fewer subsidies and benefits than their foster caregiver counterparts; and second, there needs to be a better understanding of the unique issues faced by gay and lesbian youth in the CWS which affect their permanency outcomes. Therefore, our goals for advocacy are to (1) promote kinship care permanency and financial stability, and (2) create safe environments and expand permanency options for gay and lesbian youth.

Support for Kinship Caregivers in Child Welfare Systems

There are approximately 2.7 million children being raised by their relatives in the United States (Annie E. Casey Foundation, 2012). Placing children with relative (kinship) caregivers provides many benefits to these youth. These benefits include staying with family members and remaining in their community and school system, remaining with siblings, maintaining ties to their culture, and potentially achieving overall greater stability.

There are two kinds of kinship caregivers: (1) informal caregivers, who are not legally involved in the CWS and, therefore, not eligible for subsidies for raising their children, although they can apply for benefits such as Temporary Assistance for Needy Families (TANF), Medicaid, or housing assistance, and (2) formal licensed kinship foster parents, who have been involved in the CWS and are eligible for a monthly subsidy for the care of their children, Relative Caregiver Funds and other services and supports. The majority of kinship caregivers are informal caregivers (e.g., grandparents) and therefore do not have access to monthly subsidies and may not be aware of their eligibility for other supports. However, our advocacy goal is that all kinship caregivers in CWS have access to financial assistance and other supports to ensure their financial stability and positive outcomes for children.

Supporting Permanency for Lesbian and Gay Youth

There is a growing recognition in today's society for unique support for lesbian–gay–bisexual–transgender-questioning (LGBT) youth in the CWS. LGBT children have the same rights to a safe placement as all children in the CWS, but they may fare worse due to social stigma. LGBT youth are overrepresented in the population of youth served by the CWS. Approximately 5–10 %of the general population is estimated to be gay, yet in comparison, one study of youth aging out of the CWS in three Midwestern states indicated that 23.8 % of female respondents and 10.2 % of male respondents reported a sexual orientation in a category other than completely heterosexual (National Academy of Sciences, 2011; U.S. DHHS, 2011a, 2011b). Another study found that 65 % of LGBT youth in the CWS had lived in a foster or group home, and 39 % were forced to leave this setting because of their sexual orientation or gender identity (U.S. DHHS, 2011a, 2011b). These adolescents are at high risk for verbal harassment and physical abuse in contrast to the general adolescent population (Mallon, 2006). They also experience high rates of homelessness, multiple placements, emotional trauma, and alienation from parents, sibling, and former friends.

Under the U.S. Constitution, federal and state statutes and regulations along with group care (state residential) facilities have legal responsibilities to uphold the rights of all youth in their facilities. It is expected that agencies implement these legal policies and develop services and supports that assist LGBT youth to have full rights to safety, freedom from isolation, adequate access to healthcare services and equal treatment (The Institute of Medicine (IOM), 2011).

Advocacy Action Steps for Kinship Caregivers

Many states and community agencies are taking advocacy actions and responding to the needs of both formal and informal relative caregivers. A recent report, *Stepping Up For Kids*, highlights what government and communities should do to support kinship families (The Annie E. Casey Foundation, 2012). Collective action is needed by state agencies, legislatures, the business community, faith-based organizations, and others to develop a comprehensive system of coordinated services and supports for kinship families, including safe and affordable housing, financial stability, legal representation, and access to health care. The following action steps can be accomplished by first becoming a member of your state child advocacy system. In Florida's child advocacy system a key member is the Florida Kinship Center.

Write a Letter to Congress

National advocacy organizations can stand together and write a letter to Congress that addresses the issue of adequate financial supports for kinship caregivers. The letter should recommend amendments to the Social Security Act, Titles IV-B and IV-E, which governs federal policy in child welfare, to include increased financial assistance and other supports for both foster/adoptive care and kinship/relative care parents that will enable them to appropriately and adequately provide for the safety, stability, and well-being of the children in their care. Additional recommendations would include changing policies in the TANF Block Grant to meet the actual cost of raising children, and adjusting childcare benefits and modifying policies that will align them to the needs of kinship caregivers, which vary by state. The letter can conclude by commending the Congress for their leadership and commitment to addressing the needs of children and families in the CWS and indicating a desire for timely enactment of the requests.

Help Caregivers Navigate the CWS System

The Florida Kinship Center helps relative caregivers navigate the CWS to obtain financial, legal, and additional resources as well as information they need to raise children that are placed in their home. Many relative caregivers are unaware that they may be eligible for additional supports within their own community. The Fostering Connections and Successful Adoptions Act of 2008 (Public Law 110-351) has a built-in mechanism known as Kinship Navigators that provides fiscal support to states to assist relative caregivers with finding additional resources such as after-school programs, tutoring, community SHARE programs, that will provide additional supports for the child and family. Assistance is also available to locate additional financial services and opportunities to talk with attorneys free of charge.

Organize and Mobilize the Caregivers

The Florida Kinship Care Center plays a strong role in organizing and mobilizing advocacy strategies. For example, the Center developed an online training curriculum and cooperative extension resources for kinship caregivers on how to advocate for reforms at the state and local levels. The curriculum offers valuable training sessions for kinship caregivers and includes information on understanding the legislative process and how to best prepare for meetings with state legislators and legislative staff (Florida Kinship Center, 2012).

National organizations play key leadership roles in organizing advocacy efforts at the federal level. The Child Welfare League of America provided a kinship track/platform for kinship caregivers at their 2010 national summit to equip caregivers with advocacy skills and information. Transportation was available for kinship caregivers and other attendees at the summit to go visit their U.S. Representatives.

Attend Rallies

Another state-level advocacy example is the Rally in Tally, an annual event sponsored by the Florida Kinship Center. Hundreds of kinship caregivers are bussed from their local area to the state capitol in Tallahassee for a day when the Florida Legislature is in session. The Center prepares caregivers for this event beforehand by developing a list of advocacy issues and by offering legislative advocacy training on the morning of the event. Kinship caregivers are trained to request many types of financial assistance including equal subsidies and on how TANF Block Grant funds can be better used to support kinship caregivers.

Meet with Legislators

After the training has been completed, kinship caregivers meet with legislators and their staff to discuss the advocacy issues that were identified beforehand. The Center also financially supports the participation of Florida kinship caregivers in national rallies and advocacy efforts.

Advocacy Action Steps for Lesbian and Gay Youth

Advocacy for these youth needs to be a two-pronged attack: increase permanency options by providing greater opportunities for LGBT adults to foster and adopt these children (U.S. DHHS, 2011a, 2011b) and increase training of staff that work with LGBT youth.

Advocate for LGBT Adults to Adopt and Foster Youth in CWS

State advocacy groups can improve conditions for LGBT youth by advocating for changes in states' legal definitions of marriage and cohabitation relationships as these terms apply to adoption, foster care, and kinship care (Movement Advancement Project, 2012). At the national level, the Bill of Rights protects the rights of all citizens to pursue happiness, and this has been interpreted to include marriage and family life. However, some states have passed legislation limiting marriage. Changes in states' legal definitions of marriage occur through many advocacy avenues such as repeated challenges to the legislation in court by plaintiffs and lawyers, lobbying efforts with state legislatures and state CWS agencies, and public education campaigns that lead to shifts in public opinion.

Mobilize for Training for CWS Workforce on Understanding Gay and Lesbian Youth

The National Center for Lesbian Rights and the Sylvia Rivera Law Project have issued a report, *A Place of Respect: A Guide for Group Care Facilities Serving Transgender and Gender Non-conforming Youth*, that offers guidelines for child serving agencies on how to develop and implement policies and best practices associated with LGBT youth (National Center for Lesbian Rights, 2011). The report addresses specific areas of concern such as safety in bathrooms and during body searches, verbal harassment, physical violence, and unmet healthcare needs. The guide provides step by step information to assist group care facilities in providing staff with the required skills needed for working with LGBT youth and to help ensure that LGBT youth are treated with respect and dignity. This guide could be used to develop a training curriculum that would become a required training program for state agencies that license residential facilities for CWS youth. A related action step is to advocate for resources to develop similar guides and training curriculum for LGBT youth in general foster care.

Join National Advocacy Organizations

The National Center for Lesbian Rights (NCLR) is an example of a national legal organization that promotes and defends the rights of LGBT persons and their families by advocating for legislation, public policy, and education. The NCLR also offers legal services, couching their arguments in terms of discrimination. The Center serves as a clearinghouse for local attorneys who specialize in LGBT cases, and they offer information about legal protection for children in LGBT households (www.NCLRights.org/GetHelp).

Outcomes and Next Steps

Kinship Caregivers

We have identified two advocacy goals tied to CWS reform: stronger supports for kinship caregivers and stronger support for the rights of gay and lesbian youth in foster care. One successful outcome for kinship caregivers is federal legislation, specifically the Fostering Connections and Successful Adoptions Act of 2008 (Public Law 110-351), which includes three key provisions related to kinship caregivers. This law stipulates that states must locate and provide notice to relatives within 30 days of removing children from their parents. The law also provides some federal funds for subsidized kinship guardianships, an arrangement that makes kinship caregivers the legal guardians of children and provides financial supports to the caregivers. Finally, the Act includes some funding for state-level navigation programs that assist kinship caregivers in accessing information and finding services (U.S. DHHS, 2008). However, this legislation does not provide all kinship caregivers in the CWS with fiscal stability because the resources offered are not enough to support all kinship caregivers.

Although this federal legislation affirms the rights of kinship caregivers, many other kinship caregiver issues require additional advocacy. Advocacy is needed at the national and state levels so that both formal and informal kinship caregivers have parity with the monthly stipends received by foster parents. Informal caregivers also need legislation that will assist with clarifying their legal rights to access services that address the physical health, dental care, mental health, and educational needs of their children.

Gay and Lesbian Youth

As noted earlier, a successful advocacy outcome for gay and lesbian youth in CWS is the provision of guidelines for best practices for the appropriate care of these youth, through the report *A Place of Respect: A Guide for Group Care Facilities Serving Transgender and Gender Non-conforming Youth.* Next advocacy steps are to ensure that the policies and practices recommended in the guide are mandated by state agencies, and that training curricula for workers are developed and implemented. Another necessary step is the development and implementation of similar guidelines for LGBT youth in the general foster care population.

The laws that limit rights for same-sex couples can also have an adverse impact on youth in the CWS. For example, for many years Florida law prevented LGBT parents from adopting youth in the CWS. This law was declared illegal in September 2010 (Florida Department of Children and Families v. In re: Matter of Adoption of X.X.G. and N.R.G.). Prospective parents who are LGBT now will be considered according to the same criteria as all other prospective parents. The rights of "second parent adoption," which is adoption by the nonbiological parent of the couple's child, are unresolved in Florida, and they vary in other states. Additional advocacy steps are needed at national and state levels to clarify the rights of LGBT individuals to be foster and/or adoptive parents.

Advocacy Steps That Can Be Taken by Child Welfare System Researchers

There also are advocacy steps that university-based researchers can take to improve systems. Researchers can use a variety of dissemination vehicles, including policy briefs and topical papers, which summarize research findings and implications and are directed at legislators and policymakers. For example, in the early phases of privatization in Florida, evaluation reports identified several early implementation issues that needed to be addressed. One issue was the nature of the relationship between the public agency and the child welfare lead agencies. There was confusion about whether the lead agencies were simply extensions of the public agency or equal business partners with a defined contractual relationship. The evaluation recommended that both parties in this public/private partnership needed to make fundamental shifts if privatization was to be successful. The outcome of this recommendation was that the public agency created a readiness assessment process that was implemented in each area of the state as it was privatized. These assessments were peer-led and included a review of the readiness of both the new lead agency and the local regional office of the public agency. Over time, the readiness assessment process was written into Florida statutes and continues to be used whenever a new lead agency is awarded a contract.

One challenge that the evaluation identified was the limited ability to track the effectiveness and outcomes of the expanded availability and utilization of prevention and diversion services. Not all families who received these services were being entered into Florida's statewide child welfare information system. Once this issue was identified, the evaluation team partnered with another advocacy group, the Florida Coalition for Children, to lobby for changes to the data system. Recently, Florida implemented a new component of the data system for secondary prevention cases. Data from this component will be a valuable information source in the future in order to better understand which types and amounts of prevention services and supports work best with which types of families.

Conclusions

As the examples above illustrate, advocacy is a successful avenue to create change when the CWS experiences challenges that require legislation (federal and/or state level), policy, regulations (federal, state, and/or community level), or adjustments to appropriate levels and types of funding. Advocacy action steps can directly target simple to complex policy changes, or amend existing policies within an agency. Writing campaigns and face-to-face visits can educate state officials about real situations that can be improved through policy and legislative changes.

In order to get legislation passed, advocates will need to actively complete many of the following steps:

- Contact state legislators
- Research and educate themselves on current bills related to the advocacy issues
- Seek training opportunities to enhance knowledge and skills to advocate
- Educate legislators and community about the importance of getting the bill passed
- Sign petitions that advocate for the bill
- Initiate a bill and get it signed
- Provide personal testimony to the House or Senate committee about the bill
- Connect with an advocacy group that is fighting for the same cause
- Follow the bill until it gets passed

As the CWS moves in the direction of more prevention and early intervention for at-risk families and communities, a comprehensive approach should include several other systems, such as schools, health care settings, day care and other early childhood programs, and mental health and substance abuse providers. Advocates need to call for and insist upon strong partnerships across these systems at both the state and community levels.

As the chapter illustrates, there will always be emerging issues in CWSs, such as the needs of LGBT youth that require the attention of advocacy organizations and coalitions. Everyone can do their part to increase awareness of issues in CWSs. It is the responsibility of each citizen to ensure the rights of all children, as the well-being of a society's children determines the future of that society. The potential success of those children who will become future citizens determines the success of the society as a whole.

References

Ahsan, N. (1996). The family preservation and support services program. *The Future of Children. The Juvenile Court, 6*, 157–160.

Alliance for Children and Families. (2011). The privatization of child welfare. *Alliance for Children and Families Magazine*, 3

Annie E. Casey Foundation. (2012). *Stepping up for kids: What government and communities should do to support kinship families: Policy report, Kids Count*. Baltimore, MD: The Annie E. Casey Foundation.

McCullough & Associates, Inc. (2005). *Child welfare privatization summary of national trends: A synthesis of research and framework for decisions*. Retrieved from http://www.cfsa.dc.gov/cfsa/lib/cfsa/frames/pdf/Privatization_Framework.pdf

Bass, S., Shields, M. K., & Behrman, R. E. (2004). Children, families, and foster care: Analysis and recommendations. *The Future of Children, 14*, 5–29.

Blackstone, E., Buck, A. J., & Hakim, S. (2004). Privatizing adoption and foster care: Applying auction and market solution. *Children and Youth Services Review, 26*(11), 1033–1049.

Center for Public Policy Priorities. (2005). *Privatization of Child Protective Services*. Texas: Author.

Child Abuse Prevention and Treatment Act (CAPTA) of 1974. Public Law 95–608.

Child Welfare. (2012). In *Britannica Academic Edition*. Retrieved from http://www.britannica.com/EBchecked/topic/111093/child-welfare

Craig, C., Kulik, T., James, T., & Nielsen, S. (1998). *Privatizing child welfare. (Policy Study, 248)*. Boston, MA: Institute for Children, Inc.

Florida Kinship Center: Making a difference for relatives raising children. (2012). Retrieved from May 16, 2013 http://kinshipcenter.cbcs.usf.edu/default/index.cfm/programs/training/online-training/

Freundlich, M., & Gerstenzang, S. (2003). *An assessment of the privatization of child welfare services: Challenges and successes*. Washington, D.C.: Child Welfare League of America Press.

Geen, R., & Tumlin, K. C. (1999). *State efforts to remake child welfare: Responses to new challenges and increased scrutiny*. Washington, D.C.: The Urban Institute.

Gibelman, M., & Demone, H. W., Jr. (Eds.). (1998). *The privatization of human services: Policy and practice issues*. New York, NY: Springer Publishing Company.

Houshyar, S. (2011). *Title IV-E waivers: Expanding and modifying child welfare demonstration waivers to promote flexibility and foster innovation*. First Focus. Retrieved from May 16, 2013 www.firstfocus.net.

Jones, M. L. (1999). Using the system to increase and improve adoptions: The SWAN model. *Child Welfare, 78*(5), 593–609.

Lehman, C. M., Liang, S., & O'Dell, K. (2005). Impact of flexible funds on placement and permanency outcomes for children in child welfare. *Research on Social Work Practice, 15*, 381–388. doi:10.1177/1049731505276976.

Mallon, G. P. (2006). *Lesbian and gay foster and adoptive parents: Recruiting, assessing, and supporting an untapped resource for children and youth*. Washington, DC: Child Welfare League of America.

Marsh, J. C., Ryan, J. P., Choi, S., & Testa, M. F. (2006). Integrated services for families with multiple problems: Obstacles to family reunification. *Children and Youth Services Review, 28*, 1074–1087.

Missouri Department of Social Services Children's Division. (2010). *Missouri Child and Family Services Review statewide assessment*. Jefferson City, MO: Author. Retrieved from May 17, 2013 http://www.dss.mo.gov/cd/cfsr/secondround-assessment.pdf

Movement Advancement Project. (2012). *Securing legal ties for children living in LGBT families*. Retrieved from May 16, 2013 http://www.lgbtmap.org/file/securing-legal-ties.pdf

National Academy of Sciences. (2011). *The health of lesbian, gay, bisexual and transgender people: Building a foundation for better understanding*. May 16, 2013 from http://www.iom.edu/Reports/2011/The-Health-of-Lesbian-Gay-Bisexual-and-Transgender-People.aspx

National Association of Social Workers. (2005). *Standards for social work practice in child welfare*. Washington, DC: Author.

National Center for Lesbian Rights. (2011, Spring). *A place of respect: A guide for group care facilities serving transgender and gender non-conforming youth*. Retrieved from May 16, 2013 www.nclrights.org/site

O'Brien, M. (2005). *Performance based contracting (PBC) in child welfare (Draft)*. Arlington, VA: National Child Welfare Resource Center for Organizational Improvement.

O'Brien, M., & Watson, P. (2002). *A Framework for Quality Assurance in Child Welfare*. Portland, ME: National Child Welfare Resource Center for Organizational Improvement.

Petr, C. G., & Johnson, I. C. (1999). Privatization of foster care in Kansas: A cautionary tale. *Social Work, 44*(3), 263–267.

Quality Improvement Center. (2006). *Literature review on the privatization of child welfare services*. Washington, DC: U.S. Department of Health and Human Services, Administration for Children and Families, Children's Bureau.

Shaver, M. (2006). *Performance contracting in Illinois: Using leverage to drive results*. Portland, ME: National Child Welfare Resource Center for Organizational Improvement. Retrieved from

http://muskie.usm.maine.edu/helpkids/telefiles/Performance%20Contracing%20in%20
IL-%20Paper.pdf
U.S. Department of Health and Human Services, Administration for Children and Families.
(2001). *45 CFR Parts 1355, 1356 and 1357 Title IV—E Foster Care Eligibility reviews and
child and family services state plan reviews: Final Rule. 65* Fed. Reg. 16 (proposed January 25,
2000).
U.S. Department of Health and Human Services, Administration for Children and Families.
(2008). *Fostering Connections to Success and Increasing Adoptions Act of 2008.* http://www.
childwelfare.gov/sysemwide/lawnpolicies/federal/index.cfm?event=federallegislation.
viewlegis&id=121. Accessed Sep 2012
U.S. Department of Health and Human Services, Administration for Children and Families.
(2011a). *Synthesis of findings: Title IV-E flexible funding child welfare waiver demonstrations.*
Washington, DC: Author
U.S. Department of Health and Human Services, Administration for Children and Families.
(2011b, April 6). *Information Memorandum (Log No. ACYF-CB-IM-11-03).* Retrieved from
http://www.acf.hhs.gov/programs/cb/laws_policies/policy/im/2011/im1103.htm
U.S. Department of Health and Human Services, Administration for Children and Families,
Administration on Children, Youth and Families, Children's Bureau. (1998). *Child welfare
outcomes 1998: Annual Report.* Washington, DC: Author.
U.S. Department of Health and Human Services, Administration on Children. (2010). *Child maltreatment 2010.* Washington, DC: Author.
U.S. Government Accountability Office (1997, October). *Social service privatization: Expansion
poses challenges in ensuring accountability for program results.* GAO Publication No. GAO/
HEHS-98-6. Washington, DC: Author. Retrieved from http://www.gao.gov/archive/1998/
he98006.pdf.
Unruh, J., & Hodgkin, D. (2004). The role of contract design in privatization of child welfare services: The Kansas experience. *Children and Youth Services Review, 26*(8), 771–783.
Vargo, A. C., Armstrong, M., Jordan, N., Kershaw, M. A., Pedraza, J., Romney, S., et al. (June,
2006). *Community-Based Care White Paper for State fiscal year 2005–2006.* Tampa, FL:
University of South Florida.
Watt, J. W., Porter, R., Renner, L., & Parker, L. (2007). Maintaining positive public-private part-
nerships in child welfare: The Missouri project on performance-based contracting for out-of-
home care. *Professional Development: The International Journal of Continuing Social Work
Education, 10,* 49–57.
Westat and Chapin Hall Center for Children, University of Chicago. (2002, April). *State innovations in child welfare financing.* Retrieved from http://aspe.hhs.gov/hsp/CWfinancing03/report.
pdf
Wulczyn, F. H. (July 29, 2010). *The use of child welfare waiver demonstration projects to promote
child well-being.* U.S. House of Representatives Committee on Ways and Means, Subcommittee
on Income Security and Family Support [written testimony].
Yampolskaya, S., Paulson, R. I., Armstrong, M., Jordan, N., & Vargo, A. C. (2004). Child welfare
privatization: Quantitative indicators and policy issues. *Evaluation Review, 28,* 87–1.

Chapter 13
American Indian and Alaska Native Children and Families

Diane J. Willis and Paul Spicer

Defining the Child Issue

American Indian and Alaska Native (AI/AN) children confront tremendous adversity with service systems that are under-resourced and often based on service models that are oblivious to native cultures and contexts (Gone & Trimble, 2012; Sarche & Spicer, 2008, 2012). While there is great deal of overlap between the needs of AI/AN children and families and those from other populations, here we emphasize the unique opportunities that arise for advocacy for tribes, given their direct relationship with the federal government, and for models that are informed by specific local tribal cultures. For many Americans, AI/AN issues seem to be of little contemporary relevance. AI/AN people may seem eerily absent from American society (Wilson, 1998), but AI/AN communities are rapidly growing with strong assertions of tribal sovereignty with regard to economic development, education, and health services. These dynamics shape the environment for advocacy on children's issues and provide a unique perspective on relationships between researchers and advocacy. In the case we focus on here, the work of the American Indian and Alaska Native Head Start Research Center, research was designed to respond directly to advocacy from tribal communities.

In the early nineteenth century, the goal of European Americans was to "civilize" the Indians and open more of the continent to settlers. American Indians were promised education and training in agriculture in exchange for land, but as of 1877 the

D.J. Willis, Ph.D. (✉)
Professor Emeritus, Department of Pediatrics, University of Oklahoma Health
Sciences Center, 4520 Ridgeline Drive, Norman, OK 73072, USA
e-mail: Diane-Willis@ouhsc.edu

P. Spicer, Ph.D.
Department of Anthropology, Center for Applied Social Research, University of Oklahoma,
3100 Monitor Avenue, Suite 100, Norman, OK 73072, USA

A. McDonald Culp (ed.), *Child and Family Advocacy: Bridging the Gaps Between*
Research, Practice, and Policy, Issues in Clinical Child Psychology,
DOI 10.1007/978-1-4614-7456-2_13, © Springer Science+Business Media New York 2013

appropriation for Indian education was only $20,000. In 1849, as land was becoming more scarce, the Committee on Indian Affairs "proposed that the only 'alternative to extinction' was to settle 'our colonized tribes' on government-run reservations" (Wilson, 1998, p. 289). But already by 1851 the Secretary of the Interior stated "the policy of removal—must necessarily be abandoned; the only alternatives left are to civilize or exterminate them" (Wilson, p. 289). Particularly egregious in this effort were the boarding schools, which mounted a systematic assault on AI/AN language and culture that has continued well into the twentieth century (Lomawaima & McCarty, 2006; Reyhner & Eder, 2004). Also significant were the forbidding of cultural events on reservations and denying access to culturally valued life ways. This assault, coupled with the appropriation of lands required for aboriginal subsistence, ensured that AI/ANs became, in the mid-twentieth century, "one of the most troubled minorities in America" (Wilson, p. XXVI).

In 2010, the U.S. Census Bureau reported a population of about 5.2 million AI/ANs within 565 federally recognized tribal nations. The AI/AN population tends to be younger than the general population (38 % younger than age 18 years), with a smaller number of elderly than the general population (USDHHS, 2001). About three-fourth of AI/ANs are located in the western part of the United States. Today many tribal communities are plagued by poverty and low educational attainment and dramatic health disparities (Spicer & Sarche, 2012; Willis, 2000, 2002; Willis & Bigfoot, 2003; Zuckerman, Haley, Roubideaux, & Lillie-Blanton, 2004). AI/ANs residing in tribal jurisdictions receive much of their health care through hospitals and clinics run through 12 Indian Health Service (IHS) area offices, but adequate funds for specialty services are often lacking (Dixon & Roubideaux, 2001).

In the lifetime of the first author (DJW), many AI/AN people were brought up by men and women who were sent to boarding schools. Oftentimes this resulted in impaired parenting skills and a loss of cultural heritage, contributing to child abuse and domestic violence within families (Cole, 2006). Willmon-Haque and Bigfoot (2008, 2009) report factors that contribute to the rate of child maltreatment in Indian country which include psychological, legal, economic, and social issues that impact the parents' ability to care for their children. Not surprisingly, AI/ANs are often dramatically overrepresented in reports of child maltreatment: in Alaska, AI/ANs were 43.4 % of all perpetrators of child maltreatment, in Montana 19.3 %, in North Dakota 15.8 %, and in South Dakota 43.8 % (Child maltreatment, 2010).

Domestic violence, substance abuse, and mental health among AI/ANs deserve emphasis in this context (Evans-Campbell, Lindhorst, Huang, & Walters, 2006; Oetzel & Duran, 2004; Szlemko, Wood, & Jumper-Thurman, 2006). Violence is a serious and critical health problem all over the United States but it is particularly problematic in Indian country (Oden, 2003). The rate of violence against AI/ANs is twice that of the United States as a whole, and AI/AN women experience 2–3 times more violent victimization than women of any other race (Greenfield & Smith, 1999). In 1999 the National Center on Child Abuse and Neglect reported that 79.8 % of AI girls had been sexually abused.

Kronk and Thompson (2007) reported that AI/ANs have the highest rates of methamphetamine use among all ethnic minority groups in the United States. IHS records showed a 60 % increase in treatment admissions between 2001 and 2007

(National Drug Intelligence Center, 2008). In a recent assessment, use of methamphetamine was up to 3 times higher than earlier national samples of AI/AN adolescents and about 5 times higher than the United States' population of adolescents across all races (Barlow et al., 2010). Family dysfunction and conflict coupled with frequent moves (residential instability) were factors correlated with meth use in this population. The National Institute on Drug Abuse (2009) reported that between 2006 and 2008 AI/ANs aged 12 years and older reported using meth the past year at a rate 3 times greater than the United States across all races.

Alcohol abuse also continues to be a major public health problem among AI/ANs (Spicer et al., 2003). It is known that AIs die from accidents, homicides, and suicide at a higher rate than the general US population and these causes of death are often alcohol-related or alcohol-specific (May, 1996; IHS, 2002). Alcohol also has been associated with other kinds of psychological dysfunction, PTSD, mood disorders, and suicide (Alcantara & Gone, 2007; Beals et al., 2005; IHS, 2005; Olson & Wahab, 2006). Thankfully, the news is not entirely bleak: Beauvais, Jumper-Thurman, and Burnside (2008) have noted a decrease in cocaine use/abuse and in the use of tobacco and inhalants among AI youth.

Most tragically, the suicide rate among young AI/ANs is exceedingly high. The Centers for Disease Control and Prevention (CDC, 2007) reported that AI/ANs' suicide rate for the ages 15–34 is 19.7 per 100,000, which is higher than any other age group. For AI/ANs the highest rates of suicide occur in males 20–24 years of age and the overall suicide rate is 1.8 times higher than any other race. There is a higher correlation between substance abuse and suicide for AI/ANs than found among other races, as determined by autopsy (Alcohol and Suicide, 2009).

Unfortunately, despite these very high levels of need, the publication of the Report of the Surgeon General's Conference on Children's Mental Health (Child maltreatment, 2001) identified a tremendous shortage in mental health services for children, which continues (Gone & Trimble, 2012).

Solutions

Given the broad range of disparities identified above, a number of possible solutions suggest themselves. We focus here on the need for tribal engagement for culturally appropriate intervention and workforce development for children's services. These approaches capitalize on ongoing assertions of tribal sovereignty and innovation and respond specifically and directly to calls to use evidence-based practice in a wide range of contexts.

As detailed above, AI/AN children have been subjected to a wide range of dislocating influences, and communities are rightly concerned to reverse these from the earliest possible point. A convergence of evidence underscores the possible impact of early childhood intervention for a broad range of child outcomes (Carneiro & Heckman, 2003), and many communities are especially interested in using early childhood intervention to support native language revitalization, which was undermined by the boarding school experiences described above.

In this context, Early Head Start (EHS) programs can be an important resource. This program for low-income families can start with interventions involving the pregnant mother and continue over the first 3 years of life when children can transition to Head Start preschool programs (Willis, 2003). EHS builds on longstanding commitments to Head Start in tribal communities, and has also recently been integrated with child care monies in many tribal community early childhood centers. Further opportunities arise with the new Maternal, Infant, and Early Childhood Home Visiting program, which was created by the Affordable Care Act.

Unfortunately, until the twenty-first century, AI/AN communities have not participated meaningfully in research that can support intervention development in early childhood. Indeed, AI/AN communities have been explicitly left out of national studies in early childhood funded by the Administration on Children and Families (ACF). Moreover, opportunities for the kind of culturally specific intervention development that many tribes desire are under pressure from the push to evidence-based practice (Spicer, Bigfoot, Funderburk, & Novins, 2012). Given the lack of good research on tribal early childhood intervention, a vital opportunity for advocacy has opened for tribes, which has been led by the National Indian Head Start Directors' Association.

Goal of the Advocacy Effort

The goal of the advocacy effort was based on the recommendation of the National Indian Head Start Director's Association: the need for data to be gathered specific to AI/AN children and families in the tribal communities they serve. Since previous efforts to create dedicated funding opportunities for research on AI/AN Head Start had failed, in part because of a lack of qualified investigators with the requisite relationships with tribal communities, ACF opted, instead, to create the American Indian and Alaska Native Head Start Research Center to support the development of this research capacity. In 2005, funding was awarded to the University of Colorado Denver, with the second author (PS) as the principal investigator.

This center was originally designed to create infrastructure for research on American Indian and Alaska Native Head Start by seeding campus–community partnerships. The projects in this early phase focused on workforce development and the development of culturally and linguistically appropriate materials and pedagogical approaches, again as an explicit reaction against the abuses of the boarding school era. Also central to the work was support for three junior faculty members, all American Indian women in colleges of education who were moving to early care and education after earlier work in elementary and secondary education. While this center was originally funded prior to the reauthorization of Head Start, it was soon also involved in the work that resulted from that reauthorization.

The reauthorization of Head Start in 2007 contained explicit requirements for research on tribal issues, including developing an accurate estimate of the number of children eligible for services in AI/AN communities, and inquiry into a range of issues in improving Head Start in tribal communities. This language in the reauthorization was a direct result of advocacy by the National Indian Head Start Directors' Association and the American Indian and Alaska Native Head Start Research Center was renewed for an additional 2 years of funding to respond specifically to these additional requirements (although the population estimate was developed separately). The Center was thus both created and sustained by advocacy from tribal communities, which had a direct effect on the language in the reauthorization of Head Start in 2007. In turn, the work of the Center has supported advocacy on a broad range of issues, consistent with emerging trends in community-based participatory health research in tribal communities.

Advocacy Action Steps

Our experience with the American Indian and Alaska Native Head Start Research Center points to important levers for advocacy efforts. First, advocacy organizations required skilled and available research partners who were already engaged in the work. Initial efforts to seed research on American Indian and Alaska Native Head Start failed because of a lack of investigators engaged in the work. One small research project positioned the team at the University of Colorado to be able to consult with federal staff about opportunities for a different approach to developing research on American Indian and Alaska Native Head Start. Second, partnerships with those engaged in the advocacy work were also essential in winning the award and executing the work. Members of the National Indian Head Start Directors' Association formed the core of the Center's Steering Committee, providing important insights as we prepared the application and oversight as we articulated our research and research training efforts. Several of these directors subsequently became involved in the Center's cross-site research, which responded specifically to the requirements in the reauthorization. Third, translation of the research into improvements in policy and practice requires sustained work with federal program staff and advocacy organizations. This work is ongoing, especially in the work of the new Tribal Early Childhood Research Center, the successor to the American Indian and Alaska Native Head Start Research Center at the University of Colorado, but also in the participation of program directors and investigators associated with the Center in numerous ACF advisory panels. Fourth, research must continue. The Center seeded numerous research partnerships that remain vital and active, supporting multiple new initiatives designed to improve policy and practice for AI/AN children and families.

Outcome and Next Steps

Research conducted under the auspices of the American Indian and Alaska Native Head Start Research Center emphasized a broad set of challenges in providing linguistically and culturally appropriate services, which are often represented as direct antidotes to the abuses of the boarding school era. Program directors described ongoing frustrations in implementing cultural adaptations in the context of requirements for evidence-based curricula. Several of these directors partnered with a newly funded National Center for Cultural and Linguistic Responsiveness to create "Making It Work," a guide for tribal programs interested in developing cultural programming that is consistent with the Performance Standards of Head Start. These new efforts reflect awareness in the broader Head Start community of the need for tribally specific curricula that can support tribal language and culture.

Additional work by the Center has emphasized the need for collaborative approaches to measurement. None of the measurement tools in early childhood research have been developed for tribal communities. Work on what came to be known as the cross-site study paired ethnographic research with quantitative assessments of classrooms, teachers, parents, and children. Data analyses continue in the context of the new Tribal Early Childhood Research Center at the University of Colorado, but early experience underscores the possibilities for meaningful inclusion of tribal programs in national research. Indeed, the Center's research emphasizes opportunities for national dialogues on language, culture, and pedagogy that have been lost by not previously engaging these tribal programs in national research.

Work by the Center, and especially advocacy from the program directors on the Steering Committee, has also served as a consistent reminder of the mental health challenges confronted by so many AI/AN children and families. While it is important to emphasize the strength and resilience in these communities (and the opportunities that those resources offer for improving mental health services), we have also long known about the need for increased mental health care, as documented above, as well. In the 1990s Senator Inouye and his top administrative assistant, Pat DeLeon, called for hearings on mental health issues of AI/ANs and testimony was presented by IHS and selected members of APA (Willis, 1990, 1992). The outcome of this coordinated advocacy was an increase in monies to IHS that resulted in 100 new mental health hires. But in 2009 it was noted that there is still only one psychiatrist for every 250,000 AIs, one psychologist for every 17,000 AIs and one social worker or counselor for every 3,300 AIs (Gray, 2009). So the Senate Select Committee on Indian Affairs held new hearings on suicide and mental health needs of AI/ANs where Dr. Gray, from the University of North Dakota, recommended increased funding to IHS and for the four Indians in psychology training programs to grow the number of credentialed mental health professionals. Dr. Gray also recommended increased "funding of loan repayment programs to recruit and retain qualified mental health service providers in Indian country" (p. 5).

While the results of this current advocacy remain to be seen, we are encouraged that there has been dramatic growth in the development of suicide prevention materials, addressing that specific need. For example, in 2010 SAMHSA published an evidenced-based manual "To Live to See the Great Day That Dawns: Preventing Suicide by American Indian and Alaska Native Youth and Young Adults." This program builds on the notable success of Teresa LaFromboise with her American Indian Life Skills Curriculum (LaFromboise & Lewis, 2008), which is based on social cognitive theory and guides skills training in seven areas: self-esteem, emotions and stress, communication and problem solving skills, self-destructive behaviors, suicide information, suicide intervention training, and setting goals. Research in the Zuni community demonstrated success in reducing suicidal thinking and skill improvement (LaFromboise & Howard-Pitney, 1995).

As the examples discussed above document, there is an important role for advocacy with lawmakers to affect policy and appropriations and there is a need for ongoing research that can support the kind of locally driven improvements in services that tribes have long requested. We have seen how this gave rise to an important set of studies and initiatives in Head Start, and it is likely that this will continue with the new Maternal, Infant, and Early Childhood Program, which has a set-aside for tribal programs and dedicated research funds as part of the new ACF-funded Tribal Early Childhood Research Center (which continues the work of the Head Start Research Center, but adds research on home visiting). The recent example of Circles of Care also emphasizes the value of working directly with the staff of federal programs, who often recognize the unique challenges and opportunities in AI/AN communities and are eager for partners from the academic community to assist in their efforts to create special programming (Novins & Best, 2011). This is evident, as well, in the work of the ACF-funded National Center for Cultural and Linguistic Responsiveness, which has taken on an explicit focus on AI/AN issues, including the supports for cultural programming in the classroom discussed previously, e.g., Making It Work. That said, there remain important advocacy opportunities. The work is not nearly done.

First, it is clear that IHS continues to need qualified, well trained psychologists and psychiatrists, especially to work with children. Dr. Dolores Bigfoot, who has worked with native populations in every state through her Project Making Medicine, indicates that few of the existing mental health professionals with whom she has worked utilize evidence-based practice. This occurs primarily because they have not been trained to use these treatments. The need for more highly trained mental health providers for all ages, not just adults, is a priority, especially now that we are starting to see the emergence of evidence-based practices for children that are culturally sensitive (Bigfoot & Braden, 2007; Bigfoot & Schmidt, 2006; Coteau, Anderson, & Hope, 2006; Funderburk, Gurwitch, & Bigfoot, 2005). At the same time, we also recognize the need to grow the evidence base for these and other treatments that may be uniquely fit to AI/AN contexts. As Gone and Alcantara (2007) observe, and Gone and Trimble (2012) reiterate, we need outcome studies for a broad range of interventions in tribal communities. The value of well-conducted outcome studies for advocacy cannot be overestimated.

Advocating for the needs of AI/ANs requires us to do several things. First, we need to know the population's strengths and areas in need of change. Here, basic research is essential, as are ongoing research programs and partnerships. Second, we need to team up with AI/AN leaders and national advocacy organizations. Researchers by themselves are seldom in a position to advocate for policy change. As we saw, the partnership between research and the National Indian Head Start Directors' Association was crucial in developing research that would support advocacy. Third, we should cultivate connections to Congressional members and develop brief legislative proposals that address the needs of the population. As the example of the Head Start reauthorization makes clear, congressional appropriations matter, and researchers in areas where AI/AN communities are a significant constituency can have a special impact. And, fourth, we should continue to work with program staff at the federal and state levels to make better use of the available resources over which they have discretion. Gaining an appropriation is significant; but playing a role in how it is actually spent is also significant, as we have learned in ongoing work with the ACF in the context of American Indian and Alaska Native Head Start.

Below we identify a set of specific advocacy opportunities:

1. Advocate for a nationwide reporting system especially among tribes since child abuse and neglect incidences are not collected and reported to national databases. It has been recommended that the Child Abuse Prevention and Treatment Act (CAPTA) should be amended to require the Bureau of Indian Affairs to collect this data and to require participation by tribal governments. The APA, NICWA, National Social Workers organization, the National Child Abuse organizations, and selected tribal leaders can work together to accomplish this task.

2. Increase the number of qualified mental health providers. In 2005, Joseph Stone testified before Congress on the issue of suicide and he recommended developing a "National Center for Excellence for suicide prevention in tribal communities coupled with increased funding for school-based mental health services to promote positive school environments" (p. 12, APA Monitor). Stone continues to emphasize the need for good data, collaborative suicide prevention efforts with at-risk families and communities, training mental health providers, physicians, nurses, social workers on signs and symptoms of depression and suicide, and screening of teens for depression and substance abuse.

3. Create partnerships between researchers and tribal leaders/communities. There is limited research coming out of Indian country and continued efforts must be made to overcome the distrust of tribes toward researchers and to increase the number of native investigators. The research opportunities we anticipate above all should appeal directly to the need to return benefit to AI/AN communities, increasing the possibility that research can be a viable career option for AI/AN students.

4. Increase funding to train tribal mental health and other staff at collaborating agencies to use evidence-based treatments. Bigfoot and Schmidt have developed a training program for AI/ANs at the Center on Child Abuse and Neglect at the University of Oklahoma Health Sciences Center which provides models for best practice in training the trainer in Indian country. There is probably no more urgent need than developing community capacity to respond to childhood traumatic stress.

We began this chapter with an overview of all the needs in AI/AN communities, and it is clear that, despite persistent advocacy, there remains a dearth of evidence to inform services for children and families and a lack of qualified professionals capable of delivering these services. These are the most important priorities for future work. At the same time, as the example of the National Indian Head Start Directors' Association and the reauthorization of Head Start make clear, there is tremendous untapped potential in partnerships between researchers and community leaders to support advocacy for the needs of AI/AN children and families.

References

Alcantara, C., & Gone, J. P. (2007). Reviewing suicide in Native American communities: Situating risk and protective factors within a transactional-ecological framework. *Death Studies, 31,* 457–477.

Alcohol and suicide among racial/ethnic populations—17 States, 2005–2006. (2009). *Morbidity and Mortality Weekly Report, 58,* 637–641.

Barlow, A., Mullany, B., Neault, N., Davis, Y., Billy, T., Hastings, R., et al. (2010). Examining correlates of methamphetamine and other drug use in pregnant American Indian adolescents. *American Indian and Alaska Native Mental Health Research, 17*(1), 1–24.

Beals, J., Manson, S., Whitesell, N. R., Spicer, P., Novins, D. K., & Mitchell, C. M., for the AI-SUPERPFP Team (2005). Prevalence of DSM-IV disorders and attendant help-seeking in 2 American Indian reservation populations. *Archives of General Psychiatry, 62,* 99–108.

Beauvais, F., Jumper-Thurman, P., & Burnside, M. (2008). The changing patterns of drug use among American Indian students over the past thirty years. *American Indian and Alaska Native Mental Health Research, 15*(2), 15–24.

BigFoot, D.S., & Braden, J. (2007). Adapting Evidence Based Treatments for Use with American indian and Alaska Native Children and Youth. Portland Research and Training Center on Family Support and Children's Mental Health. *Focal Point Journal, 21*(1), 19–23.

Bigfoot, D. S., & Schmidt, S. (2006). *Honoring children, mending the circle (trauma-focused cognitive behavior therapy). A training and treatment manual developed by the Indian Country Child Trauma Center.* Oklahoma City, OK: University of Oklahoma Health Sciences Center.

Carneiro, P. & Heckman, J. (2003). *Human capital policy.* IZA Discussion Paper #821. Bonn: IZA.

Centers for Disease Control and Prevention. (2007). Retrieved March 30, 2012, from www.cdc.gov/violenceprevention/suicide.

Child maltreatment (2010) Washington, DC: USDHHS, ACF.

Cole, N. (2006). Trauma and the American Indian. In T. M. Witko (Ed.), *Mental health care for urban Indians: Clinical insights from Native practitioners* (pp. 115–130). Washington, DC: American Psychological Association.

Coteau, T. D., Anderson, J., & Hope, D. (2006). Adapting manualized treatments, treating anxiety disorders among Native Americans. *Cognitive and Behavioral Practice, 13,* 304–309.

Dixon, M., & Roubideaux, Y. (2001). *Promises to keep: Public health policy for American Indians and Alaska natives in the 21st century.* Washington, DC: American Public Health Association.

Evans-Campbell, T., Lindhorst, T., Huang, B., & Walters, K. L. (2006). Interpersonal violence in the lives of urban American Indian and Alaska Native women: Implications for health, mental health, and help-seeking. *American Journal of Public Health, 96,* 1416–1422.

Funderburk, B. W., Gurwitch, R., & Bigfoot, D. S. (2005). *Honoring children, making relatives (parent child interaction therapy training manual). A training manual.* Oklahoma City: Indian Country Child Trauma Center, University of Oklahoma Health Sciences Center.

Gone, J. P., & Alcantara, C. (2007). Identifying effective mental health interventions for American Indians and Alaska Natives: A review of the literature. *Cultural Diversity and Ethnic Minority Psychology, 13*(4), 356–363.

Gone, J. P., & Trimble, J. E. (2012). American Indian and Alaska Native mental health: Diverse perspectives on enduring disparities. *Annual Review of Clinical Psychology, 8,* 131–160.

Gray, J. (2009). *Testimony for the select committee on Indian affairs.* Washington, DC.

Greenfield, L. N., & Smith, S. K. (1999). *American Indians and crime.* Washington, DC: U.S. Department of Justice, Office of Justice Statistics.

Indian Health Service. (2002). *Demographic statistics section of regional differences in Indian health 2000–2001: Tables only.* Rockville, MD: Indian Health Service.

Indian Health Service. (2005). *Facts on Indian health disparities.* Retrieved from http://www.ihs.gov/factsheets/index.cfm?module=dsp_fact_disparities.

Kronk, E. & Thompson, H. (2007). Modern realities of the "jurisdictional maze" in Indian Country: Case studies on methamphetamine use and the pressures to ensure homeland security. *The Federal Lawyer, March/April,* 48–52.

LaFromboise, T. D., & Howard-Pitney, B. (1995). The Zuni life skills development curriculum: Description and evaluation of a suicide prevention program. *Journal of Counseling Psychology, 42,* 479–486.

LaFromboise, T. D., & Lewis, H. A. (2008). The Zuni life skills development program: A school/community-based suicide prevention intervention. *Suicide & Life-Threatening Behavior, 38,* 343–353.

Lomawaima, K. T., & McCarty, T. L. (2006). *To remain an Indian: Lessons in democracy from a century of Native American education.* New York: Teachers College Press.

May, P. (1996). Overview of alcohol abuse epidemiology for American Indian populations. In G. D. Sandefur, R. R. Rindfuss, & B. Cohen (Eds.), *Changing numbers, changing needs: American Indian demography and public health* (pp. 235–261). Washington, DC: National Academy Press.

National Drug Intelligence Center, US Department of Justice. (2008). *Indian country drug threat* (Assessment DOC. ID 2008-RO958-002). Washington, DC: Author.

National Institute on Drug Abuse. (2009). *Info facts: Methamphetamine.* Rockville, MD: National Institutes of Health–U.S. Department of Health and Human Services.

Novins, D. K., & Best, G. (2011). Systems of mental health care for American Indian and Alaska Native children and adolescents. In M. C. Sarche, P. Spicer, P. Farrell, & H. E. Fitzgerald (Eds.), *American Indian and Alaska Native children and mental health: Development, context, prevention, and treatment* (pp. 189–204). Santa Barbara, CA: ABC-CLIO.

Oden, H. (Ed.). (2003). *Addressing domestic violence in Indian Country: Introductory manual.* Deluth, MN: Sacred Hoop Technical Assistance Project.

Oetzel, J., & Duran, B. (2004). Intimate partner violence in American Indian and/or Alaska Native communities. A social ecological framework of determinants and interventions. *American Indian and Alaska Native Mental Health Research, 11,* 49–68.

Olson, L. M., & Wahab, S. (2006). American Indians and suicide. A neglected area of research. *Trauma, Violence & Abuse, 7,* 19–33.

Reyhner, J., & Eder, J. (2004). *American Indian education: A history.* Norman, OK: University of Oklahoma Press.

Sarche, M. C., & Spicer, P. (2008). Poverty and health disparities for American Indian and Alaska Native children: Current knowledge and future prospects. *Annals of the New York Academy of Science, 1136,* 126–136.

Spicer, P., Beals, J., Mitchell, C. M., Novins, D. K., Croy, C. D., Manson, S., et al. (2003). The prevalence of alcohol dependence in two American Indian reservation populations. *Alcoholism, Clinical and Experimental Research, 27*(11), 1789–1797.

Spicer, P., Bigfoot, D. S., Funderburk, B. W., & Novins, D. K. (2012). Evidence-based practice and early childhood intervention in American Indian and Alaska Native communities. *Zero To Three, 32*(4), 19–23.

Spicer, P., & Sarche, M. C. (2012). *Poverty and possibility in the lives of American Indian and Alaska Native children* (The Oxford handbook of poverty and child development, pp. 480–488). Oxford: Oxford University Press.

Stone, J. (2005). *Testimony to congress on suicide in Indian country* (p. 12). Washington, DC: American Psychological Association Monitor.

Szlemko, W. J., Wood, J. W., & Jumper-Thurman, P. (2006). Native Americans and alcohol: Past, present and future. *The Journal of General Psychology, 133*(4), 435–451.

U.S. Department of Health and Human Services. (2001). *Mental health: Culture, race, and ethnicity. A supplement to mental health: Report of the Surgeon General.* Rockville, MD: Author.

Willis, D. J. (1990). *Testimony on American Indian mental health for the committee on Interior and Insular Affairs.* Washington, DC.

Willis, D. J. (1992). *Testimony on child abuse and neglect in Indian country. Committee on Interior and Insular Affairs.* Washington, DC.

Willis, D. J. (2000). American Indians: The forgotten race. *The Clinical Psychology of Ethnic Minorities, 8*(3), 1–2.

Willis, D. J. (2002). Economic, health and mental health disparities among ethnic minority children and families. *Journal of Pediatric Psychology, 27*, 305–314.

Willis, D. J. (2003). Best practices with special populations. *Clinical Psychologist, 56*(1), 1–4.

Willis, D. J., & Bigfoot, D. (2003). On native soil: The forgotten race: American Indians. In J. D. Robinson & L. C. James (Eds.), *Diversity in human interaction: The tapestry of America* (pp. 77–91). NY: Oxford University Press.

Willmon-Haque, S., & Bigfoot, D. S. (2008). Violence and the effects of trauma on American Indian and Alaska Native populations. *Journal of Emotional Abuse, 8*(1), 51–66.

Willmon-Haque, S., & Bigfoot, D. S. (2009). Violence and the effects of trauma on American Indian and Alaska Native populations. In R. Geffner, D. Griffin, & J. Lewis III (Eds.), *Children exposed to violence: Current issues, interventions and research* (pp. 48–63). New York: Routledge.

Wilson, J. (1998). *The earth shall weep: A history of Native America.* New York: Grove Press.

Zuckerman, S., Haley, J. M., Roubideaux, Y., & Lillie-Blanton, M. (2004). Access, use, and insurance coverage among American Indians/Alaska Natives and Whites: What role does the Indian Health Service play? *American Journal of Public Health, 94*, 53–59.

Part III
Illustrations of Advocacy Practices

Chapter 14
A Multilevel Framework for Local Policy Development and Implementation

Sharon Hodges and Kathleen Ferreira

Children and families deserve to have confidence that the services and supports they receive are the most effective interventions available. The concept of evidence-based and promising practices has developed as a strategy for achieving improved mental health outcomes for children and families in recent years, and the implementation of evidence-based and promising practices has grown more influential in the United States (Raghavan, Bright, & Shadoin, 2008; Tanenbaum, 2003). The term evidence-based practices (sometimes called EBPs) refers to prevention or treatment approaches that are supported by documented scientific evidence (e.g., research results from randomized or quasi-experimental designs). Promising practices are those which, although lacking a rigorous base of research evidence, show promising field-based or theoretical support. These might include locally developed services and supports intended to meet the specific strengths and needs of local populations.

Federal mental health policy has used multiple strategies to encourage the adoption of evidence-based practices that include providing databases that catalogue specific practices (e.g., NREPP, 2012), legislatively linking federal funding to evidence-based practice implementation (e.g., Maternal, Infant, and Early Childhood Home Visiting Program, 2010), providing research opportunities (e.g., IP-RISP, 2006) and providing training and technical assistance (e.g., Science of Dissemination and Implementation Conference, 2012). Less visible is the important role of local policy in the implementation of evidence-based and promising practices and its influence on positive outcomes for children and families.

What local policy infrastructure is necessary to maximize community investment in the implementation of evidence-based practices? What local policy structures

S. Hodges, Ph.D., M.B.A. (✉) • K. Ferreira, Ph.D.
Division of Training, Research, Education, and Demonstration, Department of Child and Family Studies, College of Behavioral and Community Sciences, Louis de la Parte Florida Mental Health Institute, University of South Florida, 13301 Bruce B Downs Blvd, MHC 2437, Tampa, FL 33612-3807, USA
e-mail: sphodges@usf.edu

A. McDonald Culp (ed.), *Child and Family Advocacy: Bridging the Gaps Between Research, Practice, and Policy*, Issues in Clinical Child Psychology,
DOI 10.1007/978-1-4614-7456-2_14, © Springer Science+Business Media New York 2013

support community implementation and sustainability of best practices for positive child and family outcomes? Local policy has the power to influence evidence-based and promising practice implementation by establishing prevailing standards of practice across provider agencies, by impacting the service planning and delivery decisions of local funding and administrative authorities, and by shaping expectations of community stakeholders (Hodges, Ferreira, & Israel, 2012; O'Toole & Montjoy, 1984; Percival, 2009; Proctor, 2004). More specifically, local policy supports improved child and family outcomes by ensuring that (1) interventions meet needs of an identified local population, (2) interventions are implemented as intended, and (3) services are sustainable over time (Hernandez & Hodges, 2001, 2003; Hodges et al., 2007).

This chapter will discuss the role of communities in local policy formation and will describe a policy framework for implementation of services and supports serving local children and families that is based on findings of a 3-year study of local infrastructure and field-based practice (Sustainable Infrastructure Project, 2007).[1] Policy in this case refers to courses of action adopted and pursued by local communities to implement a variety of programs and interventions including evidence-based, promising, and locally developed practices. Policy can include procedures and protocols for action as well as guidelines for decision making. The framework described in this chapter posits three levels of local policy considered critical to service implementation: provider-level, system-level, and funder-level policy. Each of these levels will be discussed, and a case study that incorporates these components will be described. In addition, the framework includes a shared value base and five core action domains that support the implementation of evidence-based and promising practices. The action domains include the Intervention Intent, Communication, Administrative Leadership, Staff Development and Support, and Evaluation domains. Students of child and family advocacy should reflect upon both professional goals and their own experiences as they consider how this framework might support improved mental health outcomes for children and family. Whether professionally or as a potential consumer of services, readers may find that their role in advocacy efforts vary over time in terms policy level and domain of action.

Policy Formation at the Local Level

Implementation of services and supports varies considerably across states and communities depending upon administrative and funding jurisdictions of states, counties, and municipalities as well as local political context. For example, an

---

[1] The Sustainable Infrastructure Project was established as a collaboration between a university research team from the Department of Child and Family Studies at the University of South Florida and a group of local intervention partners that included funders, administrative authorities, provider agencies, and families for the purpose of developing local policy to support, improve and sustain best practice in local programs. The levels and domains of the policy framework were identified through interview and observational data collected and analyzed over a 3-year period.

evidence-based or promising practice may be implemented across multiple local agencies, each having its own intra-agency administration as well as vision, mission, and goals that potentially differ from each other. In addition, the activities of these provider agencies take place in the context of other community entities such as interagency collaboratives as well as governing and funding authorities. The literature suggests that local policy formation involves community engagement at multiple levels (Percival, 2009; Ploeg, Davies, Edwards, Gifford, & Miller, 2007). Further, multilevel policy is critical because it supports cross-agency collaboration and governance and can be a determining factor in implementation success (Adelman & Taylor, 2002; Center for Mental Health in Schools, UCLA, 2004; Fagan & Mihalic, 2003; Mihalic & Irwin, 2003). Data from the Sustainable Infrastructure Project indicate that three key levels of local policy are necessary to maximize community investment in the implementation of services and supports: practice level, system level, and funder level.

Practice-Level Policy provides guidance and oversight to *intra-agency activities* of provider organizations, such as Wraparound teams, through which services are delivered directly to children and families. The implementation of evidence-based and promising practices is, perhaps, more concrete and easily observed at this level because it is the level at which children and families receive direct services. The role of practice-level policy is to provide intra-agency leadership, administration, and management to ensure that services and supports are delivered to children and families with fidelity to the program intent and implementation values.

System-Level Policy provides guidance and oversight to *cross-agency activities* of community collaboratives such as interagency children's councils and management teams. This level has direct impact on how children and families experience services because it supports the coordinated implementation of services and supports. The role of system-level policy in the implementation of evidence-based and promising practices may be less obvious to children and families because it operates at the level of service infrastructure and serves as a link between the practice and funder levels. System-level policy is particularly important when program implementation requires managing and supporting service planning and delivery across agency settings and contexts. The role of system-level policy in service implementation is to provide the cross-agency leadership, administration, and management necessary to support the consistent implementation of the intervention with fidelity to the program intent and implementation values.

Funder-Level Policy provides guidance and oversight for *community-wide activities* of community organizations that provide local governance and fiscal authority for programs being implemented. This level is likely the most abstract from the perspective of children and families because it acts to facilitate evidence-based and promising practice implementation in service of the community as a whole rather than at the level of individual provider agencies. Funder-level policy can be the responsibility of organizations such as Boards of County Commissioners, United Way and other charitable community organizations, or a variety of community-based organizations that serve as fiscal agents for local, state, and federal funds. The role of funder-level policy is to establish a definition of the intended program intervention in partnership with stakeholders and to provide guidelines necessary to support accountability in accordance with community values, needs, and program intent. The funder-level has responsibility for policy decisions that affect community-based services and supports across agencies and programs as well as establishing community-wide funding strategies and community-wide program goals and outcomes. The funder level also holds the key community responsibility for building and maintaining system infrastructure and linking an intervention to community values and principles. Funder-level responsibilities include maintaining clarity around how policy changes affect community-wide goals and outcomes and ensuring that policy changes reflect community needs and strengths.

The Role of Values in Local Policy and Advocacy

As readers reflect upon each of the policy levels described above, it is important to consider the key role that shared values play in the local implementation of services and supports. Data from the Sustainable Infrastructure Project (2007) highlight the importance of shared values and beliefs in providing a foundation for the local policy framework and support advocacy efforts related to the implementation of programs and practices that both meet local needs and build upon local strengths. Four key values could be considered critical to local policy formation:

1. Policy supports shared understanding of the intent of programs and practices across implementation levels and community stakeholders.
2. Policy ensures program consistency and quality of services and supports within and across provider agencies.
3. Policy supports the ability of provider agencies to maintain intervention fidelity while adapting to varying implementation contexts including geographic location, individualization of services and supports (including culturally appropriate adaptations), and differing provider agency contexts.
4. Policy supports the active utilization of evaluation data in decisions related to program planning and service delivery.

Because values and beliefs have the potential to guide actions taken across all levels of policy, they can have broad impact on service planning and implementation. For example, if shared values support serving children with serious mental health needs in the least restrictive, most clinically appropriate settings, then actions across policy levels should reflect a shared commitment to community-based care as an alternative to more restrictive out-of-home placements. Under such circumstances, funder-level actions would ensure adequate funding for innovative community-based programs; system-level actions would facilitate cross-agency support for programs such as community-based day-treatment programs that allow children to attend school while receiving appropriate clinical care; and practice-level actions would identify a variety of formal and informal resources that might be needed to support successful functioning in a community-based setting.

Core Action Domains

Giving consideration to the policy levels and values described above, the reader will note that successful local implementation of evidence-based and promising practices requires taking action across a complex and multilevel environment. What kinds of activities are essential to successful implementation strategies? Data from the Sustainable Infrastructure Project suggest five core action domains are useful in local implementation of evidence-based and promising practices: Intervention Intent, Communication, Administrative Leadership, Staff Development and Support, and Evaluation. These domains support focused, goal-oriented actions on the part of service planners and implementers at all levels. Each of these domains incorporates implementation strategies for each policy level. Overall, practice-level strategies should attend to intra-agency issues and concerns; system-level strategies should focus on cross-agency elements of implementation; and funder-level strategies should emphasize successful implementation of evidence-based and promising practices community-wide and support the sustainability of interventions that are meeting community need.

The *Intervention Intent Domain* involves creating specificity and shared understanding around all components of the intervention intent of a particular service or support (e.g., vision/mission, values and principles, population of focus, intervention strategies, and goals/outcomes). A shared understanding of the components of a theory of intervention is the foundation upon which other implementation strategies are built (Patton, 2008; Weiss, 1995). Mihalic and Irwin (2003) and emphasizes the importance of having clarity around program intent as a necessary component of assessing a program's effectiveness. At each level, local action related to intervention intent should support alignment of local practice with the intended vision/mission, values and principles, population of focus, strategies, and outcomes of the intervention to ensure that it is implemented in response to community need (Hodges, Ferreira, & Israel, 2012). Specific strategies include gaining clarity and shared understanding of the intent of the program for individuals involved at the practice, system, and funder levels. This can be accomplished through group activities such as program planning based on a theory of change logic model process (Hernandez & Hodges, 2003).

The *Communication Domain* involves action related to communicating aspects of the intervention across all levels of implementation. Moseley and Hastings (2005) identify communication as the center of their change process, laying the foundation for implementation. They state that the primary purpose of communication is to disseminate the details of the intervention to all stakeholders, publicize upper-management support, and renew the commitments of stakeholders. A feedback loop whereby mechanisms and formal lines of communication are maintained is critical. Practice-level action in the communication domain includes intra-agency processes by direct care staff to facilitate access and availability of services and supports for families. System-level action in the communication domain includes activities that support cross-agency understanding and collaboration within the program as well as serving as a communication source for intervention information throughout the community. Funder-level action in the communication domain includes procedures to support community-wide planning and partnership for implementing the intervention. Specific strategies within this domain might include communication of program mission, vision, goals, and outcomes through cross-agency meetings, public documents, and press releases as well as creation of a website or use of other social media to serve as a community-wide portal of information. Resulting outcomes include communication of cohesive and consistent intervention information to stakeholders throughout the community.

The *Administrative Leadership Domain* involves action related to the provision of administrative and funding support across all levels of implementation. Fagan and Mihalic (2003) indicate that administrative leadership should include priority setting, resource allocation, scheduling, and social leadership. They also emphasize that leaders should maintain a clear vision of the goals of an intervention, communicating with staff the need to embrace the values and ideas of the intervention. Administrative leadership can champion the intervention by creating buy-in and involvement in the evidence-based and promising practices being implemented. Practice-level action for administrative leadership includes establishing intra-agency management and administration processes according to program expectations such as clearly articulated policies and procedures related to service eligibility, intake and assessment processes, and guidance on the appropriate duration of services. System-level action in this domain includes facilitating cross-agency management and administration through the development of mechanisms such as cross-agency policies, contracts, and procedures. Funder-level administrative leadership action includes clear provision of funding guidelines and adequate funding to support both the intervention and its implementation. This might focus on identification of services eligible for billing to third-party payers (e.g., Medicaid) and documentation needed to ensure reimbursement.

The *Staff Development and Support Domain* involves action related to recruitment, hiring, training, coaching, supervision, and evaluation of staff (Durlak, 1998; Fixsen, Naoom, Blase, Friedman, & Wallace, 2005; Gottfredson & Gottfredson, 2002; Mihalic & Irwin, 2003). As the implementation of evidence-based practices and programs become more of a national phenomenon, staff development and support issues will likely become much more important (Fixsen et al., 2005). Practice-level action in this domain can include policies and procedures specific to intra-agency activities of recruiting, hiring, training, coaching, supervision, and staff evaluation according to program guidelines. System-level action might include cross-agency guidelines for staff development and support; and funder-level policy should attend to community-wide issues of staff development such as training on budget reporting requirements and third-party billing processes that can challenge the capacity of an individual agency or cross-agency collaborative.

The *Evaluation Domain* involves policy related to quality improvement and accountability activities. Literature on program implementation emphasizes evaluation and utilization of results as important components of successful implementation (Fagan & Mihalic, 2003; Harachi, Abbott, Catalano, Haggerty, & Fleming, 1999; Hernandez & Hodges, 2001; Mihalic & Irwin, 2003). This should include attention to the quality of implementation, particularly assessments of how a program is being implemented in comparison with its stated intent (Fagan & Mihalic, 2003). Good evaluation should generate useful feedback to guide implementation (Kubisch, Fulbright-Anderson, & Connell, 1998). Program evaluation can be compared to auditing in that there is a need to have frequent and timely examination of the integrity of the intervention, implementation, and organizational support, with the goal being to facilitate continuous improvement (Moseley & Hastings, 2005). At the practice-level, evaluation policy includes data collection and analysis related to intra-agency decision making for program improvement and participating in evaluation activities as required by other levels of implementation. This would include specific guidelines for quality assurance and data reporting requirements relevant to child and family level outcomes. System-level actions might include data collection and analyzes related to cross-agency decisions for program improvement such as training needs or gaps in the array of available services and supports. Funder-level evaluation actions might include community-wide assessments of benefits relative to costs, particularly establishing the ability of an evidence-based or promising practice to meet identified community needs at a sustainable cost.

Case Study: Local Policy in Action

To conclude this chapter, we present a case study of program implementation. This case provides an opportunity to apply the concepts presented in this chapter to local program implementation. The case narrative provides a description of implementation issues in a fictitious case management program and suggests a number of different implementation strategies that could be pursued. Using the policy framework presented in this chapter, readers will find multiple opportunities to consider procedures and protocols for action as well as guidelines for decision making. The case narrative provides readers with (1) background information on the fictitious program; (2) initial findings of an evaluation team hired to examine program implementation; and (3) discussion prompts focused on how the policy framework in this chapter can be applied to specific aspects of the case. These prompts can be completed through group discussion, written class assignment, or as part of a training activity. Following a discussion of the case, readers can choose to focus their attention on a specific action domain (e.g., Staff Development and Support or Communication) and develop strategies appropriate for each of the policy levels (practice, system, and funder) presented in the framework. The case can also be used as a tool to discuss the role and purpose of evaluation or as an opportunity to further examine the issues uncovered by the evaluation team in the case.

Background. You are a member of a multidisciplinary university-based evaluation team that has been asked to assess Community Supports, a long-standing community-based case management program that has operated for more than 15 years in the fictitious Valley County. Located in the western United States, Valley County is comprised of urban, suburban, and rural communities and has a total population of more than one million people. According to the most recent U.S. Census data, residents of Valley County are 53 % White non-Hispanic, 20 % Black, 25 % Hispanic, and 2 % classified as Other. Almost 30 % of the population falls below the federal poverty level, with concentrations of poor families exceeding 70 % in certain geographic areas of the county.

Community Supports provides case management services in both school and home settings for elementary-aged children in grades 3–5 and whom teachers and/ or other school personnel identify as at risk of school failure and have behavioral challenges. As a strategy for providing coverage across this large and diverse county, the funder contracts with five different nonprofit agencies to provide Community Supports services. Schools refer children to the Community Supports provider in their catchment area. Provider agencies are expected to conduct behavioral and psychosocial assessments for children at intake and develop a strengths-based plan with families that will link them to existing services Valley County. These services often include tutoring for the child, individual and family counseling, although case managers might also link families to services that meet a variety of other identified needs such as food banks, housing assistance, or Medicaid health benefits. The funder indicates that Community Supports case management is a short-term intervention intended to be completed within 4–6 months of the initial assessment.

Community Supports, like many long-standing community-based programs, has not been formally established as evidence based. There is, however, considerable stakeholder support for Community Supports as an established field-based practice and there is a theoretical basis for early intervention efforts that support school success. The increasing emphasis on adopting evidence-based practices presents a unique challenge for communities like Valley County. Although evidence-based practices can expand the service capacity of a community, it is challenging for communities to weigh their benefits against those of locally developed promising practices such as Community Supports.

The funder of Community Supports has asked your team to develop program planning, implementation, and evaluation strategies that support, improve and sustain best practice in Community Supports. Your team's objectives are to analyze the implementation of Community Supports and recommend how Community Supports can integrate best practice into program implementation. The funder would also like you to document lessons learned so that these results can be used to improve the implementation of other locally developed promising practices.

Initial Team Findings. You and your team conduct interviews, observations, and document review with Community Supports stakeholders at the practice, system, and funder levels. You uncover a number of challenges related to the congruence of Community Supports intervention strategies across provider agencies. Key team observations are summarized below:

- The population of children served by Community Supports varies considerably across providers. Although some providers focus services on children in grades 3–5, others serve children both younger and older than the designated population.
- Your data indicate that there is variation across Community Supports provider agencies regarding length of services. Rather than provide a short-term intervention

as is indicated by the program model, some agencies carry youth on their caseloads for up to 24 months.

- Your review of documents indicates that the primary function of Community Supports is case management and *linking* children and families to necessary services and supports. Your interview data indicate that some case managers provide direct therapeutic care and tutoring services to enrolled children.
- Community Supports providers report that other community agencies, some of them large and politically powerful, refer numerous children and youth into Community Supports who do not meet program eligibility requirements.
- Community Supports providers report that they are not clear as to the number of children they are expected to serve each year, the appropriate case load for case managers, and whether children who receive Medicaid are a priority population.
- Overall, your data indicate that the expectations for child and family outcomes are unclear (e.g., the funder tracks changes in student grades, changes in social and behavioral functioning, and satisfaction with services), and results vary considerably across Community Supports providers.

Next Steps. Consider the background information presented about Community Supports as well as the findings of your evaluation team. Use the components of the framework presented in this chapter as you complete the activities below. Remember that your goal should be in service of producing positive outcomes for children and families.

1. Identify shared values that would support more consistent implementation of Community Supports across provider agencies (Note: values should be infused across levels and action domains).
2. Identify implementation inconsistencies across the three policy levels. What strategies would you recommend for addressing these inconsistencies? (Remember: focusing recommendations on a single level is likely to be ineffective).
3. Using the five core action domains as a guide, what strategies would you recommend for strengthening the implementation of Community Supports?
4. Can you identify any ethical issues arising out of the work your team has done? If so, what are they, and how would you facilitate their resolution?
5. Overall, what advantages and disadvantages can you identify regarding the implementation of a locally developed community-based intervention compared to implementation of a nationally recognized evidence-based practice?

Conclusion

Service planning and delivery efforts should consider the important role of local policy infrastructure in achieving advocacy goals. Local policy plays a key role in ensuring that interventions serve the intended population, are implemented as intended, and are sustainable over time. This chapter provides a multilevel local policy framework that supports the implementation of evidence-based and promising practices for children and families. The action steps set forth across the core action domains and at each policy level support community implementation of evidence-based and promising practices as well as their sustainability. Ultimately, it is the role of values in local policy and advocacy that provides the foundation for local policy and supports advocacy efforts related to the implementation of programs and practices that meet local needs, build upon local strengths and produce positive child and family outcomes.

References

Adelman, H., & Taylor, L. (2002). *Safe and secure: Guides to creating safer schools—Guide 7: Fostering school, family and community involvement.* Portland, OR: Northwest Regional Educational Laboratory.

Center for Mental Health in Schools at UCLA. (2004). *An introductory packet on working together: From school-based collaborative teams to school-community higher education connections.* Los Angeles, CA: Author.

Durlak, J. A. (1998). Why program implementation is important. *Journal of Prevention & Intervention in the Community, 17*, 5–18.

Fagan, A. A., & Mihalic, S. (2003). Strategies for enhancing the adoption of school-based prevention programs: Lessons learned from the Blueprints for Violence Prevention replications of the Life Skills Training program. *Journal of Community Psychology, 31*(3), 235–253.

Fixsen, D. L., Naoom, S. F., Blase, K. A., Friedman, R. M., & Wallace, F. (2005). *Implementation research: A synthesis of the literature.* Tampa, FL: University of South Florida, Louis de la Parte Florida Mental Health Institute, The National Implementation Research Network (FMHI Publication #231).

Gottfredson, D. C., & Gottfredson, G. D. (2002). Quality of school-based prevention programs: Results from a national survey. *Journal of Research in Crime and Delinquency, 39*, 3–35.

Harachi, T. W., Abbott, R. D., Catalano, R. F., Haggerty, K. P., & Fleming, C. B. (1999). Opening the black box: Using process evaluation measures to assess implementation and theory building. *American Journal of Community Psychology, 27*, 711–731.

Hernandez, M., & Hodges, S. (2001). Theory-based accountability. In M. Hernandez & S. Hodges (Eds.), *Developing outcome strategies in children's mental health* (pp. 21–40). Baltimore, MD: Paul H. Brookes Publishing.

Hernandez, M., & Hodges, S. (2003). Building upon a theory of change for systems of care. *Journal of Emotional and Behavioral Disorders, 11*(1), 19–26.

Hodges, S., Ferreira, K., & Israel, N. (2012). "If we're going to change things, it has to be systemic:" systems change in children's mental health. *American Journal of Community Psychology, 49*(3–4), 526–37. doi:10.1007/s10464-012-9491-0.

Hodges, S., Ferreira, K., Mazza, J., Vaughn, B., Van Dyke, M., Mowery, D., et al. (2007). *Phase I report (Developing sustainable infrastructure in support of quality field-based practice series, FMHI # 248–2).* Tampa, FL: University of South Florida, Louis de la Parte Florida Mental Health Institute, Department of Child and Family Studies.

IP-RISP. (2006). Interventions and practice research infrastructure program. National Institute of Mental Health. Retrieved May 8, 2012, from: http://grants.nih.gov/grants/guide/pa-files/PAR-06-441.html.

Kubisch, A. C., Fulbright-Anderson, K., & Connell, J. P. (1998). Evaluating community initiatives: A progress report. In A. C. Kubisch, K. Fulbright-Anderson, & J. P. Connell (Eds.), *New approaches to evaluating community initiatives: Theory, measurement and analysis* (Vol. 2, pp. 1–13). Washington, DC: The Aspen Institute.

Maternal, Infant, and Early Childhood Home Visiting Program. (2010). Health Resources and Service Administration. Retrieved May 8, 2012, from: http://mchb.hrsa.gov/programs/homevisiting/

Mihalic, S. F., & Irwin, K. (2003). Blueprints for violence prevention: From research to real-world settings—factors influencing the successful replication of model programs. *Youth Violence and Juvenile Justice, 1*(4), 307–329.

Moseley, J. L., & Hastings, N. B. (2005). Implementation: The forgotten link on the intervention chain. *Performance Improvement, 44*(4), 8–14.

NREPP. (2012). National Registry of Evidence-Based Programs and Practices. Substance Abuse and Mental Health Services Administration. Retrieved May 8, 2012, from: http://www.nrepp.samhsa.gov/

O'Toole, L., & Montjoy, R. (1984). Interorganizational policy implementation: A theoretical perspective. *Public Administration Review, 44*(6), 491–503.

Patton, M. Q. (2008). *Utilization-focused evaluation*. Thousand Oaks, CA: Sage.

Percival, G. (2009). Exploring the influence of local policy networks on the implementation of drug policy reform: The case of California's Substance Abuse and Crime Prevention Act. *Journal of Public Administration Research and Theory, 19*(4), 795–815.

Ploeg, J., Davies, B., Edwards, N., Gifford, W., & Miller, P. E. (2007). Factors influencing best-practice guideline implementation: Lessons learned from administrators, nursing staff, and project leaders. *Wordviews on Evidence-Based Nursing, 4*(4), 210–219.

Proctor, E. (2004). Leverage points for the implementaion of evidencce-based practice. *Brief Treatment and Crisis Intervention, 4*(3), 227–242.

Raghavan, R., Bright, C. L., & Shadoin, A. L. (2008). Toward a policy ecology of implementation of evidence-based practices in public mental health settings. *Implementation Science, 3*, 26.

Science of Dissemination and Implementation: Research at the Crossroads. (2012). Conference sponsored by the National Institutes of Health, March 19–20, 2012. Retrieved May 8, 2012, from: http://conferences.thehillgroup.com/obssr/di2012/about.html

Sustainable Infrastructure Project. (2007). *Developing sustainable infrastructure in support of quality field-based practice*. Tampa, FL: University of South Florida, College of Behavioral and Community Sciences, Louis de la Parte Florida Mental Health Institute, Department of Child and Family Studies. Retrieved May 8, 2012, from: http://cfs.cbcs.usf.edu/projects-research/detail.cfm?id=375

Tanenbaum, S. (2003). Evidence-based practice in mental health: Practical weaknesses meet political strengths. *Journal of Evaluation in Clinical Practice, 2*, 287–301.

Weiss, C. (1995). Nothing as practical as good theory. In J. P. Connell (Ed.), *New approaches to evaluating community initiatives: Concepts, methods and contexts* (Vol. 1). Washington, DC: Aspen Institute.

Chapter 15
When Evidence and Values Collide: Preventing Sexually Transmitted Infections

Brian L. Wilcox and Arielle R. Deutsch

In the following pages, we will lay the groundwork for, and then recount, an advocacy effort focused on adolescent reproductive health, one that specifically addressed state school board policy around the delivery of school-based services to prevent sexually transmitted infections (STI). We begin with some background regarding STI among adolescents, along with a summary of what is known about effective prevention models. As we turn to the advocacy case study we will switch to the first-person narrative form, as the first author undertook this effort, and the story is more readily told in this manner.

Sexually Transmitted Infections and Adolescents

In the past 20 years there have been marked improvements in some aspects of adolescent sexual health in the United States. However, even with these improvements, the United States lags behind other industrialized nations on many indicators of sexual health, and it is obvious that adolescent sexual health is an area in need of attention. While rates of unintended pregnancies among adolescents have shown encouraging declines since the late 1980s, some other aspects of adolescent reproductive health have not shown similar improvements. Foremost among the troublesome trends is the very high rate of sexually transmitted infections among adolescents. If these infections were merely annoyances that could be easily identified and treated, with no lasting complications, concern for the high levels of infections

B.L. Wilcox, Ph.D. (✉)
Center on Children, Families and the Law, University of Nebraska,
206 S. 13th Street Suite 1000, Lincoln, NE 68588-0227, USA
e-mail: bwilcox@unl.edu

A.R. Deutsch, Ph.D.
Department of Psychological Sciences, University of Missouri, Columbia, MO, USA

A. McDonald Culp (ed.), *Child and Family Advocacy: Bridging the Gaps Between Research, Practice, and Policy*, Issues in Clinical Child Psychology,
DOI 10.1007/978-1-4614-7456-2_15, © Springer Science+Business Media New York 2013

would be unwarranted. Unfortunately, among adolescents, many STI go unidentified and untreated, and result in serious health consequences, particularly for females.

To understand the problem of STI among adolescents, it helps to understand some basic characteristics of adolescent sexual behavior, as the common defining characteristic of all STI is that they are *sexually transmitted*. Slightly less than half of all teenagers in the United States report having had sexual intercourse, with percentages ranging from 46 % in the Youth Risk Behavior Survey (YRBS) (Centers for Disease Control and Prevention, 2010) to 43 % in the National Survey of Family Growth (NSFG) (Centers for Disease Control and Prevention, 2011a). This rate has slowly been declining for the past 20 years; by comparison, 51 % of females and 60 % of males reported ever having had sexual intercourse in 1988. Much of this decline occurred prior to 2002. The proportion of youth reporting having had sexual intercourse has not changed significantly from 2002 to 2006–2010 for either males or females. The prevalence of having ever had sexual intercourse is higher among some ethnic minority groups than others. Black males are more likely to have had sex compared to their White and Hispanic peers, and Hispanic males are more likely to have had sex compared to white males. For females, black adolescents are more likely to have had sexual intercourse compared to their white and Hispanic peers, while white adolescents are more likely to have had sex compared to Hispanic youth, although these ethnic group differences are not always significant (CDC, 2011a). The average age at which teens first have sex is 17, which is comparable to the average age of onset in other industrialized countries (Darroch, Singh, & Frost, 2001). However, this again can vary by ethnic group: black adolescents, particularly males, are more likely to have first sexual intercourse before age 13 compared to their Hispanic or White peers. Most teenagers report having had few sexual partners; 26 % of females and 29 % of males report having more than one sexual partner (CDC, 2011a), while 13.8 % of youth report having had four or more sexual partners (CDC, 2010). This rate is higher for older, male, and black adolescents.

A smaller percentage of adolescents are considered "sexually active," that is, those reporting having had intercourse recently. Approximately 30 % of teenagers report having had sex at least once in the past 3 months (CDC, 2010, 2011a), with older adolescents more likely to be sexually active than younger adolescents, and black adolescents more likely than Hispanic or white adolescents. However, variations exist by gender and ethnicity: ethnic differences among female adolescents are much less pronounced than ethnic differences among male adolescents (CDC, 2011a).

These behavioral data provide important insights into the potential risk for exposure to STI, as it is well understood that adolescents who initiate sexual activity at very early ages, and engage in sex frequently with multiple partners are at especially high risk (Aral & Holmes, 1990). Reducing rates of these behaviors becomes one of the goals of adolescent STI preventative interventions.

Compared to adults, adolescents are disproportionately affected by STI. Although youth make up only 25 % of the sexually active population, it is estimated that they account for half of all new cases of STI per year (Weinstock, Berman, & Cates, 2004). Not only is this a serious health issue, but an economic one as well. In the year 2000 alone, the estimated economic burden for treatment of STI among youth was $6.5 billion dollars (Chesson, Blandford, Gift, Tao, & Irwin, 2004). For many STI, including chlamydia, gonorrhea, and the human papillomavirus (HPV), the adolescent age group annually makes up the highest proportion of all individuals who are diagnosed, and seroprevalence studies likewise indicate that rates for these STI are higher in adolescents than adults (CDC, 2008, 2011b). In 2010, rates of chlamydia for adolescents between the ages of 15 and 19 were 3,378.2 per 100,000 for females and 774.3 per 100,000 for males. Rates for gonorrhea among adolescents in 2010 were 570.0 per 100,000 for females and 253.4 per 100,000 for males (CDC, 2011b). The most prevalent STI in the United States, HPV, also hits teens particularly hard. Approximately 35 % of youth between ages 15 and 19 have had an HPV infection (CDC, 2011b), a virus linked to both genital warts and several forms of cancer, especially ovarian cancer (CDC, 2011c). While there is no test for the presence of HPV among males, rates of treatment for complications from HPV are significantly higher among females than males. These data underscore the serious gender disparities regarding STI rates. Young females are more susceptible to infection, and experience far more serious complications, than their male age mates. There are also ethnic differences in STI rates: chlamydia and gonorrhea disproportionally affect black female youth ages 15–19, compared to either black males or white females.

Youth ages 13–19 made up only approximately 5 % of the new HIV cases reported in 2009 (CDC, 2011d). Black male teens are disproportionately diagnosed with HIV compared to their peers; in 2009 73 % of teens diagnosed with HIV were black, compared to 13 % Hispanic and 12 % white youth. Males accounted for 77 % of cases among adolescents in 2009 (CDC, 2011e). Most transmission in teens is due to male-to-male sexual contact. In 2009, 90.8 % of new cases were due to male–male contact, 4.6 % due to heterosexual contact, and 2.5 % due to male–male contact paired with injection drug use.

Longitudinal studies indicate that the incidence of some STI have increased over time. For HIV/AIDS, while incidence has decreased between 1997 and 2006 for females, it has increased among males ages 15–19, doubling from 1.3 to 2.6 per 1,000 individuals (CDC, 2009). Other STI rates, including chlamydia and HPV, have also increased among teens. The incidence of gonorrhea has largely stabilized since 1997, after a 20-year trend of decreasing. Syphilis, while increasing among teens between 2004 and 2009 (reflecting a general increasing trend globally), decreased slightly in 2010 (CDC, 2011b).

While global comparisons for most STI are difficult to make due to differences in screening and reporting, analyses indicate that compared to other western industrialized countries (including Canada and all of Europe), the United States has the highest rate of teenagers currently living with HIV/AIDS (UNICEF, 2011). Similar trends are found for other STI, although these comparisons are not as recent (Panchaud, Singh, Feivelson, & Darroch, 2000).

In summary, many STI can be considered to be epidemic among US adolescents. Incidence rates are higher for teens than for adults in many cases, and available evidence suggests that these rates are higher for US teens than for youth in other similar countries. The health toll of STI is considerable, especially for females, who face increased risk for a variety of cancers, pelvic inflammatory disease, ectopic pregnancy, and infertility (Eng & Butler, 1997). And, as previously noted, the economic burden of STI among adolescents is extremely high. Clearly, existing public health policy and practice has yet to yield a highly successful response to this hidden epidemic.

Preventing Adolescent STI: What Are Our Options? What Are Communities Trying?

In the mid-1990s, a committee was convened by the Institute of Medicine (a group chartered by the National Academy of Sciences) to examine the nature of the STI epidemic, catalogue and evaluate current prevention and treatment approaches in the US, and offer recommendations to guide public health-related programs, practices, policymaking, and research. In their report (Eng & Butler, 1997), the committee described the most promising preventative approaches. Not surprisingly, given the behavioral underpinnings of STI, most prevention efforts are built around the goal of changing a set of behaviors that either increase (risk behaviors) or decrease (protective behaviors) the risk of infection. For example, preventative interventions often attempt to reduce an array of sexual risk behaviors highly associated with increased rates of STI. These include (a) early onset of sexual intercourse, (b) high frequency of intercourse, (c) high number of sexual partners, (d) sex with high-risk partners, and (e) failure to use a barrier contraceptive method (Aral, 1994). As many such interventions are grounded in behavior change models such as the Theory of Reasoned Action or the Health Belief Model (National Cancer Institute, 2005), they also focus on altering participants' perceptions of risk and behavioral intentions. A good deal of research indicates that young Americans significantly underestimate their level of risk for STI (Ethier, Kershaw, Niccolai, Lewis, & Ickovics, 2003), so getting adolescents to develop more accurate perceptions regarding their STI risk is one key to motivating changes in behavioral intentions and actual behavior, although this is insufficient in and of itself to produce such changes.

Beyond behavioral approaches to reducing the risk for STI, there have been some successes on the biomedical front, but they are limited. To date, vaccines have been developed for only two of the major STIs: Hepatitis B and HPV. The relatively recent development of the HPV vaccine represents a significant achievement, given that the vaccine appears to prevent the major HPV subtypes responsible for cervical cancer and most cases of genital warts. Nevertheless, uptake of the vaccine remains relatively low: a recent report based on data from the 2010 National Immunization Survey-Teen found that only 34.8 % of teen girls had received all three doses of the vaccine (Dorell et al., 2012).

While an array of behavioral intervention approaches has been developed to target adolescents, the model that has the potential to reach the largest percentage of teens is the school-based intervention. Individual interventions, while often effective, reach a miniscule portion of the population, and nonschool, community-based interventions have shown promise but have never been widely implemented. Schools, as the saying goes, are where youth can be found; thus, the remainder of this section will focus on school-based interventions.

During the height of the HIV epidemic, a large percentage of schools across the country, with assistance from the federal Centers for Disease Control, developed curricula to address HIV and other STI. In some cases these curricula were freestanding units offered as part of some required course. More often, the HIV/STI prevention material was folded into existing sex education units within health courses. When asked about STI knowledge, most adolescents report that the majority of their information was obtained at school (American Social Health Association, 1996), as part of sex education courses or units. Sex education is a natural place to embed STI information, given that many of the methods used to reduce STI risk also reduce teen pregnancy risk, which is often a central goal of sex education curricula.

The obvious challenge to situating STI prevention within schools, and with sex education curricula, is that sex education in schools emerged as a hot button political issue in the 1980s. It was the battle over competing visions of STI and sex education that precipitated the advocacy effort later described in this chapter.

Prior to the advent of the HIV epidemic, sex education was only sporadically available in US schools, and often consisted in little more than a few lectures (often with the genders sent to separate classrooms). Even this minimal focus of sex and sexuality in the schools was enough to engender substantial controversy in communities, but for the most part the controversy sat in the background. However, the HIV epidemic brought calls for an increased focus on adolescent sexual health in the schools, and as the implementation of HIV and sex education curricula grew more widespread, so did the reactions from social conservatives who opposed these curricula on a variety of grounds, which will be discussed later. In response to this clash of viewpoints, social conservatives shifted their strategy and began developing and promoting a very different approach to sex education, one that was centered first and foremost around the promotion of sexual abstinence as a means to prevent teen pregnancies and STI (Luker, 2006; Moran, 2000). The "abstinence-only" movement received considerable support from political conservatives in Washington, DC, and the movement grew (for a brief history, see Wilcox, 1999). We now have a bifurcated "system" of sex education in the United States, with some young people receiving abstinence-only curricula and others receiving comprehensive sex education.

Abstinence-only education promotes sexual activity only within a marital relationship, emphasizing that this is the only certain way to prevent STI and pregnancy. There is little, if any, discussion of contraception or birth control, as abstinence-only proponents argue that such discussion could encourage (unsafe) premarital sexual activity. Most curricula that discuss condoms place the primary emphasis on their failure rate, and do not advocate their use to prevent infections. Comprehensive sexual education also emphasizes that abstinence is the best way to prevent unwanted pregnancies and STI, although there is also discussion about how to reduce STI risk while engaging in sexual activity by using condoms correctly. Proponents of comprehensive sexual education argue that such programs target both adolescents who will choose to remain abstinent as well as those who choose to (or may already have started to) engage in sexual activity (Kirby, 2008). Until very recently, most federal and state government funding was exclusively for abstinence-only sex education programs, thus influencing the choice between abstinence-only and comprehensive sex education programs for many school districts (Kantor, Santelli, Teitler, & Balmer, 2008). Over the past 15 years, a number of rigorous evaluations have generated a growing body of literature examining elements of the effectiveness of these contrasting models.

Comprehensive Sex Education

There is a growing set of studies suggesting that well-constructed and implemented comprehensive sex education programs can produce a variety of positive sexual health outcomes for youth, including reducing rates of risky sexual behaviors that are linked to STI. Kirby's (2008) analysis of 48 studies examining comprehensive sex education outcomes documented that two thirds of the programs had at least one positive sexual health outcome. These included delaying intercourse initiation, reducing the number of sexual partners, and increasing condom use and/or contraceptive use. A number of these programs (15 out of 24) had more than one positive outcome for reducing sexual risk. Finally, virtually all improved at least one factor influencing sexual health and behavior from the following: increased sexual health knowledge, more positive attitudes towards condoms and contraception, greater accuracy of risk perception, increased sexual efficacy (e.g., ability to refuse unwanted sex, engage in protective measures against STI/HIV and pregnancy), and better ability to communicate effectively with others about sexuality. A weakness of the collected evaluations is that none examined the actual impact of the program on rates of STI.

While comprehensive sex education shows promise in producing positive sexual health behaviors, attitudes, and intentions related to STI, how the programs are developed and implemented is important. Kirby (2007) documented 17 character-istics of effective sexual education programs, involving how the curricula are developed, curriculum content, and curriculum implementation. Effective interven-tions focus on the needs and characteristics of both the individuals targeted and the community's values and resources. Effective programs build skills designed to directly prevent STI and/or pregnancy, rather than deter teens from engaging in sexual intercourse.

While critics of comprehensive sex education argue that these programs present mixed messages about sexual behavior, addressing as they do both the value of abstain-ing from sexual intercourse and the virtues of safe sexual behaviors such as condom use, research also strongly supports the contention that comprehensive sex education does not promote sexual activity or hasten adolescents' sexual initiation, as some critics argue. Numerous reviews of the relevant research, including those by the Institute of Medicine (Eng & Butler, 1997) and National Campaign to Prevent Teen and Unplanned Pregnancy (2011b), point to the potential held by well-designed and implemented school-based comprehensive STI/sex education programs for reducing STI.

Abstinence-Only Sex Education

While federal support for abstinence-only sex education began with the 1981 Adolescent Family Life Act (AFLA), this demonstration program was miniscule in comparison to what has largely supplanted it. In 1996, as part of the welfare reform legislation passed by Congress, conservatives inserted a new funding stream for grants to states to support abstinence-only programs. Since 1996, federal support for abstinence-only education has expanded considerably. Over $1.5 billion have been spent on abstinence only education over the past 25 years by the federal government (SIECUS, 2009). This investment was somewhat surprising, given that none of the evaluations conducted of programs funded under AFLA showed any evidence of effectiveness in delaying onset of sexual activity. More recent highly rigorous evaluations of abstinence-only programs have also failed to find benefits from the programs. The legislation creating the program mandated a careful randomized experimental evaluation of a set of the most promising abstinence-only programs. The study, conducted by Mathematica Policy Research (MPR), found no evidence that the programs produced sustained attitudinal changes supportive of abstinence, and no evidence of even short-term change in any sexual behaviors (Trenholm et al., 2007). One of the few effects of these programs was that youth held misconceptions about the effectiveness of condoms in preventing STI. A recent review by Kirby (2008) concludes, with respect to abstinence-only programs, that there is little evidence that they achieve any of their program goals, namely, delaying sexual initiation, increasing sexually active teens' return to abstinence, or decreasing the number of sexual partners. Rates of early initiation of sexual intercourse and condom use are comparable for teens who participate in an abstinence-only program when compared to an untreated control group of their peers.

Similar findings were documented in evaluations of a genre of abstinence-only programs that emphasize virginity pledges (programs in which teens sign an agreement to delay sex until marriage). Bearman and Bruckner (2001) found that only in cases where a minority of students (approximately 30 %) in their school took a virginity pledge did doing so delay the initiation of sexual intercourse. If too many or too few students pledged virginity until marriage, there was no effect. Furthermore, although pledgers in the study did delay intercourse for a longer period of time than their peers, they were less likely to use condoms when they did engage in sex. The fact that the pledgers had STI rates comparable to their peers, even though they had fewer partners and were sexually active for shorter periods of time, indicates that pledging failed to create protective health outcomes (Bruckner & Bearman, 2005).

In summary, there is mounting evidence that comprehensive approaches to school-based STI/sex education can reduce a wide array of behaviors related to increased risk for STI and alter risk perceptions and behavioral intentions supportive of these protective behaviors. A few studies have found that well-crafted interventions can reduce rates of STI among participants, but the majority of studies have focused on behavior change and have not assessed the actual impact on STI. On the other hand, there is no evidence suggesting that abstinence-only programs produce lasting changes in attitudes or risk behaviors, and some evidence that they may have limited iatrogenic effects, leading participants to undervalue the effectiveness of condoms and consequently engage in unprotected sex once they become sexually active.

An STI Prevention Advocacy Effort: Precipitating Events and Goals

While I (Wilcox) was sitting in my university office one afternoon, two phone calls came through in rapid succession. A senior staff member from the State of Nebraska's Department of Health and Human Services and the director of education from the local Planned Parenthood affiliate called to announce that the State Board of Education had just proposed to officially endorse "abstinence-only HIV/STI education." In doing so, the state would make itself ineligible to receive grant funding for school-based HIV/STI prevention activities from the Centers for Disease Control, funds that the state had been receiving for a number of years. CDC required that funded efforts be evidence based, and believed strongly that abstinence-only programs failed to meet this criterion. The requests from both callers were straightforward: "you need to do something about this!" Both callers knew I had conducted research on the effectiveness of abstinence-only and comprehensive sex education programs, that I was a member of the National Campaign to Prevent Teen and Unplanned Pregnancy's Research and Effective Programs Task Force, and that I was serving on the Technical Advisory Workgroup for the MPR national evaluation of abstinence-only programs. As the local research resource on interventions related to adolescent reproductive health, they felt I might bring useful information to the discussions that would precede the process required to adopt a new STI prevention education policy. As a psychologist who had spent nearly 8 years involved in policy analysis and advocacy work with the American Psychological Association, I was drawn to the challenge like a moth to a flame.

Most advocacy efforts are proactive in nature. That is, the advocacy efforts are built around goals to create, expand, or improve services for a population in need. This effort, in contrast, was reactive; the overarching goal of the advocacy undertaking was to prevent the termination of existing policy (comprehensive STI education) and the establishment of new policy and related programs (abstinence-only STI policy and programs). We somewhat jokingly referred to our goal as "preventing the prevention of prevention."

State school board policymaking is, in contrast to legislative policymaking, a relatively closed process. School board members, unlike legislators, do not have a readily defined constituency with whom they regularly interact. Few citizens can name a single member of their state school board. While state school board meetings are open to the public, meetings are sparsely attended, and news coverage of state school board activities rarely occurs in advance of final action. In those rare instances where any coverage occurs, the reporting rarely makes reference to the votes cast by individual board members. Given this context, it seemed that the short-term strategy would necessitate an appeal to the board's members to consider an array of evidence related to the assumptions underlying their proposed policy change. Failing here, my colleagues and I felt, we might need to use other advocacy tools, such as direct appeals to the public and to key influential media sources.

As the researcher in the group, my task was relatively clear. I was expected to bring evidence to the board's deliberations in order to evaluate claims regarding the effectiveness of abstinence-only STI prevention programs and their critiques of comprehensive STI prevention programs. My expectations regarding the likely success of this strategy were modest: I knew from previous experience that policy-makers often give greater weight to their personal values than to empirical evidence when dealing with subjects where public values diverge markedly. I also knew that several new board members were social conservatives who had run stealth campaigns with the express purpose of getting elected so that they might tackle policy issues, such as school vouchers and sex education, which were of interest to their constituencies. Despite my doubts, we agreed that establishing a base of evidence in support of our position would be crucial regardless of the ultimate direction of the advocacy effort.

Advocacy in Action I: Sometimes You Lose

As expected, the State Board of Education posted an announcement on their website of their intention to hear public comments on their proposal to adopt guidelines for state school-based STI prevention programs built around abstinence-only principles. These guidelines, it bears noting, would only be advisory to local school districts. No school would be compelled to adopt them. Nevertheless, this policy action was likely to have two significant effects on STI prevention programs in the state. First, if passed, it would energize the small but vocal abstinence-only proponents in many communities and support their efforts to alter local school district STI prevention programs. Second, passage would immediately result in the loss of CDC STI prevention grants to the state, which would weaken existing programs even if they continued to adhere to a comprehensive model.

In preparation for the hearing, I developed a set of "fact sheets," each addressing a criticism of comprehensive programs or an argument supporting abstinence-only programs, as well as two more general background fact sheets dealing with adolescent sexual risk behaviors and STI among youth. In the case of these last two fact sheets, I included as much Nebraska-specific data as possible, as one argument being made by opponents of the existing comprehensive guidelines was that the entire issue of STI among youth was overblown.

My testimony, and the first set of fact sheets, focused primarily on the following four claims by the abstinence-only proponents: (1) parents oppose the discussion of condoms in schools and are generally opposed to comprehensive sex education approaches; (2) discussing condom use, and contraceptive use more generally, with youth increases the likelihood that they will engage in sexual activity; (3) abstinence is the only 100 % effective means of preventing STI; and (4) abstinence-only education is effective in delaying sexual activity.

Parental opposition. Fortuitously, several polls of parents had been conducted by groups such as the Kaiser Family Foundation, ABC News, and National Public Radio over the prior 5 years specifically asking parents about their support for or opposition to school-based instruction regarding condom use and safer sex techniques. In all cases, significant majorities (79–95 %) of parents reported that they felt that schools should give safer sex information, including information about proper condom use, to teen students, including those who were not yet sexually active. In response to a related question, significant majorities of parents (81–65 %) expressed a preference for comprehensive sex education when contrasted with abstinence-only approaches.

Talk of condoms leads to sexual activity. Again, fortuitously, this argument had been examined within the context of a number of studies of the effects of comprehensive sex education programs. Reviews of this literature by the World Health Organization (Grunseit & Kippax, 1993), the National Campaign to Prevent Teen Pregnancy (Kirby, 2007), and the Institute of Medicine (Eng & Butler, 1997) independently concluded that the inclusion of information about condom and contraceptive use in STI and sex education programs did not hasten the onset of sexual activity among participants. Moreover, all three reports stated that substantial evidence indicated that well-designed and implemented comprehensive programs had been demonstrated to delay the onset of first intercourse. And parents appear to agree with the researchers: a 1999 Kaiser Family Foundation poll found that 78 % of parents rejected the notion that messages about safe sex increase the likelihood that teens will initiate sexual activity. This finding was corroborated in an analysis using parent data from the National Longitudinal Survey of Adolescent Health, in which only 4 % of parents agreed with the statement that talking with their teens about birth control might encourage them to have sex (Miller, 1998).

Only abstinence is 100 % effective. In this instance, I initially surprised my audience, along with those testifying in support of abstinence-only programs, by agreeing the abstinence is, indeed, the only 100 % effective means of preventing any negative consequences that might result from engaging in sex. The statement is patently true, but only when abstinence is practiced 100 % of the time. I went on to note that intentions to remain abstinent have a remarkably high failure rate. I cited several types of evidence to buttress this claim. First, data demonstrate that the majority of Americans initiate sex during adolescence, and this has been true for many decades. The notion that even the most effective abstinence promotion intervention imaginable could shift this statistic by more than 10 % flies in the face of what we know about the impact of interventions on complex social behaviors such as sex. I cited the findings from the Bearman and Bruckner (2001) study, noted earlier, which found that the vast majority of teens taking abstinence vows failed to remain abstinent. Second, I argued that we simply have no evidence that abstinence-only interventions can produce major changes in the rate of adolescent sexual behavior. And if a large percentage of teens will eventually engage in sexually activity while still adolescents, it would seem ill-advised to not prepare them with the knowledge and skills to protect their sexual health and make sound decisions about their sexual lives.

Evidence for abstinence-only interventions. Finally, I noted that not only do we not have concrete evidence that abstinence-only programs can delay sex and prevent STI, but we have mounting evidence that the programs are ineffective, and some hints that a singular focus on abstinence might even increase exposure to STI. Citing the MPR national evaluation of abstinence-only programs (Trenholm et al., 2007) and the Bruckner and Bearman (2005) study of the effects of virginity pledges on STI, I concluded that the most rigorous evaluations available find no evidence that abstinence-only interventions result in changes in sexual attitudes, intentions or abstinence-related sexual behaviors. On the basis of the best evidence available, I argued, the Board of Education had no grounds for making the proposed policy change.

At the end of the day, I had the evidence on my side but I didn't sway the vote. By a one-vote margin, the Board of Education rescinded existing STI education guidelines and replaced them with recommendations steeped in an abstinence-only ideology.

Advocacy in Action II: Sometimes You Win

One of the first lessons I learned when I began my adventures working in policy settings is that neither defeats nor victories are necessarily permanent. Policy debates that might seem to have been settled often reappear on the policy agenda as the social and political context changes. A loss at one point in time can turn into a victory later.

Following the vote of the State Board of Education, a group of advocates met to conduct of postmortem review of why we'd failed, and what next steps we might take. We concluded that we'd failed because the decision makers we'd made our appeal to were simply uninterested in evidence. They'd come to their positions on the Board intent on developing and making policies consistent with their values, and had little interest in whether evidence supported or contradicted those values. Policymaking is an inherently political process, even within state boards of education. Rational appeals were unlikely to sway them, so we needed to look in a different direction to achieve a change in policy. Perhaps there was a way to use the evidence clearly favoring our case to change the balance of power.

We turned to the media, and specifically to the two largest newspapers in the state. Our reasoning was that by shining a light on the actions of the Board of Education—actions that our evidence indicated were inconsistent with public opinion— we might be able to pressure the board to reconsider their actions or convince the public to vote out those board members who had supported the policy change at the next election. Our hope that was if the two major papers picked up the issue, smaller papers and other media outlets, including television, might follow in their footsteps.

All of us had previous experience in writing opinion pieces, or op-eds, for newspapers. Writing an op-ed is a bit of an art, and quite a challenge, especially when trying to summarize research evidence for a public audience in just a few paragraphs, and also describing the policy context and offering recommendations for action. Our efforts paid off, however, as both newspapers published pieces written specifically for them.

Our next task was a bit more audacious: we scheduled meetings with members of the editorial page staffs of the two papers, and made a pitch for them to write editorials regarding the action of the State Board of Education. I brought them all of the research summaries and fact sheets that I'd prepared for the Board of Education hearing, and emphasized state-specific data regarding adolescent STI rates and risky sexual behavior, along with the information contrasting the efficacy of comprehensive versus abstinence-only intervention approaches. My colleagues emphasized the political aspects of the process, noting that several of the board members had run stealth election campaigns, never mentioning their plans to alter an array of school board policies.

Much to our surprise and delight, both papers soon published editorials blasting the State Board of Education for their actions. Both papers have generally conservative editorial viewpoints on most issues, but their editors were swayed by the logic underlying our arguments. The editorials criticized the Board of Education for placing politics ahead of reason and sound public health practice, and argued that the Board's actions, if not overturned, could well put the state's youth in harm's way. The papers took hold of this issue, and when the Board of Education failed to rescind their action, the papers singled out the members supporting the abstinence-only policy and endorsed candidates running for their seats. The following year, one of these board members resigned rather than face reelection, and three others were defeated. Shortly after the new Board was seated, they rescinded the abstinence-only policy guidelines.

Lessons Learned and Next Steps

Those of us involved in this advocacy effort came away from the process having learned a variety of lessons. First, we came to appreciate the aforementioned point about neither victories nor losses being permanent in the policy arena. Policymaking is a process, and there are opportunities to reverse losses throughout the course of that process. Additionally, policy issues are rarely settled in any permanent sense, and if the advocate maintains a sufficiently long time perspective, the odds are that policymakers will revisit the issue on their own, or that advocates may find that the political context has shifted sufficiently to increase their chances for success. In this instance, we lost our efforts to directly sway the opinions of the policymakers, but we succeeded when we took the case to the public. But in all honesty, when we began this effort, we had not envisioned that success would come in this fashion.

One clear implication of this first lesson is that advocates must avoid becoming discouraged when initial policy actions don't go their way. There will be other opportunities, but the advocate must think broadly with respect to where those opportunities might exist. Had we locked our focus on one small element of the policymaking apparatus (i.e., the State Board of Education), we might have had to wait much longer for the Board's ideological makeup to shift far enough to overturn the abstinence-only policy. By shifting our focus to the media and the public, we were able to change the Board's political makeup fairly quickly and overturn their earlier action. A second implication is advocates must avoid overconfidence when things do go their way. Wins can later become losses just as readily as the reverse, and vigilance is required to protect those wins from later reversal.

Given this first lesson, those of us involved in this advocacy effort formed a loose coalition that meets twice annually to share information about adolescent reproductive health policy. Each of us monitors various state agencies and tracks relevant federal policy as part of an effort to assure that we can act, or react, quickly when opportunities for or threats to sound reproductive health policymaking present themselves. We've developed good relationships with staff in the key state agencies, such there is a great deal of good will and trust.

A second lesson, not a new one but one that certainly was brought home by this episode, is that evidence can not be expected to sway the minds of all policymakers, no matter how clear it may be to those of us who produce the evidence. As previously noted, policymaking is, first and foremost, a political process, and policymakers must weigh a variety of factors in reaching any policy decision. Among those factors are public values and political ideology. Sawhill (1995), an economist who served as director of the White House Office of Management and Budget during the Clinton administration, and who is president of the National Campaign to Prevent Teen and Unplanned Pregnancy, voiced the issue quite clearly. "When research and values collide, values will always win. Analysts who ignore this fact are wasting their time" (p. 12). Her message, however, is not as pessimistic as the foregoing comment suggests, as she goes on to note that "over the long run, however, the scribblings of some researcher, filtered through the media and elite opinion, has at least the potential to push public values in new directions" (p. 12). We can't say for certain whether our scribblings, as interpreted and communicated by the media, led to a change in public values, as we suspect that most members of the public shared our concerns and the key values underlying them. Nevertheless, it was by appealing to the public, via the media, that we won this round.

References

American Social Health Association. (1996). Teenagers know more than adults about STDs, but knowledge in both groups is low. *STD News, 3*, 1–3.

Aral, S. O. (1994). Sexual behavior in sexually transmitted disease research: An overview. *Sexually Transmitted Disease, 21 (March–April Supplement)*, S59–S64.

Aral, S. O., & Holmes, K. (1990). Epidemiology of sexually transmitted diseases. In K. Holmes, P. A. Mardh, P. F. Sparling, & P. J. Wiesner (Eds.), *Sexually transmitted diseases* (pp. 181–193). New York: McGraw-Hill.

Bearman, P., & Bruckner, H. (2001). Promising the future: Virginity pledges and first intercourse. *The American Journal of Sociology, 106*, 859–912. doi:10.1086/320295.

Bruckner, H., & Bearman, P. (2005). After the promise: The STD consequences of adolescent virginity pledges. *Journal of Adolescent Health, 36*, 271–278. doi:10.1016/j.jadohealth.2005.01.005.

Centers for Disease Control and Prevention. (2008). *Sexually transmitted disease surveillance.* Atlanta, GA: CDC.

Centers for Disease Control and Prevention. (2009). Sexual and reproductive health of persons aged 10–24 years - United States 2002–2007. MMWR No. SS-6. Atlanta GA: CDC.

Centers for Disease Control and Prevention. (2010). *Youth risk behavior surveillance—2009* (Surveillance Summaries, MMWR No. SS-5). Washington, DC: U.S. Government Printing Office.

Centers for Disease Control and Prevention. (2011a). *Teenagers in the United States: Sexual activity, contraceptive use, and childbearing, 2006–2010 National Survey of Family Growth* (DHHS Publication No. (PHS) 2012–1983). Washington, DC: U.S. Government Printing Office.

Centers for Disease Control and Prevention. (2011b). *Sexually transmitted disease surveillance 2010.* Atlanta, GA: CDC.

Centers for Disease Control and Prevention. (2011c). *Genital HPV infection fact sheet.* Retrieved April 23, 2012, from http://www.cdc.gov/std/HPV/STDFact-HPV.htm.

Centers for Disease Control and Prevention. (2011d). *HIV among youth.* Retrieved April 23, 2012, from http://www.cdc.gov/hiv/youth/pdf/youth.pdf.

Centers for Disease Control and Prevention. (2011e). *HIV surveillance in adolescents and young adults.* Atlanta, GA: CDC.

Chesson, H. W., Blandford, J. M., Gift, T. L., Tao, G., & Irwin, K. L. (2004). The estimated direct medical cost of sexually transmitted diseases among American youth, 2000. *Perspectives on Sexual and Reproductive Health, 36*, 11–19. doi:10.1363/3601104.

Darroch, J. E., Singh, S., Frost, J. J., & The Study Team. (2001). Differences in teenage pregnancy rates among five developed countries: The roles of sexual activity and contraceptive use. *Family Planning Perspectives, 33*, 244–250. doi:10.2307/3030191.

Dorell, C., Stokley, S., Yankey, D., Jeyarajah, J., MacNeil, J., & Markowitz, L. (2012). National and state vaccination coverage among adolescents aged 13–17 years—United States, 2011. *Morbidity and Mortality Weekly Report, 61*(34), 671–677.

Eng, T. R., & Butler, W. T. (Eds.). (1997). *The hidden epidemic: Confronting sexually transmitted diseases.* Washington, DC: National Academy Press.

Ethier, K. A., Kershaw, T., Niccolai, L., Lewis, J. B., & Ickovics, J. R. (2003). Adolescent women underestimate their susceptibility to sexually transmitted infections. *Sexually Transmitted Infections, 79*, 408–411. doi:10.1136/sti.79.5.408.

Grunseit, A., & Kippax, S. (1993). *Effects of sex education on young people's sexual behavior.* Geneva: Global Programme on AIDS, World Health Organization.

Kantor, L. M., Santelli, J. S., Teitler, J., & Balmer, R. (2008). Abstinence-only policies and programs: An overview. *Sexuality Research and Social Policy, 5*, 6–17. doi:10.1525/srsp.2008.5.3.6.

Kirby, D. (2007). *Emerging answers 2007: Research findings on programs to reduce teen pregnancy and sexually transmitted diseases.* Washington, DC: National Campaign to Prevent Teen and Unplanned Pregnancy.

Kirby, D. (2008). The impact of abstinence and comprehensive sex and STD/HIV education programs on adolescent sexual behavior. *Sexuality Research and Social Policy, 5*, 18–27. doi:10.1525/srsp.2008.5.3.18.

Luker, K. (2006). *When sex goes to school: Warring views on sex—and sex education—since the sixties.* New York: Norton.

Miller, B. C. (1998). *Families matter: A research synthesis of family influences on adolescent pregnancy.* Washington, DC: National Campaign to Prevent Teen and Unplanned Pregnancy.

Moran, J. P. (2000). *Teaching sex: The shaping of adolescence in the 20th century.* Cambridge, MA: Harvard University Press.

National Campaign to Prevent Teen and Unplanned Pregnancy. (2011). *What works 2011–2012: Curriculum-based programs that help prevent teen pregnancy.* Washington DC: NCPTUP.

National Cancer Institute. (2005). *Theory at a glance: A guide for health promotion practice.* Washington, DC: U.S. Government Printing Office.

Panchaud, C., Singh, S., Feivelson, D., & Darroch, J. E. (2000). Sexually transmitted diseases among adolescents in developed countries. *Family Planning Perspectives, 32,* 24–32. doi:10.2307/268145.

Sawhill, I. V. (1995). The economist vs. madmen in authority. *Journal of Economic Perspectives, 9*(3), 3–13. doi:10.1257/jep.9.3.3.

Sexuality Information and Education Council of the United States (SIECUS). (2009). *What the research says...Abstinence-only-until-marriage programs.* New York: SIECUS.

Trenholm, C., Devaney, B., Fortson, K., Quay, L., Wheeler, J., & Clark, M. (2007). *Impacts of four Title V, Section 510 abstinence education programs.* Princeton, NJ: Mathematica Policy Research.

United Nations Children's Fund. (2011). Opportunity in crisis: PReventing HIV from early adolescence to young adulthood. UNICEF: NY.

Weinstock, H., Berman, S., & Cates, W. (2004). Sexually transmitted diseases among American youth: Incidence and prevalence estimates, 2000. *Perspectives on Sexual and Reproductive Health, 36,* 6–10. doi:10.1363/360064.

Wilcox, B. L. (1999). Sexual obsessions: Public policy and adolescent girls. In N. G. Johnson, M. C. Roberts, & J. Worell (Eds.), *Beyond appearances: A new look at adolescent girls.* Washington, DC: American Psychological Association.

Chapter 16
Lessons from the Legislative History of Federal Special Education Law: A Vignette for Advocates

Grace L. Francis and Rud Turnbull

Assume you are a doctoral student in a discipline serving individuals with disabilities and their families. Assume your major advisor, Professor Shelly Keats, received an invitation to testify before a Congressional committee that is preparing a bill to reauthorize (re-enact) the Individuals with Disabilities Education Act (IDEA). The committee members want to know about the types of interventions and services they should require educators to use.

Dr. Keats asks you to prepare a memorandum on how to be an effective advocate. More than that, she asks you to be prepared to testify in her stead, because she will be unable to do so herself, having surgery long-scheduled for that day. What strategies should you use to be an effective advocate for the students covered by the law and their teachers and other professionals? You know that Congress, in the 2004 reauthorization, declared that special educators should use evidence-based practices (IDEA, 2004). You also know that Dr. Keats has developed a nationally significant line of research about assessment and intervention to improve students' behavior. You and she strongly believe that scientific evidence is the most persuasive evidence of all.

You are unsure how to prepare your testimony, so you ask another professor, Dr. Harry Thomas. He is experienced in testifying before Congress' committees. He asks you: "Should changes in policy be grounded in only research?" You answer, "Yes." Then he turns the question around. "What, he asks, is the connection between research and policy? If research should affect policy, then should policy also affect the kind of research you and your professors do?"

G.L. Francis, Ph.D. (✉) • R. Turnbull, L.L.M., L.L.B., J.D.
Beach Center on Disability, University of Kansas, Lawrence, KS 66045-7534, USA
e-mail: glucyf6@gmail.com; rud@ku.edu

A. McDonald Culp (ed.), *Child and Family Advocacy: Bridging the Gaps Between Research, Practice, and Policy*, Issues in Clinical Child Psychology, DOI 10.1007/978-1-4614-7456-2_16, © Springer Science+Business Media New York 2013

Stunned by the turn of events—your advisor's assignment, her absence from testifying, your unaccustomed and frightening role, and the other professor's questions—you ask yourself two questions. First, as a future professional in the field of disability research, what evidence can I use to be persuasive? Second, what skills can I use to be effective?

To prepare, you decide to read IDEA's legislative history. You also decide to talk with an experienced disability advocate. From reading the legislative history, you hope to learn the effect that research had when Congress enacted the law in 1975 and amended it later. From talking with the advocate, you hope to learn some strategies for testifying. You believe that research has played a powerful role, but you also have a hunch that other factors had their effects, too. So, you begin your research, wanting to be the best advocate you can be.

Advocacy

This scenario repeats itself whenever young professionals, seeking to improve the quality of life of individuals and families affected by disabilities, have to enter the "forensic" arena—the place where there is power to effect change—instead of remaining within their research offices or laboratories. Upon entering this forensic arena, these professionals become advocates.

What is an "advocate?" Webster's Collegiate Dictionary defines the term as "one who "pleads the cause of another" and "maintains a cause or proposal;" to "advocate" means to "plead in favor of" (Mish, 2004, p. 19). The authors of this book define child advocacy as follows:

> Advocacy involvement spans differing levels from service activities in school and communities, to grass-roots groups organizing for community social justice and change, to political lobbying, and to testifying before legislative bodies on behalf of quality life issues for children's growth and development. The advocacy work in the legislative arena is focused on public programs and social services, based on solid child development research, that assure safe and healthy (physical and mental) development for children and their families.

In disability policy, advocates have included members of Congress or a state legislature; expert witnesses not affiliated with an organization; representatives of various professional or family/parent organizations; individuals with disabilities (self-advocates); and individuals who have family members with disabilities.

As the list of advocates suggest, there is more to advocacy than research. To demonstrate that point, we review some legislative history of the federal special education law. Although we pull from a legislative history to highlight effective approaches of advocacy, the approaches we highlight in this chapter are generally universal to most advocacy efforts.

From our review, you will learn that advocates use various types of evidence and strategies when presenting evidence. In short, you will have answers to the two questions the student in our scenario asked: what type of evidence is persuasive, and how can a witness present evidence in the most compelling way? But before having those answers, you need to know something about the way advocacy has worked with respect to the federal special education law, the Individuals with Disabilities Education Act (IDEA), originally called the Education of All Handicapped Children Act. (We do not review IDEA's entire legislative history.)

Congress passed the Education for All Handicapped Children Act in 1975, as Public Law 94–142. It authorized federal assistance to the states to educate children with disabilities, ages 6–21. Congress later amended it to authorize federal aid to the states to educate preschool children, aged 3–6, and then to educate infants and toddlers, birth to three. The most recent amendments were in 1997, when Congress renamed the law as the Individuals with Disabilities Education Act (Public Law 105–107), and in 2004 (Public Law 108–446).

Two-Part Advocacy: What and How

What kind of advocacy persuaded Congress in 1975, 1997, and again in 2004 to enact and then reauthorize this important federal law? The answer lies in the legislative record. The record makes it clear that two types of advocacy prompted Congress to act. The first has to do with the types of evidence that witnesses produced. The question here is: What kind of evidence did Congress rely on? The second has to do with the strategies the witnesses pursued in presenting their evidence. The question here is: How did the witnesses present their evidence?

The "What" Type of Evidence

This type of evidence consists of research, statistics, and facts that courts have trusted when ordering state and local education agencies to educate students with disabilities. This evidence consists of facts that can be independently confirmed. These facts are "hard" data. These are the "what" of advocacy. People may disagree about how to interpret these facts, but they are unable to deny the existence of the facts.

The "How" Type of Evidence

This type of advocacy involves using strategies and techniques to present the "what" type of evidence. These are the means that advocates use, the ways to present factual evidence in the most persuasive manner possible. Although these strategies cannot be independently confirmed or proven, they are affective styles of making the point that the evidence itself backs up. These are the "how" of advocacy.

As you will learn later in this chapter, advocates who combine the "what" and "how" are apt to be more effective than advocates who use only one type of evidence and presentation. We now turn to the legislative record to buttress this assertion. Before we do, however, we must tell you that we also rely on the personal experiences of the second author of this chapter, Rud Turnbull. As is appropriate and relevant, we offer evidence and strategies he used as witness in hearings before Congressional committees.

Turnbull is a nonpracticing lawyer, policy researcher, professor, consultant, and advocate. Turnbull's son Jay (1967–2009), who had intellectual and a related developmental disability, inspired him to become an advocate on the behalf of individuals with disabilities and their families. In the scenario at the beginning of this chapter, Turnbull's testimony is "the firsthand experiences of an veteran disability advocate" our young professional seeks learn from. For the sake of brevity, we paraphrase Turnbull's testimony. (His testimony is available in the published Reports by the Committees of the House of Representatives or Senate before which he testified, or as reprinted in scholarly journals.)

The "What" Type of Evidence

Witnesses used four types of "what" evidence: (a) research and reports, (b) statistics, (c) anecdotal statements and assertions, and (d) previous legislation. Table 16.1 provides examples of these four types of evidence.

Research and Reports

Witnesses used national research studies and reports to support their positions. In 1975, for example, Kate Long, a teacher from West Virginia, used recent data to illustrate some shortcomings of the current educational system. She cited inadequate assessment procedures, parental exclusion from tests, subjective school judgments, and misclassification as problems that a federal law should address (Education for All Handicapped Children, 1975). Years later, in 2003, Douglas Carnine, a senior researcher at the University of Oregon's National Center to Improve the Tools of Educators, referred to the science of neurology to make his point that Congress should authorize state aid for programs of early special education:

> If you look at the images in the left hemisphere of the brain before scientifically based instruction, there is little activity during reading. After 65 hours of intensive scientifically based instruction, there is substantial activity in the left hemisphere resembling that of successful readers. (IDEA: Focusing on Improving Results for Children with Disabilities, 2003, p. 13).

What if Ms. Long and Dr. Carnine had made statements they could not support by reference to facts? That would have made their testimony less persuasive. Consider, for example, the experience of Larry Lorton, a school administrator from Caroline County, Maryland, when testifying in favor of all-day kindergarten special education. Encouraged by his testimony, a member of Congress asked Mr. Lorton whether he could isolate all-day kindergarten as the "important factor" (p. 35) in children's education. Mr. Lorton did not have the research to back up his claim: "the reality is that

Table 16.1 Evidence used by witnesses in Congressional Hearings for P.L. 108-779 and P.L. 94-142

Public law	Witness	Type of evidence	Evidence
P.L. 94-142	Kate Long	National report	I would like to point particularly to the Children's Defense Fund report, "Children Out of School in America" (which notes) inadequate assessment procedures…parental exclusion from tests, …. subjective school judgments… misclassification (that) often occurs. Current methods of identifying children with disabilities lack validity or reliability. (O.T.)
P.L. 108-779	Douglas Carnine	National reports	It is not surprising that longitudinal data from the National Institute of Child Health and Human Development (NICHD) show clearly that the majority of children who are poor readers at age nine or older never read at grade level with their peers and continue to have reading difficulties into adulthood. (W.T.)
P.L. 108-779	Cindy Oser	National report	More than four decades of knowledge about early childhood development, which has been integrated into a widely acclaimed report from the National Research Council and Institute of Medicine entitle, *From Neurons to Neighborhoods: The Science of Early Childhood Development*, can help inform the re-authorization process. (In reference to the benefits of early childhood intervention). (W.T.)
P.L. 108-779	Douglas Carnine	National research	Such dramatic changes have been documented through brain images. If you look at the images in the left hemisphere of the brain before scientifically based instruction, there is little activity during reading. After 65 hours of intensive scientifically based intervention, there is substantial activity in the left hemisphere resembling that of successful readers… (O.T.)
P.L. 94-142	Richard Dowling	National research	We took a comprehensive survey of the speech and hearing consultants in the 50 State departments of education… we were very disappointed with the results… the consultants reported widely differing classifications for handicapped. Current methods of identifying children with disabilities lack validity or reliability. (O.T.)
P.L. 108-779	Dianne Talarico	Non-cited Research	Recent research shows that a lack of kindergarten readiness is the single most significant reason for the achievement gap between children of poverty and their high socioeconomic counterparts. We need to ensure that the early intervention programs under IDEA Part C reach as many children as possible. (O.T.)

(continued)

Table 16.1 (continued)

Public law	Witness	Type of evidence	Evidence
P.L. 108-779	Larry Lorton	Local Statistics	The black bars show the climb of our local special education budget, and the stacked lighter bars show the state and federal contributions and revenues to our budget. The gap between the two is what we pick up locally. Special education is what it is. The services are not optional. They have to be delivered. (O.T.)
P.L. 94.142	Francis McIntyre	State statistics	Approximately 40% of the handicapped children in Maryland are not receiving programs or services that can be considered appropriate, or are receiving no program at all. (O.T.)
P.L. 94.142	Albert T. Pimentel	National statistics	The Bureau of Education for the Handicapped (reported) that only 22% of preschool aged children were participating in some kind of educational program…S.6 would make it possible for 78% of these children to be involved in some education program. (O.T.)
P.L. 94.142	Jennings Randolph	National statistics	Although educational services to handicapped children have improved since the early 1960s and the number of children being served has increased, and while the Federal efforts under the Education of the Handicapped Act increased from 25 million in 1964 to approximately 200 million this year, there are still 3.9 million children waiting for the fundamental equal educational opportunity. (O.T.)
P.L. 94.142	Dudley Koontz	National statistics	We must carefully consider those recent statistics published by the Bureau for the Education of the Handicapped, which point out that barely one-half of school aged children and less than one-fourth of preschool age children are receiving special education. (O.T.)
P.L. 94.142	Fred Burke	Anecdotal (personal)	Based on our experience in New Jersey, where we have already developed procedures to involve parents in the determination of IEPs, I can attest to their administrative workability. (O.T.)
P.L. 94.142	Albert T. Pimentel	Anecdotal (personal)	We know from personal experience where the physical, psychosocial, and economic obstacles lie as one attempts to maneuver through an education system usually not designed with handicapping conditions in mind…it is essential that the proposed legislation exactly spell out that this money is earmarked for special education. State educational agencies have not, when faced with many different demands for their educational dollar, provided adequately for special education in the past, and we have no reason to believe that they will do… (O.T.)

P.L. 108-779	Harriet Brown	Anecdotal (personal)	We definitely need to eliminate the requirement for procedural safeguards for parents every time we have a meeting. Our parents tell us that they can wallpaper their houses with all of the procedural safeguards. There are critical times that they need a reminder, and I think we should still give that to them… (O.T.)
P.L. 94-142	Frederick J. Weintraub	Anecdotal (assertion)	It becomes a Catch 22 logic to say we cannot serve children until personnel are developed. It is frankly difficult to develop the personnel until there is a clear mandate to serve the children. (O.T.)
P.L. 108-779	Douglas Carnine	Anecdotal (assertion)	I encourage the committee to allow the development of ways of finding out if children are actually benefiting so our prevention investment does pay off. (O.T.)
P.L. 108-779	Harriet Brown	Anecdotal (assertion)	Right now, we have a referred test and place model for special education. Any time a child is referred, it is a cry for help from the teacher. If there were some specific information and guidelines, I think it would help all of us. (O.T.)
P.L. 108-779	Douglas Carnine	Legislation	Under the current regulations, the discrepancy formula is the basis for determining when a child will be eligible for special education services for a learning disability. The formula makes eligibility for services dependent on a discrepancy between an IQ in the normal range and an achievement level that is generally two or more years below grade level. (O.T.) The No Child Left Behind Act (NCLB) passed last year creates a strong incentive for schools to support a response to intervention approach to identifying and serving students with learning disabilities. For the first time in U.S. history, all students with disabilities must be included in the state accountability system. (W.T.)
P.L. 108-779	Todd Platts	Legislation	The concern I have is when that transition occurs, that with the way the law is written, it does not allow a very seamless transition. It is kind of like starting over, because you are in the new system. (O.T.)

Note: This table references selected forms of evidence used by witnesses in written testimonies (W.T.) and oral testimonies (O.T.)

we cannot isolate that particular variable with the results that we get from our children on assessments" (p. 35). Mr. Lorton was unable to provide data to support his assertion. We may never know whether his failure to cite research discredited his statement to the Committee, but we may caution that it is unwise for a witness to make bold statements without being able immediately to cite research to back up assertions.

Research is persuasive. It wins skeptics by providing reliable sources of research and data to support their positions. It adds to a witness' credibility, but only if the witness can cite it when asked to prove an assertion. Research is, however, not the only kind of compelling "what" evidence. Statistics are powerful because they make issues more tangible and relatable.

Statistics

Consider the evidence that Dudley Koontz, representing the Consortium Concerned with the Developmentally Disabled, gave in 1975, to support his advocacy: "We must carefully consider those recent statistics published by the Bureau for the Education of the Handicapped, which point out that barely one-half of school aged children and less than one-fourth of preschool age children are receiving special education" (Education for All Handicapped Children, 1975, pp. 83–84). Similarly but with respect to the 2004 reauthorization, Larry Lorton, who could not cite research about the efficacy of prekindergarten special education, was otherwise effective because he used statistics to demonstrate that his school district, and others like it, needed federal funds to educate students with disabilities. Referring to a chart depicting fiscal statistics, he testified as follows:

> The black bars show the climb of our local special education budget, and the stacked lighter bars show the state and federal contributions and revenues to our budget. The gap between the two is what we pick up locally. Special education is what it is. The services are not optional. They have to be delivered. (IDEA: Focusing on Improving Results for Children with Disabilities, 2003, pp. 15–16)

Here, then, is a caution about advocacy: be prepared to cite data and to illustrate statistics. Given that you may have only a few minutes to make your key points (Congress allows a witness a bare 5 min of uninterrupted testimony), make your points succinctly, illustrate them with graphs, and be prepared to cite the basis for your points, either in your oral testimony or in the written testimony that you later provide. And, if you can, supplement the research and statistics with anecdotes and real-life stories.

Anecdotal Statements and Assertions

Anecdotal evidence, including personal stories and assertions, are persuasive because they put a personal face on your testimony. For example, when Fred Burke, the Commissioner of Education in New Jersey, was testifying in 1975, he assured members of Congress that parents' participation in educational decision-making would not keep educators from doing their job, as experts: "Based on our experience in New Jersey, where we have already developed procedures to involve parents in the determination of IEPs, I can attest to their administrative workability" (Education for All Handicapped Children, 1975, p. 298). Similarly, in the 2003 hearings, Harriet Brown, director of Early Special Education Policy and Procedures in Florida, used feedback she received from parents to support her argument that Congress should grant some relief to educators when they join parents in making decisions: "We definitely need to eliminate the requirement for procedural safeguards for parents every time we have a meeting. Our parents tell us that they can wallpaper their houses with all of the procedural safeguards." (IDEA: Focusing on Improving Results for Children with Disabilities, 2003, p. 11).

An additional type of anecdotal evidence includes personal assertions. Albert Pimentel, representing the Coalition of Citizens with Disabilities, used his knowledge about states' expenditures in special education to make the point that Congress, when enacting the 1975 law, should include provisions to prevent misuse of funds: "State educational agencies have not, when faced with many different demands for their educational dollar, provided adequately for special education in the past, and we have no reason to believe they will do so" (Education for All Handicapped Children, 1975, p. 292).

Witnesses also used anecdotal assertions to advocate for policy that would drive research and result in systems change. For example, Doug Carnine, testifying as a researcher in 2003, asserted that the federal law should influence the type of research that he and his colleagues should carry out to improve early childhood education: "I encourage the committee to allow the development of ways of finding out if children are actually benefiting so our prevention investment does pay off" (IDEA: Focusing on improving results for children with disabilities, 2003, p. 34). He was making the same point that Fred Weintraub, representing the Council for Exceptional Children, made in 1975, namely, that policy must impel professional development: "It becomes a Catch 22 logic to say we cannot serve children until personnel are developed. It is frankly difficult to develop the personnel until there is a clear mandate to serve the children" (Education for All Handicapped Children, 1975, p. 313).

During his time as a witness, second-author Turnbull also employed anecdotal evidence. On several occasions when he testified in Congress as a parent representing a parent association (The Arc), he "put a human face" on his testimony by acknowledging that members of the committee have brothers or sisters who have disabilities, or by describing his son, who had disabilities. When testifying before a Senate committee holding oversight hearings on the Rehabilitation Act Amendments of 1972, he buttressed his credibility by linking his work to the interests of the members of the committee before which he was testifying:

> Senator Harkin, I know from having been on your staff that you have a brother who is deaf. Senator Kennedy, I know from having been a Kennedy Public Policy Fellow that you have a sister with an intellectual disability. Gentlemen, my son Jay has an intellectual disability, autism, and a rapid-cycling emotional-behavioral disorder. Together, we have intimate knowledge of the challenges families and individuals face.

Anecdotal evidence and personal assertions can be engaging, powerful, and effective. That is especially true when an advocate supports anecdotes and assertions with research and statistics. If you do that, you will be relying on three different types of "what" evidence. If, in addition, you can cite existing law or court cases to support your points, you will be even more persuasive.

Existing Legislation

That is what Doug Carnine did when testifying in 2003. He was advocating for a change in the standards and procedures that schools must follow in order to classify a student as having a specific learning disability. He first referred to the 1997 special education act: "Under the current regulations, the discrepancy formula is the basis for determining when a child will be eligible for special education services for a learning disability." He then referred to the federal general education act: "The No Child Left Behind Act ... creates a strong incentive for schools to support a response to intervention approach to identifying and serving students with learning disabilities." (IDEA: Focusing on Improving Results for Children with Disabilities, 2003, p. 12).

As useful as it is to refer to present law, it is also useful to rely on decisions of federal or state courts that require federal or state legislatures to support special education. For example, witnesses in the 1975 hearings were able to cite three decisions that they said justified or even required Congress to enact the Education of All Handicapped Children Act (P.L. 94–142). In one case, *Mills v. D.C. Board of Education* (1972), a federal court ordered the District of Columbia Board of Education to educate students with disabilities, holding that the Board's failure to do so denied the students their constitutional right to due process. In another case, *PARC v. Commonwealth* (1972), a federal court also held that the state violated students' constitutional right to equal treatment (access to education). These decisions imposed huge costs on states and justified advocates in arguing that Congress could relieve the states financially and thereby assist them in complying with the constitution (Turnbull, Stowe, & Huerta, 2007).

In summary, research, statistics, anecdotes and personal assertions, and existing laws or court decisions are the "what" that advocates used to persuade Congress to enact and then reauthorize the federal special education law. They are, however, only one part of effective advocacy. The other is the "how" of advocacy—the ways in which advocates put forward their case in a compelling, engaging, and memorable fashion.

The "How" Type of Advocacy

Having discussed the types of evidence that witnesses used to persuade Congress, we now discuss the strategies they used in presenting their evidence. These strategies include (a) establishing credibility, (b) clarifying key points, (c) using powerful and engaging language, (d) interpreting, anticipating, and collaborating with others' positions, (e) recognizing broad implications, (f) sharing stories, (g) citing research, and (h) using demonstrative evidence. Table 16.2 provides examples of how witnesses used these strategies.

Credibility

Many witnesses began their testimony by establishing their credibility, stating why they are testifying and their qualifications to testify. Professional witnesses cited the number of years they worked as researchers or administrators and their professional accomplishments. Similarly, witnesses from professional organizations often named the organization they represented and referred to the organization's mission. For instance, Eva Johnson, a member of the education committee of The National Association for Retarded Children (now, The Arc), began her 1975 testimony by stating, "I speak for the education committee of the National Association for the Retarded Citizens. The national association is supported by some 1,500-plus ARCs throughout the Nation in our 50 states" (Education for All Handicapped Children, 1975, p. 87).

When testifying to committees that had members from Kansas, Turnbull identified himself as the father of a son with multiple disabilities and, simultaneously, as a professor in special education and law; he thus coupled his personal and professional credentials, using essentially this approach:

> Not only am I Jay's father, but I also am the Beach Distinguished Professor in special education and courtesy professor of law. Senator Dole, being from Kansas, you know Ross and Marianna Beach. They have supported the research center I codirect. My son works there.

On the other hand, witness also made sure to indicate areas where they were not experts, thereby supporting their credibility as authorities on the topics they *are* authorities in. For example, when asked a question by the committee, Dr. Carnine was sure to preface that his answer "should not be taken with much weight," because the topic was out of his primary area of expertise (IDEA: Focusing on Improving Results for Children with Disabilities, 2003, p. 26). Restating and clarifying key points is another useful strategies good advocates employ.

Key Points

Clarifying key points is a wise strategy to ensure that the committee understands the most essential pieces of your testimony. Witnesses clarified key points using several methods, including underlining key sentences and bulleting recommendations in their written testimony. While testifying, witnesses clarified key points by restating their main ideas and providing succinct summaries of large amounts of evidence. They frequently sequenced main ideas by using terms such as "first," "second," and "third" to indicate main points in summaries. They also referred to graphics such as charts and graphs while testifying to highlight key points.

Table 16.2 Strategies used by witnesses in Congressional Hearings for P.L. 108-779 and P.L. 94-142

Public law	Witness	Type of strategy	Strategy
P.L. 94-142	Eva Johnson	Credibility	I speak for the education committee of the National Association for Retarded Citizens. The national association is supported by some 1,500-plus ARC's throughout the Nation in our 50 states. (O.T.)
P.L. 108-779	Harriet Brown	Credibility	I began my special education career as a college student in Virginia... After graduate school I worked for twelve years in the Chicago Public Schools as speech-language pathologist... (O.T.)
P.L. 108-779	Douglas Carnine	Credibility	I am not really an expert in this area, so my comment will be brief and should not be taken with much weight. (O.T.)
P.L. 94-142	Kate Long	Credibility	My name is Kate Long.... I am currently finishing a book concerning the problems of implementing legislation at the local school system. (O.T.)
P.L. 108-779	Dianne Talarico	Key points	There are three key recommendations regarding the reauthorization of IDEA that I would like to make today... (O.T.)
P.L. 108-779	Larry Lorton	Key points	If I can call your attention very briefly to page 4 of my written testimony, you can see the breakdown of where our special education children lie. (O.T.)
P.L. 108-779	Douglas Carnine	Key points	If you look at the images in the left hemisphere of the brain before scientifically based instruction, there is little activity during reading. (O.T.)
P.L. 108-779	Douglas Carnine	Powerful language	Most of the learning disability community agrees that the IQ-achievement discrepancy formula needs to go. It is ineffective, inefficient, irrational, immoral, and indefensible. The opportunity to put millions of students on a better trajectory toward academic success is before you now. Now is the time. (W.T.)
P.L. 94-142	Frederick J. Weintraub	Powerful language	Imagine yourself as a parent of a handicapped child, or a handicapped child... (You say) "I am here to receive my education" (and) you are told you cannot receive your education or you are assigned to an inappropriate class. (O.T.)

P.L.	Witness	Strategy	Quote
P.L. 94-142	Frederick J. Weintraub	Powerful language	One of the major problems of the handicapped is the multitude of delivery agencies. The consequent behavior reminds me of the TV program "Chico." They are always saying, "It is not my job, man." (O.T.)
P.L. 108-779	Douglas Carnine	Others' positions	As with any other research enterprise, implementing the research-based practice on a broad scale is difficult (referring to bringing RtI to scale). (W.T.)
P.L. 108-779	Dianne Talarico	Others' positions	I absolutely support everything that Ms. Brown said…And it is interesting, because I shared with her an IEP from our local school district. And, you know, she rolled her eyes and shook her head, and that is what I did when I saw it. (W.T.)
P.L. 94-142	Charles Mathias	Others' positions	Reviewing statements which were presented before this subcommittee yesterday, it appears that the overwhelming weight support the bill. (O.T.)
P.L. 94-142	Francis McIntyre	Others' positions	The argument against (universal education) is that handicapped children are denied services because they cost more money…the conclusion is that the handicapped child is less than equal as a human being. (O.T.)
P.L. 94-142	Carl Megel	Broad implications	Employing handicapped people has grown tremendously in the last 10 years… there is a need for education… the education of all children cannot be delayed. (O.T.)
P.L. 108-779	Douglas Carnine	Broad implications	I think if you did away with the IQ-discrepancy formula and allowed earlier intervention, over the next 10 years, you would reduce the severity of learning disabilities in probably hundreds of thousands of children. (O.T.)
P.L. 108-779	Douglas Carnine	Stories	My wife is a retired special education teacher. She called me last night, and she said, "This testimony you're giving today is maybe the most important thing you've ever done." (O.T.)
P.L. 108-779	Joe Wilson	Stories	Two of our sons went through the IEP process. One just graduated from law school and the other is a junior in college. So it (IDEA) is successful, but the paperwork is extraordinary. (O.T.)
P.L. 108-779	Douglas Carnine	Research	The President's Commission on Excellence in Special Education reported that "…when aggressive reading programs are implemented with accountability for results LD identifications are reduced." (W.T.)
P.L. 94-142	Frederick J. Weintraub	Research	I would refer the committee to the study by Nicholas Hobbs for the Secretary of HEW on the whole issue of labels… as long as resources are limited, we are going to have to label people. (O.T.)

Note: This table references selected strategies used by witnesses in written testimonies (W.T.) and oral testimonies (O.T.).

For example, Turnbull distinguished one point of his testimony from another by saying, "First," and then making his point, and "Second," and doing the same, until he had made all of his points. That strategy made it easy for him to summarize his testimony and thereby repeat his key points: "Mr. Chairman, I want to summarize. My first point was... My second was..." and so on. Succinct and clear language is an absolutely essential component to making your points clear. Powerful and engaging language is another strategy that can help clarify your main points and make them memorable as well.

Powerful and Engaging Language

Doug Carnine was especially artful at using compelling language to stress action on the behalf of Congress and create a sense of urgency. In the following example he used strong language and alliteration to grab the committee's attention:

> Most of the learning disability community agrees that the IQ-achievement discrepancy formula needs to go. It is ineffective, inefficient, irrational, immoral, and indefensible. The opportunity to put millions of students on a better trajectory toward academic success is before you now. Now is the time. (IDEA: Focusing on Improving Results for Children with Disabilities, 2003, p. 66).

Years before, Frederick J. Weintraub, representing the Council for Exceptional Children, used imagery to engage members of Congress on the subject of the least restrictive environment, "Imagine yourself as a parent of a handicapped child, or a handicapped child... you are told you cannot receive your education or you are assigned to an inappropriate class" (Education for All Handicapped Children, 1975, p. 312). Mr. Weintraub also engaged his audience by relating the issue of children with disabilities being disserved by disjointed agencies to a popular TV show of the time: "(the issue) reminds me of the TV program *Chico*. They are always saying, 'It is not my job, man'" (p. 309).

When testifying before a committee concerning abuses in state institutions for persons with developmental disabilities and trying to persuade Congress to enact a law that would authorize the U.S. Department of Justice to investigate state institutions, Turnbull recounted episodes of abuse that he had uncovered as a member of an institution's independent patient protection committee, testifying substantially as follows:

> Mr. Chairman (Sen. Birch Bayh) you are a lawyer in your home state in Indiana. I am sure you must know the old saying: when a lawyer has the facts he argues the facts; when he has the law, he argues the law; and when he has neither, he screams like hell. Well, I have some horrific facts. They should cut to the jugular of the matter before you. I have little law, which is why I am testifying to get some law. And I'm about to scream like hell.

As these witnesses demonstrated, language is a powerful tool that can spark interest in your testimony and make your remarks memorable. Simple tools such as imagery and humor can engage listeners and humanize issues. However, novice advocates must be aware of over- or misusing strong language, as it may dissuade decision-makers. It is, however, always useful to recognize others' testimony.

Others' Positions

In 1975, Francis McIntyre, director of the Maryland Department of Education, effectively supported his position that all children deserve an equal right to a free and appropriate education by interpreting the argument that educating students with disabilities is too costly an endeavor for a federal law to fund: "The argument against (P.L. 94–142) is that handicapped children are denied services is because they cost more money...the conclusion is that the handicapped child is less than equal as a human being" (Education for All Handicapped Children, 1975, p. 147). By addressing the underlying message of "it costs too much," Dr. McIntyre exposed it as an argument that children with disabilities are not worth educating—that they are inferior and underserving.

Similarly, effective advocates sometimes forecast arguments that other advocates are likely to make, thereby preemptively weakening their adversaries' points. For example, Doug Carnine acknowledged that he recognized potential complications with implementing a recently developed research-based strategy, Response to Intervention (RtI), as a means for identifying whether a student has a specific learning disability. Having acknowledged implementation challenges, he then was in a position to address them and, in doing so, diminish them.

In the same vein, Dianne Talarico, superintendent of a school district in Ohio, aligned her testimony with another witness' to strengthen her position:

> I absolutely support everything that Ms. Brown said. I am glad that she got to cover an area that I could not...I shared with her an IEP from our local school district. And, you know, she rolled her eyes and shook her head, and that is what I did when I saw it (IDEA: Focusing on Improving Results for Children with Disabilities, 2003, p. 22).

The strategy of collaborating or aligning your position with other advocates works well when the witnesses on the same "panel" (group of witnesses want the same outcome). When testifying about the reauthorization between the 1997 and 2004 laws, Turnbull said in effect:

> Mr. Chairman, my colleague just gave you some compelling research showing why Congress should act on the matter before you. I agree with her and want to supplement her point with some additional points of my own.

As an advocate, you must always be ready to defend your position, and others' positions may help you do that. Whether you are interpreting, recognizing, or collaborating with others' positions, you gain support for your claim. But effective advocates do not stop there; they acknowledge and then address the broad implications of their position.

Broad Implications

Decision-makers are almost always concerned about the long-term impacts and the cost-effectiveness of proposed policies. In an effort to demonstrate the long-term impact that P.L. 94–142 could have on the national economy, Carl Megel, representing the American Federation of Teachers, told Congress in 1975 that "employing handicapped people has grown tremendously in the last 10 years... the education of all children cannot be delayed" (Education for All Handicapped Children, 1975, p. 329). Likewise, Doug Carnine pointed out the implications of changing the procedures and standards for identifying children who have specific learning disabilities: "If you did away with the IQ-discrepancy formula and allowed earlier intervention, over the next 10 years, you would reduce the severity of learning disabilities in probably hundreds of thousands of children" (IDEA: Focusing on Improving Results for Children with Disabilities, 2003, p. 63).

Describing the implications of your position can help skeptics see past many immediate barriers such as upfront cost or issues related to systems capacity-building. It is, however, not the only one. Storytelling is another strategy used by advocates that may help win over individuals on the "opposing team" by humanizing policies and their implications.

Stories

As a supplement to research, personal stories can be persuasive. That is especially so when an advocate must persuade individuals who are unfamiliar with a specific population (e.g., individuals with disabilities) or the implications of a particular policy for individuals with disabilities, families, teachers, students without disabilities. Stories infuse emotion, making legislation more relatable. Furthermore, well-told stories are memorable and can make a lasting impression.

Larry Lorton used this strategy as he framed his positions with rich descriptions of his school, including personal stories of teachers and students. Relatedly, Doug Carnine engaged the committee by describing a conversation he had with his wife, a retired special education teacher, the night before the hearing: "(she said) 'This testimony you're giving today is maybe the most important thing you've ever done.' Her heart was broken as a special education director seeing children not being able to receive services they need..." (IDEA: Focusing on Improving Results for Children with Disabilities, 2003, p. 14).

Like the advocates for P.L. 94–142 and IDEA, Turnbull also used storytelling in his advocacy work. In 1995 he was invited to talk with President Clinton, Attorney General Reno, and Treasury Secretary Rubin about the effect of the federal antidiscrimination law, the Americans with Disabilities Act, that Congress enacted and President George H.W. Bush signed in 1990.

Mr. President, General Reno, and Secretary Rubin: When my son was born with an intellectual disability, the doctors told me to institutionalize him. I did not. When he was in school, educators told my wife and me he would never be able to work outside of a workshop. We told them they were wrong. When he graduated, they said he'd have to move into a group home. We again told them they were wrong. Today, Mr. President, our son Jay lives in his own home and works at the University of Kansas. Today, he is paying your salary by the taxes he pays! That's what good law makes possible.

The President said nothing, but, in his usual charismatic way, made a fist and raised his hand over his shoulder in a boxer's punch, signaling how deeply he took the point. Some nearly 50 persons with disabilities and other advocates for them, assembled to hear a few people speak with the President, broke out in spontaneous applause. The President smiled. Every advocate needs allies. Storytelling is one method to gain allies. Citing research is another.

Cite Research

Witnesses for P.L. 94–142 and IDEA strategically referred to and interpreted research to support their positions. For instance, Dr. Carnine used information from a national report by The President's Commission on Excellence in Special Education to support his position on evidence-based instruction: "(the report stated that) 'when aggressive reading programs are implemented with accountability for results LD identifications are reduced'" (IDEA: Focusing on Improving Results for Children with Disabilities, 2003, p. 63). As we mentioned earlier, this strategy is most effective when sources are cited either in an oral or written testimony. So is another strategy, namely, evidence that demonstrates the point you are making.

Demonstrative Evidence

Witnesses did not use this effective advocacy strategy when Congress dealt with the federal special education law. However, coauthor Turnbull witnessed the use of demonstrative evidence when Congress was deciding whether to authorize the Assistive Technology for Individuals with Disabilities Act (Tech Act, 1988), which sanctioned funds to assist states to create statewide assistive technology systems.

Having drafted the "Tech Act" and convened hearings about it, the committee that sponsored the act arranged for a two-day demonstration of technology. The demonstration was held in the lobby of the Hart Senate Office Building. The lobby is huge, about a quarter the size of a football field. It was full of booths displaying all sorts of assistive technology. The most persuasive of all technologies, however, was a motorized scooter and several sophisticated motorized wheelchairs. These enabled persons with disabilities to maneuver quickly in most types of crowd conditions and up and down low-rise stairs and ramps. A senior member of Congress,

who was then in his late 80s and who was highly influential with the most conservative members of his party, approached Turnbull, who at that time was a member of
the staff of the Senate committee. "Senator," Turnbull said, "why don't you take a
ride in that scooter to see what it does?" The Senator agreed, motored around the
lobby several times, returned to the staff member and said, "Well, damn, that was
great. I'm signing on and getting a lot of other senators to do so, too." The point is:
demonstrate what can happen, and it may well happen.

Conclusion

What's the take-home lesson of this chapter? It is that there are two aspects of advocacy: the "what" and the "how." Effective advocates use (a) research and reports, (b)
statistics, (c) anecdotal statements and assertions, and (d) existing legislation or
court cases. These are the "what" of advocacy.

Effective advocates also use the "how" approach. They (a) establish their credibility, (b) clarify their key points, (c) use powerful and engaging language; (d) interpret, anticipate, and collaborate with others' positions, (e) acknowledge and address
the broad implications of policy they wish to create, (f) share stories, (g) cite
research, and (h) use demonstrative evidence.

Now, let's revisit our story about an eager but intimidated budding advocate, and
let us assume that the novice has created Tables 16.1 and 16.2 as examples of "what"
and "how" strategies.

*You have completed your research on the legislative history of the original fed-
eral special education law and subsequent reauthorizations. You have had a conversation with an experienced advocate to learn about his experiences testifying as a
witness before Congress. You now meet with your professor, Dr. Shelly Keats, and
with the other professor, Dr. Harry Thomas.*

"In a nutshell," Dr. Keats tell you, "what did you learn? We are eager to hear."

*"Yes, that's true, but keep it brief. Give us the essence of it. I'm a busy man," says
Thomas, provoking an admonishing stare from his colleague.*

*"Well, I learned that advocacy means advancing a cause. In the research I did,
it was the right of students with disabilities to a free appropriate education in the
least restrictive environment. I learned that research is important, but that is not all
I learned." Here, Dr. Keats smiles and nods approvingly.*

*"I found out that experts need allies, and the more those allies are the people
affected by the law and research, the better. That means bringing families, individuals with disabilities, and administrators into the picture."*

*"Is that all?" says Dr. Thomas, obviously provoked that you have not mentioned
other people.*

*"Oh, of course not," you respond, "I'm sure you know I place a great deal of
importance on those special insiders, the people in Congress who are speaking to
their peers." Dr. Thomas smiles. You have scored a point with him. But he wants more.*

"What's the relationship between policy and research," he asks. "All you have done so far is to tell me about the people. What about the significance of their being allies?"

"Professor Thomas, I am glad you asked," you say, returning his skeptical gaze with a confident smile. "Research shapes policy. And in turn policy affects the research. Just look at Dr. Carnine's and Mr. Weintraub's testimony."

Here, Dr. Keats interrupts. "You two are about to run this conversation into the late night if I don't interrupt. Harry," she says, looking at her colleague, "you said you wanted to keep this discussion short. Let me give you a hand."

Turning to you, she asks, "Did you learn anything about the type of testimony a witness can provide?"

"Oh, did I ever," you answer. "There are 4 types of evidence: research and reports, statistics, anecdotal statements and assertions, and references to existing laws."

You take a deep breath, for you just answered Dr. Keats in a single breath.

"And there's more. It's important how witnesses testify. They have to be credible, use clarifying and engaging language, interpret and anticipate others' testimony and collaborate with others when they can, recognize the broad implications of their testimony, tell stories, cite research, and provide demonstrative evidence."

Professor Thomas taps Dr. Keats on the elbow. They exchange glances, smile, and, as if in chorus, say, "Well done, young scholar. Well done."

References

Education of All Handicapped Children Act. (1975). Pub. L. No. 94–142, 20, U.S.C. § 1400.

IDEA: Focusing on improving results for children with disabilities: Hearing before the Subcommittee on Education Reform of the Committee on Education and the Workforce, (Serial 108–9), 108th Cong. (2003).

Individuals with Disabilities Education Act (IDEA), (as amended in 2004). Pub. L. No. 108–446, 20, U.S.C. § 1400.

Mills v. District of Columbia Bd. of Ed., 348 F. Supp. 866 (D.D.C. 1972).

Mish, F. C. (Ed.). (2004). *Merriam-Webster's collegiate dictionary: The words you need know* (10th ed.). Springfield, MA: Merriam-Webster.

Pennsylvania Association for Retarded Children (PARC) v. Commonwealth., 343 F. Supp. 279 (1972).

Technology Related Assistance for Individuals with Disabilities Act of 1988 (Tech Act) (P.L. 100–407), 29 U.S.C. Secs. 3001 *et seq.*

Turnbull, H. R., Stowe, M. J., & Huerta, N. E. (2007). *Free appropriate public education: The law and children with disabilities* (7th ed.). Denver: Love.

Chapter 17
The Promise of Family Engagement: An Action Plan for System-Level Policy and Advocacy

Kathleen Ferreira, Sharon Hodges, and Elaine Slaton

In its blueprint for mental healthcare reform, the President's New Freedom Commission outlined a plan for system transformation that prioritized consumer and family-driven care (2003). This federal policy position came on the heels of the Surgeon General's Report on Children's Mental Health (1999), advocating an integrated service system model that is inclusive of family engagement. Children's mental health policy affects children, youth, and families at both the individual treatment level and the system level. The individual level refers to the ways in which direct care staff members interact with individual youth, families, and their support systems in the planning and delivery of services and supports (Rosenblatt, 1998). In contrast, the system level refers to the structural, administrative, and fiscal organization of a continuum of services and supports including linkages between child-serving agencies such as mental health, child welfare, juvenile justice, and education in a community-based setting (Rosenblatt, 1998). Although the past 20 years have marked significant expansion in the role of families in individual treatment-level decision making (Hoagwood, 2005), consistent and meaningful engagement of families in system-level policy action has been much more difficult to accomplish. Knitzer and Cooper (2006) note considerable variation across states related to family advocacy as well as value-driven conflict around family empowerment in system-level decision making.

K. Ferreira, Ph.D. (✉) • S. Hodges, Ph.D., M.B.A
Division of Training, Research, Education, and Demonstration, Department of Child and Family Studies, College of Behavioral and Community Sciences, Louis de la Parte Florida Mental Health Institute, University of South Florida, 13301 Bruce B. Downs Boulevard, MHC 2433, Tampa, FL 33612, USA
e-mail: ferreira@usf.edu

E. Slaton, M.S.A.
Slaton Associates, LLC, Tampa, FL, USA

A. McDonald Culp (ed.), *Child and Family Advocacy: Bridging the Gaps Between Research, Practice, and Policy*, Issues in Clinical Child Psychology,
DOI 10.1007/978-1-4614-7456-2_17, © Springer Science+Business Media New York 2013

Throughout this book, authors have described a number of advocacy efforts specific to a broad array of child and adolescent issues. For example, McCabe et al. (this volume) detail their approach to advocacy for children's mental health through multi-sector stakeholder collaboration. This chapter will focus specifically on the role of families in system-level policy and advocacy efforts for children and adolescents with mental health challenges. In children's mental health, family-run organizations are often the structural mechanisms used to coordinate and impact advocacy efforts at the system level. Although the focus of this chapter is children's mental health, the framework provided could be applied to adult mental health, primary healthcare, or other consumer advocacy organizations and efforts.

Historically, the degree to which families have been engaged in the mental, emotional, and behavioral health care of their children has varied considerably, as have perceptions by professionals across different service sectors as to what constitutes an appropriate family role. This chapter will consider the impact of family advocacy in children's mental health and will present an action plan for family engagement in child mental health policy and advocacy at the service system level. The chapter will provide a policy framework that identifies goals of system-level family engagement and specific action steps grounded in the structures, processes, relationships, and values of family engagement. Specific examples of successful family engagement in the system-level processes of policy change and advocacy efforts at the local, state, and federal levels will be described. The policy impact of these efforts will also be discussed.

Throughout this chapter, the terms "family" and "family-driven care" are used. It is important to note that in the context of family advocacy and family-driven care, the term "family" is broad, and its meaning is often unclear. Does family refer to biological parents, siblings, or extended family? How is this different from the term "consumer" that is often used in adult mental health advocacy efforts? For the purpose of this discussion, the term "family" as it relates to "family-driven care" will refer to an individual who is a primary caregiver for a child or youth with mental, emotional, or behavioral challenges (USDHHS, 2002). This will include biological parents, stepparents, adoptive parents, foster parents, surrogate parents, extended family members, or other caregivers. It should be noted that although children and youth are *consumers* of mental health services, their status as minors means that their decision-making authority is limited, and adult caregivers generally serve in the primary decision-making role for these consumers. It should also be acknowledged that many biological parents are no longer in primary decision-making roles because they have lost custody or have been forced to relinquish custody in order to access services for their children or youth (Friesen, Giliberti, Katz-Leavy, Osher, & Pullmann, 2003).

The Changing Role of Families in Children's Mental Health

The literature indicates that the role of families within mental health service systems has seen much change over the last century. In the early to mid-twentieth century, families of youth with mental health challenges had a particularly difficult time engaging in the treatment process because family members were perceived as a primary cause of the behavioral and emotional challenges of their children (Duchnowski & Kutash, 2007; Friesen & Koroloff, 1990; Friesen & Stephens, 1998). In fact, Friesen and Koroloff (1990) note that the pattern of ignoring the role of families in the treatment process was not accidental "but is related at least in part to deep-seated beliefs about the nature and cause of emotional disorders in children" (p. 14). This perspective began to change in the 1950s as families began to be regarded as *passive recipients of interventions* (Duchnowski & Kutash, 2007; Friesen & Stephens, 1998). The 1980s reflected a significant shift in thinking and activity as families were actively engaged as *partners in the treatment process* (Bryant-Comstock, Huff, & VanDenBerg, 1996; Duchnowski & Kutash, 2007; Friesen & Stephens, 1998; McManus & Friesen, 1986), a role that is still very much a part of the current model of treatment.

The 1990s to present day have reflected a more strengths-based approach to serving children and families, increased collaboration with families, and expansion of the role of families beyond their role in the treatment planning process for their individual children. The purposeful expansion of family involvement is commonly reflected in case management activities, peer-to-peer support and advocacy, training, and mediation (Friesen & Stephens, 1998; Hoagwood, 2005; Kutash, Duchnowski, Green, & Ferron, 2011). The field of children's mental health is also seeing the role of families in evaluation and research gain momentum, particularly when empowerment evaluation and participatory action research is used.

The broad timeline above reflects the changing role of families from old theories of the mother as pathogen to newer approaches that include families as partners in the treatment process, advocates, evaluators, and leaders in children's mental health initiatives. Although subtle changes in the perceptions of families had taken place earlier, activities in the 1980s significantly impacted the role of families in the field of children's mental health. What has been the impetus for these significant changes in the field? What impact has public policy had on advancing the role of families in children's mental health? A brief discussion of research and advocacy activities, funding support, and policy influences sheds light on some of the driving forces for this change.

Among significant drivers of public policy change, the Substance Abuse and Mental Health Services Administration and National Institute on Disability and Rehabilitation Research provided funding for the Research and Training Center (RTC) on Family Support and Children's Mental Health at Portland State University in 1984; the RTC's 1986 *Families as Allies* conference provided one of the first conferences on the role of families in improving services, supports, and family advocacy; and the RTC's *Next Steps* meeting in 1988 focused exclusively on core child and family issues. These events emphasize significant milestones in the advancement of the role of families in the children's mental health field (Bryant-Comstock et al., 1996). Activities to support families further gained traction in 1988 with grants through the Children and Adolescent Service System Program to develop statewide family networks, and in 2005 with the Children's Mental Health Initiative funding requirement that each community hire a lead family contact as it develops a system of care for youth with serious emotional disturbance (USDHHS, 2005). In addition, the creation of the National Federation of Families for Children's Mental Health in 1989, an organization developed specifically to provide advocacy for families of children and youth with mental health challenges, highlighted a myriad of issues faced by families of youth with emotional and behavioral challenges. The role of family-run organizations has primarily been to provide information, support, and advocacy to the families of children and youth with mental health needs.

Further, policy influences such as the Surgeon General's Report (1999) and the President's New Freedom Commission (2003) strongly supported consumer and family-driven services. Most recently, the Patient Protection and Affordable Care Act (2010) has emphasized the important role of consumers in healthcare access and service delivery. Although families have become more involved as advocates in the individual treatment of children and youth with emotional or behavior challenges, their role in system-level policy and advocacy efforts related to children's mental health services and supports is still developing.

The Importance of Family Engagement in Policy and Advocacy

The developments described above indicate a shift in expectations for family engagement at both the individual treatment and system levels. It is important to consider two perspectives underlying this expanded role —one is centered on outcomes and the other is grounded in values.

Outcomes Consideration

One justification for increasing family engagement is that such involvement improves outcomes. Comprehensive examinations of family engagement in individual treatment planning for youth with mental health challenges demonstrate improved treatment retention, satisfaction, and levels of active participation in service planning (Hoagwood, 2005) and improvements in school behavior for their children, including decreases in expulsions, suspensions, and detention referrals (Osher, Xu, & Allen, 2006). Further, research shows that empowerment of families at the individual treatment level leads to improved service system knowledge, self-efficacy, and sense of control in their lives (Bickman, Heflinger, Northrup, Sonnichsen, & Schilling, 1998; Taub, Tighe, & Burchard, 2001). Yet, what outcomes might be expected when families are engaged in decision making, policy development, and advocacy efforts at a broader system level?

The outcomes of *system-level* family engagement are more evident in primary healthcare and developmental disabilities than in the field of children's mental health, where research on family engagement at the system level is somewhat limited. Literature shows that consumer engagement in policy and advocacy in primary healthcare has produced demonstrably positive results in improving healthcare quality (Arnold, 2007; Hurley, Keenan, Martsolf, Maeng, & Scanlon, 2009; Leape et al., 2009), health outcomes (Baker et al., 2005; Barratt, 2008; Hurley et al., 2009; Légaré, Ratté, Gravel, & Graham, 2008; Lorig et al., 2001), and patient satisfaction (Baker et al., 2005). Some have made significant contributions with their single story, such as the Beckett family, whose advocacy efforts led to the *Katie Beckett Waiver*, changing healthcare coverage for those with long-term disabilities who wish to receive nursing care at home (Johnson, 2000).

In children's mental health, there are likely multiple reasons for the dearth of research on outcomes resulting from family engagement. One reason may be that system-level policy and advocacy is often carried out through family-run organizations, and the immediacy and political sensitivity of their efforts make them difficult to document. However, family advocates involved in organizations such as the National Federation of Families for Children's Mental Health (http://www.ffcmh. org) argue that family-run organizations have improved outcomes through system-level advocacy by engaging thousands of diverse families, gathering and synthesizing their input, and strategically undertaking activities that serve to inform the creation, passage, funding, and monitoring of local, state, and federal policy. Family advocates also indicate that because people tend to share more intimate information with trusted colleagues with whom they share common experiences, beliefs, and values, family-run organizations have access to information otherwise unavailable. In addition to information gleaned through relationships, family-to-family service provision, support groups, and conferences, family-run organizations often gather data using online surveys. This structured information gathering supports proactive activities such as educating legislators about issues of importance or making specific requests of program administrators as well as providing real-time response to pending legislation. Family-run organizations have the capacity to distribute plain language notice of the draft legislation to their constituents in several languages, including links to online survey requests for family input. One such action described by a member of a statewide family-run organization indicated that they were able to provide their legislator with response to pending legislation from more than 19,000 families within 24 h. This simple activity changed the course of the legislation.

Values Consideration

In addition to research indicating that family engagement leads to positive outcomes for children with mental health challenges and families, many would argue that regardless of outcomes, family engagement in decision making at any level is simply a right that families should have. The right of families to be engaged at both the individual and system levels might best be understood as a form of citizen participation in the democratic process. Core to democratic tradition, citizen participation has been defined as "[citizen] deliberation on issues affecting one's own life" (Fischer, 2000, p. 1). The direct connection of policies and programs to the people impacted benefits society by giving meaning to democracy, legitimizing policy development and implementation, and adding local knowledge to the discourse (Fischer, 2000). Local knowledge, in the case of family engagement, is defined not exclusively by geography, but by the common experiences and expertise of families raising children with mental health challenges.

In children's mental health, the position that families have the right to be engaged and that their inclusion is the appropriate ethical response has been supported by many in the field noting that principles of empowerment provide a value that essentially makes the link to outcomes superfluous (Croft & Beresford, 1992; Dunst & Trivette, 1987; Linhorst, Eckert, & Hamilton, 2005; National Association of Social Workers, 2008).

In sum, family engagement in system-level children's mental health policy and advocacy efforts should be considered essential in order for policy to serve the needs of those most directly impacted. The public discourse around children's mental health must be informed by the expertise of those who have witnessed firsthand what does and does not work for children in their care to ensure positive outcomes result from policy implementation. Thus, family engagement is critical to the formation, implementation, and evaluation of all policies impacting children with mental health challenges and their families.

A Framework for Engaging Families in Policy and Advocacy

The examples of family engagement described above illustrate a small sample of successful activities that may occur when families are engaged in system-level policy and advocacy efforts. It is less clear how system-level family engagement can be successfully fostered. A framework for supporting family engagement is critical to integrating families into the policy process. The framework presented below is derived from findings of a 5-year national study of the development and implementation of collaborative interagency service systems for children and youth with mental health challenges[1] and a sub-study on the role of families in system-level service planning and delivery.[2]

The initial study, Case Studies of System Implementation (CSSI), used a multi-site embedded case study design to examine systems change in six system-of-care communities throughout the country. Key points of investigation included examination of facilitators and impediments to reducing system fragmentation and strategies for providing less restrictive community-based services and supports. Data from document review, semi-structured key informant interviews, meeting observations,

---

[1] *Case Studies of System Implementation*, a 5-year study jointly funded through the National Institute on Disability and Rehabilitation Research and the Substance Abuse and Mental Health Services Administration. http://rtckids.fmhi.usf.edu/cssi/default.cfm.

[2] *Actualizing Empowerment: Developing a Framework for Partnering with Families in System Level Service Planning and Delivery.* http://logicmodel.fmhi.usf.edu/resources/PDF/ActualizingEmpowermentSymposium3_21_11.pdf

Fig. 17.1 Framework for
system-level family
engagement

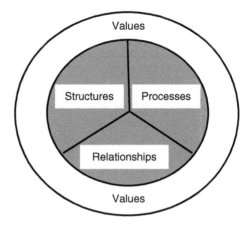

and surveys were coded to identify themes related to systems change strategies. This analysis yielded a cross-site theme regarding the role of families in service planning and delivery decisions. In particular, the data suggested that family-run organizations played a pivotal role in accomplishing and sustaining systems change, prompting further examination of this topic. A secondary analysis of data was conducted to look in greater detail at how these systems engaged families in policy-level decision making. Data included 307 documents, 268 transcribed interviews with key informants, and 41 sets of observation notes. Findings from this secondary analysis suggest that strategies for engaging families in system-level policy and advocacy can be divided into four core components of action that are critical to accomplishing family-driven care at the local, state, and federal levels. These findings were validated through a series of focus groups conducted with family members and system leaders. The four components of action include structures, processes, relationships, and values. It should be noted that although the policy framework described in this chapter presents an example of advocacy efforts within the field of children's mental health, these core action components have the potential to impact a broad array of advocacy efforts.

In system development, changes to one part of a system impact other parts of the system and the functioning of the system as a whole (Hodges, Ferreira, & Israel, 2012). The graphic in Fig. 17.1 is intended to illustrate the interrelatedness of the four action components. Findings indicate that when engaging family members in system-level policy and advocacy efforts, structures, processes, and relationships are critical components and essentially equal in importance. However, data indicate that a *shared value* for the importance of family engagement is foundational and must be infused into the structures, processes, and relationships that support family engagement in system-level policy and advocacy. Definitions of each of these action components are useful in understanding the framework and will be provided below.

Structures

Structures can be understood as the specified roles, responsibilities, and authorities that establish organizational boundaries and enable an organization to perform its functions. Findings from the study reflect the importance of the presence of a family-run organization in providing information, support, and training for families as well as leadership and advocacy related to policy action. Research data indicate that family-run organizations could successfully partner with formal service providers by engaging in activities as diverse as training, evaluation, budgeting, and political advocacy. These family-run organizations were locally developed, politically and financially autonomous, and respected as equal partners with the formal agencies within their systems. The reader will note that in terms of policy action, data suggest the presence of a family-run *organization* is important as opposed to the involvement of individual unaffiliated family members. An engaged and well-organized family-run organization may influence policy by allowing a large number of families or consumers to have a highly active, coordinated advocacy effort and a unified voice in policy, whether at the local, state, or federal level. Data indicate that the absence of a formal family-run organization made the sustainable impact of family advocacy more difficult to achieve.

How can families have impact on policies affecting the lives of children with mental health challenges? Including families on formal interagency governance or policy boards increases the likelihood that families will meaningfully impact policy and advocacy efforts by creating a critical presence, and the inclusion of multiple family members helps ensure that a variety of family perspectives are represented. Compensating family members for their participation acknowledges that their time is meaningful and helps to create equality across all members of the board. Further, data indicate that when family members serve as representatives of formal family-run organizations on governing boards, their presence brings more influence.

In regard to the development of family-run organizations, system partners demonstrate their support of family members in the policy process when they work with families to develop the family-run organization. It is important to note, however, that autonomy of the family-run organization, both politically and financially, allows the organization to focus on support, advocacy, and training for families without fighting competing priorities of a larger organization.

Processes

Processes are defined as the methods and procedures for carrying out organizational activities and often involve sequences or sets of interrelated activities that enable an organization to perform its functions. A key study finding was that system partners engage in activities to create collaborations with and help build capacity of the family-run organization. Collaborative activities might include joint evaluation and quality assurance activities, strategic planning, joint decision making around funding, collaborative grant writing, copresenting at state and national conferences, and cross-agency problem-solving and conflict resolution as well as shared training activities. An additional study finding was that family-run organizations initiate multiple processes to build capacities of families, build the capacity of the organization, and strengthen collaborations with system partners. These activities may include training and coaching family members in preparation for governance, policy board, and interagency council meetings; active participation in governance and policy meetings; conducting targeted outreach to system partners to strengthen collaborations; and evaluation and dissemination activities related to children's mental health services and supports.

Relationships

Relationships are trust-based links creating connectedness across people and organizations. A key finding related to relationships is that the *process of relationship building* is a critical characteristic of family engagement in system-level policy and advocacy. In fact this broad relationship building is more critical than developing relationships with only a small group of specific individuals. For example, rather than focusing only on connecting with the director of the child welfare agency, members of the family-run organization conduct ongoing outreach to a broad array of individuals within the agency, working constantly to develop new relationships. Strengths-based interactions used to develop relationships between family members and formal providers are in stark contrast to the adversarial relationships that are often observed in children's mental health, and they reflect team-based planning and problem-solving processes that are far more inclusive of families. Relationship building is a one-on-one, continuous process that is viewed as a long-term commitment between families and formal providers. It is important to note that although many stakeholders benefit from the inclusion of families' perspectives and collaboration, study findings indicate that members of family-run organizations have accepted an enormous amount of responsibility for developing positive relationships with agencies.

Values

Values are defined as an ideal accepted by an individual or group. A key study finding in systems that successfully engaged families in system-level policy and advocacy was the presence of a *shared value* for family involvement that resulted in a *shared commitment* to making this happen. It should be noted that some child-serving agencies might not embrace system-level family engagement, at least in the beginning. It is important to consider that disparate mandates across agencies may create opposing perspectives or experiences with families (e.g., juvenile justice or child welfare partners may have different expectations related to participation of families than those of mental health entities). Data indicate that in systems that have successfully engaged families, system leaders work to infuse a core value for system-level family engagement across system partners using both the outcomes and values arguments. The expectation that families would be involved in system-level decision making and collaborative activities and that the family-run organization *is* and *should be* an equal partner with child-serving agencies has become embedded as a core system value.

Action Steps for Achieving Family Engagement in System-Level Policy and Advocacy

Each component of the framework described above yields action steps that system stakeholders may undertake to promote system-level family engagement in policy and advocacy efforts. These action steps may be carried out by individuals in positions of authority within the system, members of the family-run organization, and other stakeholders within the system such as direct care providers, members of faith-based or other community-based organizations. Action steps to support each of the four action components are described below. The reader will then be asked to apply this information to a real-world situation.

Action Steps: Structures

Action steps that support family engagement in children's mental health policy and advocacy at the local, state, and federal levels include developing structures that solidify their roles and responsibilities. Examples of action steps used to impact structure include:

- Formal interagency governance and policy boards with authority at the local, state, and federal levels could ensure that their mission and vision statements, bylaws, policies and procedures, logic models, and strategic plans reflect the inclusion of families and clearly articulate their roles and responsibilities
- Formal interagency governance and policy boards could develop and maintain permanent positions for family members in their membership, and these boards could include multiple and varying family members to gain multiple perspectives
- Family members who participate in governance and policy boards, strategic planning activities, and other system-level policy planning activities could be compensated for their time
- Family-run organizations could articulate a commitment to policy and advocacy work in their mission statements and develop strategic plans that reflect this mission
- Family-run organizations could maintain connections with other local, state, and national chapters for support, technical assistance, policy information, and inclusion in policy and advocacy efforts

Scenario *Your best friend's 10-year-old child has been having academic and behavioral challenges and was recently diagnosed with Attention Deficit Hyperactivity Disorder (ADHD) and an Anxiety Disorder. Your friend is trying to access services and supports for her child and family. You recently heard a story on your local public radio station about Supporting Families, a local family-run organization that provides resources and support for families of children and youth with mental health challenges. Considering the discussion on structures above, what information would you want to know about the organization? How could you find out more information about what supports it provides? How could you help your friend get connected to this resource?*

Action Steps: Processes

Action steps that support family engagement in children's mental health policy and advocacy at the system level include identifying and implementing processes that strengthen collaboration across all partners, including families. Action steps:

- System leaders could encourage family attendance and active participation in governance and policy meetings
- System stakeholders could include families in collaborative activities with other agency partners—activities such as training, grant writing, joint decision making around funding, cross-agency problem solving, and copresenting at state and national conference and meetings
- System leaders and staff within provider agencies could provide family-run organizations with training and technical assistance in organizational management, grant writing, evaluation/quality assurance activities, working toward 501C3 status in order to support their autonomy and long-term sustainability
- System leaders could collaborate on policy change to allow the family-run organization to become part of the provider network and have reimbursable activities
- Family-run organizations could work to prepare families for meaningful participation in governance and policy boards and interagency meetings
- Family members could attend governance and policy board and interagency meetings and actively participate
- Family-run organizations could develop skills needed to run an organization, including training in organizational management, grant writing, evaluation activities, and becoming effective trainers
- Family-run organizations could engage in strategic outreach with formal system partners, focusing on developing collaborations, problem solving, and relationship building

Scenario *You were recently hired as the director of a program that provides Parent Child Interaction Therapy (PCIT) to treat young children who have experienced trauma. What processes can you facilitate to: create collaborations with other local provider agencies and family-run organizations, develop a referral process for trauma services, and engage in community-wide education and outreach related to trauma?*

Action Steps: Relationships

Relationships are an important factor in promoting family engagement in policy and advocacy efforts for children's mental health. Action steps that support relationship building:

- System stakeholders, in particular system leaders and members of the family-run organization, could model strengths-based interactions with family members and across agency partners. This modeling demonstrates to system partners how to work with families in an expanded role
- System stakeholders could include families at every opportunity of system development and implementation
- System leaders could make a long-term, shared commitment to support the family-run organization (including assisting them in becoming financially and politically autonomous)
- System stakeholders could acknowledge and prepare for relationship building to be a long-term investment because it takes time to develop relationships, especially due to staff turnover in agencies and family-run organizations

Scenario *You are the newly elected President of the Board of Supporting Families, the local family-run organization. What strategies do you use to approach system leaders about developing collaborations with their agencies? How will you work to develop relationships between your family-run organization (and its members) and direct care staff of provider agencies? How will you demonstrate a commitment to the work of system partners? How will you communicate what your organization has to offer as a partner?*

Action Steps: Values

The concept of Values is not one that generally connotes concrete action steps; however, there are activities that can help to infuse the shared value for families in system-level policy and advocacy efforts. Action steps:

- System leaders could regularly articulate the expectation that families be involved in governance and policy decisions and collaborative activities
- System stakeholders could model collaboration with families and the family-run organization, ensuring family voice at all levels of governance, even when this means stopping and rescheduling meetings when families are not represented
- All system stakeholders could regularly engage in self-reflection, exploring new ways in which families can be involved in system-level policy and advocacy efforts
- Family-run organizations could identify at least one system leader who is a "champion" for family engagement in system-level policy and advocacy and work with them to promote family-driven care with system partners
- Family-run organizations could work to demonstrate to system partners the benefits of teaming with the family-run organization

Scenario *You were recently hired as a case manager for a local agency that serves children and families involved in the child welfare system. Your agency director regularly talks about family driven care and providing strengths-based services, but you are not quite sure what she means. What steps could you take to better understand these values and apply them to your daily work with children and their families?*

Policy Impact of System-Level Family Engagement

This chapter has provided a framework and action steps to support family engagement in system-level policy and advocacy efforts in the field of children's mental health. What is the impact of family engagement in system-level policy and advocacy efforts in the field of children's mental health? Based on study findings, we suggest the following:

1. *Family engagement increases community awareness of children's mental health issues and reduces of stigma.* Public dissemination of information about mental health disorders in children and youth and dissemination of system outcomes data by family advocates—especially when conducted with formal system partners—demonstrates a team-based effort to work together to improve the lives of youth with mental health challenges and their families. Further, family members' strengths-based, rather than adversarial, interactions with these community partners help to create a positive perception of families struggling with these issues. Social media campaigns on mental health awareness, public information events, press conferences, and other activities at the local, state, and national levels help to put a face to the many challenges these families experience. In turn, this community awareness helps to create an environment in which policies and budgets are likely to be more responsive to real needs because policymakers are better informed about the lives of children and youth with mental health issues and their families
2. *Family engagement improves the service system's ability to respond to community need.* A strong family voice contributes to gaining a clearer understanding of the issues of children's mental health at local, state, and federal policy levels. This has the potential to impact setting of priorities for legislative or funding initiatives or making changes to priorities based on emerging issues. In addition, engagement of families allows for direct input on effective ways to address the needs of children and youth with mental health challenges and their families
3. *Family engagement improves service system sustainability.* The engagement of families, especially in the context of a family-run organization, can support a service system by advocating for children's mental health funding, infrastructure, services, and supports. This is particularly evident as they partner with formal service providers in grant writing, evaluation, and quality assurance activities as well as through direct education of policymakers, legislators, and committee members. In addition, as independent family-run organizations develop services that are cost reimbursable, their own sustainability becomes less dependent, less of a burden, on the rest of the system and their services may reduce tension on a system straining to meet the needs of the community

Conclusion

The framework and action steps presented in this chapter emphasize the importance of families in policy and advocacy efforts at local, state, and federal levels, but particularly highlight the powerful presence that family-run *organizations* can have on policy and advocacy. Family-run organizations have long focused on the delivery of information, support, and advocacy to families raising children with mental health challenges. They have the ability to: (a) ensure authentic representation of the collective population of families raising children with mental health challenges in policy and advocacy; (b) provide a clear focus using strategies to maximize their influence; and (c) simultaneously ensure creditability with both policy makers and the public at large to have the most impact.

The framework presented in this chapter reinforces the notion that the involvement of families in system-level policy and advocacy requires collaborative action and the commitment of formal service providers, community stakeholders, and families. Ultimately, the engagement of families as significant contributors to and collaborators in system-level policy and advocacy is both a value and responsibility that we must each assume.

References

Arnold, S. B. (2007). Improving quality health care: The role of consumer engagement *Issue Brief 1*. Princeton, NJ: Robert Wood Johnson Foundation.

Baker, D. W., Asch, S. M., Keesey, J. W., Brown, J. A., Chan, K. S., Joyce, G., et al. (2005). Differences in education, knowledge, self-management activities, and health outcomes for patients with heart failure cared for under the chronic disease model: The improving chronic illness care evaluation. *Journal of Cardiac Failure, 11*(6), 405–413. doi:10.1016/j.cardfail. 2005.03.010.

Barratt, A. (2008). Evidence based medicine and shared decision making: The challenge of getting both evidence and preferences into health care. *Patient Education and Counseling, 73*(3), 407–412. doi:10.1016/j.pec.2008.07.054.

Bickman, L., Heflinger, C. A., Northrup, D., Sonnichsen, S., & Schilling, S. (1998). Long term outcomes to family caregiver empowerment. *Journal of Child and Family Studies, 7*(3), 269–282. doi:1062-1024/98/0900-0269$15.00/0.

Bryant-Comstock, S., Huff, B., & VanDenBerg, J. (1996). The evolution of the family advocacy movement. In B. A. Stroul (Ed.), *Children's mental health: Creating systems of care in a changing society* (pp. 359–374). Baltimore, MD: Paul H. Brookes.

Croft, S., & Beresford, P. (1992). The politics of participation. *Critical Social Policy, 35*, 20–44. doi:10.1177/026101839201203502.

Duchnowski, A. J., & Kutash, K. (2007). *Family driven care: Are we there yet?* Tampa, FL: University of South Florida, The Louis de la Parte Florida Mental Health Institute, Department of Child & Family Studies.

Dunst, C. J., & Trivette, C. M. (1987). Enabling and empowering families: Conceptual and intervention issues. *School Psychology Review, 16*, 443–456. Retrieved from http://www.nasponline.org/publications/spr/sprmain.aspx

Fischer, F. (2000). *Citizens, experts, and the environment: The politics of local knowledge*. Durham and London: Duke University Press.

Friesen, B. J., Giliberti, M., Katz-Leavy, J., Osher, T., & Pullmann, M. D. (2003). Research in the service of policy change: "The custody problem". *Journal of Emotional and Behavioral Disorders, 11*(1), 39–47. doi:10.1177/106342660301100106.

Friesen, B. J., & Koroloff, N. (1990). Family-centered services: Implications for mental health administration and research. *Journal of Mental Health Administration, 17*(1), 13–25. doi:10.1007/BF02518576.

Friesen, B. J., & Stephens, B. (1998). Expanding family roles in the system of care: Research and practice. In M. H. Epstein, K. Kutash, & A. J. Duchnowski (Eds.), *Outcomes for children and youth with emotional and behavioral disorders and their families: Programs and evaluation best practices* (1st ed., pp. 231–259). Austin, TX: Pro-ED.

Hoagwood, K. E. (2005). Family-based services in children's mental health: A research review and synthesis. *Journal of Child Psychology and Psychiatry, 46*, 690–713. doi:10.1111/j.1469-7610.2005.01451.x.

Hodges, S., Ferreira, K., & Israel, N. (2012). "If we're going to change things, it has to be systemic:" Systems change in children's mental health. *American Journal of Community Psychology.* Advance online publication. doi:10.1007/s10464-012-9491-0.

Hurley, R. E., Keenan, P. S., Martsolf, G. R., Maeng, D. D., & Scanlon, D. P. (2009). Early experiences with consumer engagement initiatives to improve chronic care. *Health Affairs, 28*(1), 277–283. doi:10.1377/hlthaff.28.1.277.

Johnson, B. H. (2000). Family-centered care: Four decades of progress. *Families, Systems & Health, 18*(2), 137–156. doi:10.1037/h0091843.

Knitzer, J., & Cooper, J. (2006). Beyond integration: Challenges for children's mental health. *Health Affairs, 25*(3), 670–679. doi:10.1377/hlthaff.25.3.670ersity.

Kutash, K., Duchnowski, A. J., Green, A. L., & Ferron, J. (2011). Supporting parents who have youth with emotional disturbances through a parent-to-parent support program: A proof of concept study using random assignment. *Administration and Policy in Mental Health and Mental Health Services Research, 38*, 412–427. doi:10.1007/s10488-010-0329-5.

Leape, L., Berwick, D., Clancy, C., Conway, J., Gluck, P., Guest, J., et al. (2009). Transforming healthcare: A safety imperative. *Quality & Safety in Health Care, 18*(6), 424–428. doi:10.1136/qshc.2009.036954.

Légaré, F., Ratté, S., Gravel, K., & Graham, I. D. (2008). Barriers and facilitators to implementing shared decision-making in clinical practice: Update of a systematic review of health professionals' perceptions. *Patient Education and Counseling, 73*(3), 526–535. doi:10.1016/j.pec.2008.07.018.

Linhorst, D. M., Eckert, A., & Hamilton, G. (2005). Promoting participation in organizational decision making by clients with severe mental illness. *Social Work, 50*(1), 21–30. Retrieved from http://www.naswpress.org/publications/journals/sw.html

Lorig, K. R., Ritter, P., Stewart, A. L., Sobel, D. S., William Brown, B., Jr., Bandura, A., et al. (2001). Chronic disease self-management program: 2-year health status and health care utilization outcomes. *Medical Care, 39*(11), 1217–1223.

McManus, M., & Friesen, B. J. (1986). *Parents of emotionally handicapped children: Needs, resources, and relationships with professionals.* Portland, OR: Research and Training Center on Family Support and Children's Mental Health, Regional Research Institute, Portland State University.

National Association of Social Workers. (2008). *Code of ethics of the National Association of Social Workers (revised).* Washington, DC: Author. Retrieved from http://www.socialworkers.org/pubs/code/code.asp.

Osher, T., Xu, Y., & Allen, S. (2006, May–June). *Does family engagement matter? Findings from the Family-Driven Study.* Presentation at the 2006 Joint National Conference on Mental Health Block Grant and National Conference on Mental Health Statistics, Promoting Recovery through Transformation: Integrating Consumers and Families with Planning and Data, Washington, DC.

Patient Protection and Affordable Care Act of 2010, § H.R. 3590 (2010). Retrieved from http://frwebgate.access.gpo.gov/cgi-bin/getdoc.cgi?dbname=111_cong_bills&docid=f:h3590enr.txt.

President's New Freedom Commission on Mental Health. (2003). *Achieving the promise: Transforming mental health care in America, Final Report* (Pub. No. SMA-03-3832). Rockville, MD: Department of Health and Human Services.

Rosenblatt, A. (1998). Assessing the child and family outcomes of systems of care for youth with serious emotional disturbance. In M. Epstein, K. Kutash, & A. Duchnowski (Eds.), *Outcomes for children and youth with behavioral and emotional disorders and their families* (pp. 329–362). Austin, TX: PRO-ED.

Taub, J., Tighe, T. A., & Burchard, J. (2001). The effects of parent empowerment on adjustment of children receiving comprehensive mental health services. *Children's Services: Social Policy, Research, and Practice, 4*(3), 103–122. doi:10.1207/S15326918CS0403_1.

U.S. Department of Health and Human Services (USDHHS). (1999). *Mental health: A report of the Surgeon General. Chapter 3: Children and mental health.* Rockville, MD: Substance Abuse and Mental Health Services Administration, Center for Mental Health Services, National Institutes of Health, National Institute of Mental Health.

U.S. Department of Health and Human Services (USDHHS). (2002). *Cooperative agreements for the comprehensive community mental health services for children and their families program guidance for applicants (GFA) No. SM-02-002.* Washington, DC: Substance Abuse and Mental Health Services Administration Center for Mental Health Services.

U.S. Department of Health and Human Services (USDHHS). (2005). *Cooperative agreements for the comprehensive community mental health services for children and their families program request for applications (RFA) No. SM-05-010.* Washington, DC: Substance Abuse and Mental Health Services Administration, Center for Mental Health Services.

Part IV
History of Division 37

Chapter 18
The Evolving Legacy of the American Psychological Association's Division 37: Bridging Research, Practice, and Policy to Benefit Children and Families

Georgianna M. Achilles, Sandra Barrueco, and Bette L. Bottoms

> *Never doubt that a small group of thoughtful,*
> *committed citizens can change the world.*
> *Indeed, it is the only thing that ever has.*[®]
>
> Margaret Mead

Psychology has so much knowledge to offer to society, via a multitude of service and practice efforts. But it takes carefully orchestrated advocacy to ensure that our knowledge and services reach those who need it, especially children and families in distressed circumstances. Few understand this so well as members of the American Psychological Association's Division 37: The Society for Child and Family Policy and Practice, and its Section on Child Maltreatment. Division 37 was conceptualized 30 years ago, amid escalating national and international concern about the considerable mental health needs of children and families. Today the Division translates research into policy and action, developing and improving programs and services, and advocating for children and families at the local, state, and federal levels to prod those in power to allocate funds for research and services. The Division promotes the research, practice, and training relevant to child maltreatment and the

G.M. Achilles, Ph.D. (✉)
Midstep Centers for Child Development, 454 Rolling Ridge Drive, State College, PA 16801, USA
e-mail: gma@midstep.com

S. Barrueco, Ph.D.
The Catholic University of America, 620 Michigan Aveune, N.E., Washington, DC 20064, USA

B.L. Bottoms, Ph.D.
University of Illinois, Chicago, IL, USA

A. McDonald Culp (ed.), *Child and Family Advocacy: Bridging the Gaps Between Research, Practice, and Policy*, Issues in Clinical Child Psychology, DOI 10.1007/978-1-4614-7456-2_18, © Springer Science+Business Media New York 2013

mental health issues faced by victims. It has addressed various other stressors that impact children and families such as divorce and custody, foster care, drug- and HIV-exposure, homelessness, systemic racism, and other emerging agendas through the work of dedicated members who work tirelessly on task forces and committees. Since its inception, Division 37 members have diligently pursued the mission "to apply psychological knowledge to advocacy, service delivery, and public policies affecting children, youth, and families."

Early Division History

Division 37 was initiated in the 1970s under the tenacious leadership of Gertrude "Trudie" Williams and Milton Shore, who united various APA members interested in encouraging advocacy and influencing policy related to child and youth development. Although other APA divisions had previously engaged in child and family-relevant activities through their research- or practice-focused endeavors, thus addressing the first two aims of APA's general mission ("to advance psychology as a science and profession"), Division 37 was among the first to endorse a primary focus on APA's third and final aim: to promote "health, education, and human welfare" (APA, 2013, Article I—Objects; Routh & Culbertson, 1996).

The Divisions' founding sparked controversy about redundancy with other child-oriented divisions as well as its proposed child advocacy interests, which were seen as inconsistent with APA's scientific mission. The Division's founding was approved only after modifying the name from *Division of Children and Youth* to *Division of Children and Youth Services*, promoting confusion about whether its concerns lie primarily in the child clinical domain. Unrest about the goals and strategies was also evident within the budding Division.

However, clarity began to emerge through efforts of individuals such as Gary Melton, whose vision and energy helped set the Division on course for promoting child advocacy. As the first editor of the Division's newsletter he set an important precedent by providing in-depth discussions that were pertinent to the Division's interests. Further, he focused the Division activities through efforts such as proposing a set of task forces with clearly stated themes and objectives related to public policy and the methods for disseminating their findings to relevant audiences; orienting early career psychologists towards policy-related scholarship; and creating monograph discussions of child and family policy. He encouraged collaboration across divisions and proposed Division awards to recognize psychologists and non-psychologists whose advocacy work on behalf of children was exemplary. Melton served on the executive committee for twelve consecutive years, cultivating a style of operation and inspiring a foundational programmatic agenda.

The strong advocacy and policy focus seen in Melton's (1986) edited book on adolescents and abortion and Weithorn's (1987) volume on psychologists' involvement in child custody determinations was maintained and strengthened over time. In 1991, the Division adapted its mission statement to not only include *advocacy*, but also to list *advocacy* prior to *service delivery*. These changes, accompanying a growing portfolio of experiences in advocacy and service activities, placed the Division in a unique and strong position to respond to increasing mental health challenges facing children, youth, and families.[1]

Recent Division History

In 2007, the Division changed its name to the *Society for Child and Family Policy and Practice*. The new name was thought to better reflect the Division's current mission and welcome members from a broad range of disciplines. Advocacy was not added to the name, even though members share the belief that it, along with training, are essential elements of the Division's mission. The new name aptly reflects other important aspects of the Division's mission, which is "the application of psychological knowledge to advocacy, service delivery, and public policies affecting children, youth, and families. The Society advances research, education, training, and practice through a multidisciplinary perspective" (APA, n.d.b). Further, as stated in the Division's by laws, the Division's purposes are: "(1) To provide a recognized and designated organizational entity in APA to be concerned specifically with professional, scientific, and public interest issues relative to services and service delivery structures for children, youth, and families; (2) To advance and integrate the professional efforts of psychologists who work with children, youth, and families in different perspectives and settings; (3) To promote the application of developmental and ecological theory and research as a basis for development of prevention and intervention efforts with children, youth, and families; (4) To emphasize the importance of adequate education and training in service and investigative approaches related to children, youth, and families, and to the individuals, groups, and organizations who are in positions of influence in their lives; (5) To provide a systematic forum for the presentation of policy, clinical, and research findings in the area of services to children, youth, and families at APA meetings; (6) To provide a vehicle for relating psychological knowledge and integrating it with other fields (e.g., anthropology, law, pediatrics) and dimensions (e.g., employment, education, recreation, family planning), dealing with the total welfare of children, youth, and their families; (7) To provide a mechanism for child, youth, and family advocacy in order to bring about those social changes consistent with psychological knowledge that will promote the well-being of children, youth, and families; and (8) To stimulate the development of research initiatives on professional and policy issues concerning children, youth, and families by highlighting what is known and what needs to be known about these issues."

---

[1]For additional details on the early history of Division 37, see Routh and Culbertson (1996) in *Unification through division: Histories of the American Psychological Association*.

A Call to Action: Why Division 37 Is Needed

During the past 2 decades, numerous reports have documented the conditions contributing to unprecedented levels of serious mental health issues among our youth. The case for what is now recognized as a crisis in children's mental health is detailed in landmark federal documents such as *Mental Health: A Report of the Surgeon General* (U.S. Public Health Service, 1999), the *Report of the Surgeon General's Conference on Children's Mental Health* (US Public Health Service, 2000), the *Blueprints for Change: Research on Child and Adolescent Mental Health* (National Institutes of Health, 2001), and the *President's New Freedom Commission on Mental Health* (2003). Together, these reports examine research in biology, neurology, human development, and psychology and conclude that an alarming gap between research and practice currently limits the development of responsive social policies, and that there is a need for action to integrate these domains. The urgency of this need is underscored by the fact that child and adolescent mental illnesses are now estimated to affect 16–20 % of youth in our nation (National Research Council and Institute of Medicine, 2009), yet the vast majority of youth have limited access to treatment (Masi & Cooper, 2006). Untreated mental health problems are associated with short- and long-term problems such as chronic mental illnesses, substance abuse, school dropout, early parenthood, incarceration, and diminished quality of life (NIMH, 2001). These consequences take an enormous emotional and economic toll on our youth, their families, and society at large. As such, there have been additional calls by top researchers to focus policy efforts on prevention, as highlighted in the report *Preventing Mental, Emotional, and Behavioral Disorders Among Young People: Progress and Possibilities* (National Research Council and Institute of Medicine, 2009).

Likely contributing to the present level of need are the insufficiencies and instabilities of our managed care and welfare systems (Morris & Gennetian, 2006; Powell & Dunlap, 2005), along with the limited availability of treatments that have already garnered empirical support (Huang, Mcbeth, Dodge, & Jacobstein, 2004; Kutash & Rivera, 1995). There is special concern about the sociocultural relevance of many current treatments for the increasingly diverse and impoverished population of children of the twenty-first century (Crockett, 2003; Tolan & Dodge, 2005). As this group is least likely to use therapeutic services yet disproportionately absorbs the impact of multiple-stress environments (NIMH, 2001), the stage has been set for an explosion of mental health difficulties and a concomitant need for policy, funding, and services targeted at children, youth, and families. The stakes are high. As noted by Mary Jane England, Chair of the National Advisory Mental Health Council Workgroup on Child and Adolescent Mental Health Intervention Deployment, "Our ability to create a promising future for the country depends, in part, on our ability to ensure that all children have the opportunity to meet their full potential and to live healthy, productive lives. Meeting this challenge will require the work of many people. The research community must partner with families, providers, policymakers, and Federal agencies providing children's services, as well as other stakeholders, to create a knowledge base on interventions and services that is usable, disseminated, and sustained in the diverse communities where children and their families live. Equally important to this effort is the need to develop the capacity of the field. A new generation of truly interdisciplinary researchers must be trained to strengthen the science base on child and adolescent mental health research and bridge the gaps within and across research, practice, and policy" (NIMH, 2001, p. iii).

England's recommendation (NIMH, 2001) resonates with the purpose of Division 37 to improve the circumstances and futures of youth, their families, and communities through research, advocacy, service delivery, and public policy development. The Division has targeted these goals through a remarkable and interrelated set of activities including (a) building and maintaining a strong, organized infrastructure and an informed and active membership; (b) communicating and disseminating research to inform policy and services; (c) establishing professional development, training, and recognition programs; and (d) promoting divisional, interdivisional, and interdisciplinary collaborations focused on research, clinical outreach, and advocacy.

Infrastructure and Leadership: Secure Foundations for an Active Membership

Division 37 leaders and members have invested considerable effort in building the procedural framework, resources, and infrastructure needed to support members in child and family advocacy-oriented activities. The division functions under the leadership of the Executive Committee, which comprises 10 elected officers with voting rights: President, Past-president, President-elect, Secretary, Treasurer, Council Representative, Section on Child Maltreatment President, and 3 Members-at-Large. Other nonvoting, appointed officers of the Division include Graduate Student Representative (since 2000), Editor of the *Advocate* newsletter, Fellows Chair, Membership Chair, various chairs of committees and task forces, and liaisons to other organizations. In 2005, the Division also established an Undergraduate Student Representative position, optionally appointed by the President.

Each year, Presidents choose a theme for their initiatives. These have included the following: Edward Zigler: "Children, Youth, and Families"; Cynthia Shellenbach: "Fostering Resilient Children, Youth, and Families"; Karen Saywitz: "Developmental Psychology and the Child Witness"; Shelia Eyberg: "Dissemination of Mental Health Information to Parents and Teachers of Young Children in Head Start"; Brian Wilcox, who eschewed an explicit theme and focused on the Division's financial health and sustainability; Richard Abidin: "Children's Mental Health: Access Issues, Issues in the Delivery of Culturally Competent and Effect Treatments"; Luis Vargas: "Access, Engagement, and Intervention in the Delivery of Mental Health Services to Underserved and Culturally Diverse Children, Youth, and Families"; Bette Bottoms: "Improving Policy and Services through Research-based Advocacy"; Anne McDonald Culp: "Advocating for Prevention Programs and the Promotion of Positive Mental Health in Children"; Carol Falender: "Collaboration; Advancing

Thinking and Practice of Evidence-Based Treatments for Minority Children, Youth, and Families; and Expanding Advocacy Training on Children's Issues"; and Patrick Tolan: "Advancing Children's Mental Health by Emphasizing the Value of Collaboration." The division's most recent presidents include Carolyn Schroeder, Sandra J. Bishop-Josef, and Karen Budd. At this writing, the President is Michael Roberts and the President-elect is John E. Lochman.

The Section on Child Maltreatment

Division 37 has one section, the Section on Child Maltreatment, which was established to act as a catalyst for advocacy and research related specifically to child maltreatment. In the early to mid-1990s, amidst a climate of nationwide distress over escalating rates of child abuse, increasing levels of poverty, and declining federal support for social programs, Diane J. Willis directed the APA's Coordinating Committee on Child Abuse and Neglect to pioneer three working groups focused on child abuse issues: prevention and treatment, the legal system, and education and training. Their findings underscored the need to create an entity to champion child abuse issues in an exclusive and ongoing way. Willis approached a receptive Division 37 executive committee and President (Jan Culbertson) about this idea, and in 1994, the Section on Child Maltreatment was established with the mission to "advance scientific inquiry, training, and professional practice in child maltreatment, to provide up-to-date information about maltreatment, and to encourage networking and collaboration across Divisions/Sections in the area of child maltreatment." As Chair of the new Section, Willis wrote its original bylaws and led a Coordinating Committee of devoted child advocates with expertise in child maltreatment (including Barbara Boat, Barbara Bonner, Jan Culbertson, Dennis Drotar, Jeff Haugaard, Karen Saywitz, Cynthia Schellenbach) into its first official meeting at which the first Executive Committee was elected (consisting of a President with a 2-year term, President-Elect, Past-President, Treasurer, Secretary, and three Members-at-Large). Over the next 3 years, the first dedicated President, Jeffrey Haugaard, further developed the bylaws and appointed an Advisory Board of 20 widely known researchers, clinicians, and advocates in child maltreatment.

Today, the Section on Child Maltreatment is one of only two groups within the APA that focuses *exclusively* on issues related to child maltreatment (the other being a related special interest group within Division 56, Trauma Psychology). Most Section members are also Division members, illustrating the large role the Section plays in attracting and maintaining the membership of the Division as a whole. This is not surprising, given the centrality of child maltreatment to understanding children's mental health issues. Section members have conducted research, disseminated information, and organized trainings on the prevalence, causes, and prevention of child maltreatment, and on issues that arise when child victims enter the legal system. As discussed below, the Section has led the division in sponsoring congressional briefings, amicus briefs, and interdisciplinary conferences related to child maltreatment. In so doing, Section members have heightened awareness of child maltreatment and the needs of victims in public, professional, and political domains. Such advocacy activities have been possible because of the Section's Social Policy Committee, formed in 2000 under Gail Goodman's leadership to enhance the Section's policy work.

Communicating and Disseminating Research to Inform Policy and Services

Most recently, Division 37 has expanded synergistic communications among its members and society, by way of meetings and conferences, newsletters, and peer-reviewed publications.

Meetings, Conferences, and Electronic Communication

The Executive Committee meets in person semi-annually, at the APA convention and at a midwinter meeting often held in Washington, DC to facilitate connections with APA. The Section on Child Maltreatment Executive Committee also meets at the APA convention. The annual APA convention allows a range of opportunities for members to congregate and connect. It is a central event for the Division and Section, which do not have a separate dedicated conference as do some other larger divisions. The Division and Section sponsor a hospitality suite, social hours, symposia, poster sessions, business meetings, and award speeches.

Symposia are important forums for information dissemination. Key symposia have included "Linking Juvenile Delinquency and Child Maltreatment: Causes, Correlates, and Consequences"; "From Proof to Practice: Does Research Change Policy and Practice in Children's Services?"; and "Promoting Resiliency in Children and Families in the Wake of Hurricane Katrina." The Division expands its approximately ten symposium offerings by sometimes sponsoring cross-cutting interdivisional symposia with other child-relevant divisions. For example, while President, Bette L. Bottoms organized a cross-cutting symposium, "Psychology and Children: Translating Research into Better Policy and Services," involving divisions 37, 7, 16, 54, 27, 53, and Division 37 Past Presidents Gerry Koocher, Gail Goodman, and Brian Wilcox. While President, Carol Falender organized "Children's Mental Health: Innovations in Evidence-Based Treatment for Ethnic Minority Children and Adolescents," involving divisions 37, 12, 16, 37, 48, and 53. Both symposia formed the basis for issues of the *Child and Family Policy and Practice Review.*

The Division has expanded its outreach by cosponsoring conferences organized by other like-minded organizations. For example, in 1998, the Division cosponsored the conference "Violence Against Children in the Family and Community: A Conference on Causes, Developmental Consequences, Intervention and Prevention," which led Penelope Trickett and Cynthia Schellenbach into a Division 37/27 collaboration that culminated in their edited book, *Violence Against Children in the Family and Community.* The Division also cosponsored the *Florida Conference on Child Health Psychology* in 2001, and the Section on Child Maltreatment cosponsors and/or contributes to numerous cross-disciplinary conferences, trainings, and colloquia on interpersonal violence issues, with organizations such as the American Professional Society on the Abuse of Children (APSAC), the American Bar Association, and the American Psychology-Law Society (APA Division 41).

In 2000, the Division dedicated one of its Member-at-Large positions to "Communications and Technology," which has led to "virtual" meetings among members. Web-based chat rooms allow members to discuss child-relevant interests such as "Policy and Research in Child Rehabilitation Psychology," "Interventions for Depressed Youth" and "Issues Facing Children in the Legal System." A Division 37 electronic listserv functions to keep members informed about child and family issues, conference events, and policy developments. It is frequently used by Division presidents to communicate with the membership and by members of the Public Interest Government Relations Office to notify members of pending legislation in need of psychological input and action.

Newsletters

One of the most important channels of communication for Division members has been its publications. Its newsletter was established in 1978 under the direction of Seth Kalichman. Milton Shore and Suzanne Sobel published the first seven newsletters; when Gary Melton became editor in 1980, he created more a formal organizational framework. As the subsequent editor from 1983 to 1985, Donald Wertlieb formatted the newsletter to a newspaper style. Jan L. Culbertson then developed it to resemble its current format, originally including more advocacy-related topics in a "point—counterpoint" debate-style fashion. It was renamed the *Child, Youth, and Family Services Quarterly* in 1990 and then *The Child, Youth and Family Services Advocate* ("The Advocate") in 2000, mirroring the increasing transparency the division has placed on its public interest activities. The newsletter has evolved over the years, from early single-themed issues that included comprehensive literature reviews related to current policy and needed policy changes, to today's newsletter format that informs the membership about diverse substantive topics as well as organizational business issues. Across these transformations, it has always continued to be a comprehensive resource intended to keep readers current on research, service, and policy developments central to child and family well-being, as well as to encourage translating this knowledge into advocacy and practice. For example, articles focus on nutrition, Head Start, child welfare, child abuse and other such areas. Each issue often includes columns from Division leaders, members, and guest writers reviewing cutting-edge academic research and policy reports in articles such as "Socially Supportive Interviewing of Child Eyewitnesses" and "Advocating for Prevention Programs and the Promotion of Positive Mental Health for Children." In 1998, a regular column featuring the latest policy and advocacy developments in Washington, DC was added. Past newletters can be accessed at: http://www.apa.org/divisions/div37/child_maltreatment/child_newsletter.html.

The Section on Child Maltreatment regularly contributes to the *Advocate* with columns by its President and Graduate Student Representative, but the Section also has its own newsletter which spun off from the division's newsletter in 1997. It includes articles relevant to various aspects of abuse and recurring features such as the "Case Notes" column, launched by Bette Bottoms and focused on the implications of legal decisions related to child maltreatment and psychology, and the "Best Practices" column, launched Anthony Mannarino and focused on clinical best practices related to child maltreatment.

Peer-Reviewed Publications

A prime goal of Division 37 has always been to provide peer-reviewed publication outlets for materials relevant to child advocacy. Growing from an initiative during David Wolfe's presidency, between 1998 and 2002, the Division published and distributed to its membership more than 20 issues of its own peer-reviewed journal, *Children's Services: Social Policy, Research, and Practice,* edited by Michael Roberts. Articles reflected the Division's mission and ranged from Grasley, Wolfe, and Wekerle's (1999) discussion of a community-based program aimed to decrease violence in youth's relationships to Holden and Brannan's (2002) special issue disseminating the national evaluation of the Comprehensive Community Mental Health Services for Children and Their Families Program. Although it filled an important niche in the field, *Children's Services* was ultimately discontinued in 2003 due to the financial strain it placed on the Division. The final issue, cosponsored with the Section on Child Maltreatment, focused on the link between childhood maltreatment and later life juvenile delinquency (Quas, Bottoms, & Nuñez, 2002).

The resulting void was filled in 2005 with a semi-annual publication called the *Child and Family Policy and Practice Review*, edited and reviewed by Division presidents and their appointees. In some ways, this publication was a reincarnation of the initial single-themed *Child, Youth, and Family Services Quarterly*. For example, the inaugural issue, edited by Luis Vargas, "Cultural Diversity and Mental Health," highlighted the importance of appreciating diversity in mental health issues and of attending to the needs of underserved people. The issue represented the multicultural themes that are inherent in many of today's division activities. Later issues included Bette Bottoms' and Patricia Hashima's "Psychology and Children: Translating Research into Better Policy and Services," and Anne Culp's "Practice, Research and Policy Agendas for Healthy Family America: A Program Designed to Prevent Child Maltreatment." The publication of the *Review* ceased at the end of 2008 with Carol Falender's retrospective issue containing articles by Division presidents from every 5 years since 1985. In 2006, on behalf of the Division and the Section, Bottoms and Quas (2006) edited an issue of the *Journal of Social Issues* entitled, "Emerging directions in child maltreatment research: Multidisciplinary perspectives on theory, practice, and policy." The volume was dedicated to the very real needs of actual child maltreatment victims, after a decade that was at times more focused on debates about false reports and whether some forms of child sexual abuse are actually harmful (for discussion, see Goodman, 2006 and Ondersma et al., 2001).

The Section on Child Maltreatment has also sponsored an important series of publications describing model undergraduate, graduate, and professional curricula on child abuse and neglect. The first two, *Information on Child Maltreatment in the Undergraduate Curriculum* and *Including information on Child Maltreatment in the Graduate Curriculum*, resulted from one of Jeff Haugaard's presidential initiatives and were published in 1995 in cooperation with APA's Public Policy Directorate. In 2000, the trilogy was completed with a high school curriculum, *An Introduction to Child Maltreatment: A Five-Unit Lesson Plan for Teachers of Psychology in Secondary Schools*, with Cindy Miller-Perrin serving as editor (Miller-Perrin, 2000). Miller-Perrin and Malloy (2007) recently published an updated compendium of all the guides, the *Curriculum Guide for Instruction in Child Maltreatment*. These products, which can be accessed at http://www.apa.org/divisions/div37/resources.html, allow the Section and Division to reach hundreds (perhaps thousands) of students at the undergraduate and graduate level by providing packaged curricula that teachers who are not experts themselves can use to teach students about psychology-relevant issues facing children.

Professional Development, Training, and Recognition Programs

Division 37 and its Section on Child Maltreatment consider training and professional development to be of central importance. Building on national training guidelines endorsed by the Hilton Head Conference on Training Clinical Child Psychologists in 1985 (Roberts, Erickson, & Tuma, 1985), the Division is actively engaged in the development and dissemination of models and programs that strengthen the training of psychologists who provide services for youth (Roberts et al., 1998; Roberts & Task Force, 1996). The Division and Section have also developed vehicles for providing education on issues relevant to children, youth, and families for students, early career and established professionals, and the public at large. Finally, the Division and Section provide financial and monetary awards to support researchers in the field.

Student Training

The Division is deeply invested in cultivating the talents and interests of students and has established a highly visible support structure for this purpose. The Division offers students a special reduced-fee membership category and even free membership at times, believing that engaging students at the beginning of their careers will lead to an enduring commitment to the Division and, more importantly, to its purpose. The annual conference offers a student reception, mentorship and research presentation opportunities. Graduate student representatives edit a student page on the website and write a regular column in the Division's newsletter, aimed at educating students about how to become involved in advocacy and about policy-relevant pre- and postdoctoral training and career opportunities within academic, governmental, and nonprofit organizations. Undergraduate student representatives also contribute a newsletter column, "Spotlight on Undergraduates," which highlights an undergraduate involved in research or advocacy related to the Division's mission.

The Section on Child Maltreatment has also been dedicated to student training since its inception, as reflected in (a) its student representative position, (b) its 1997 roundtable discussion on training and education in child maltreatment at the annual APA conference (Nightingale & Portwood, 1997), (c) its maintenance of an Internship Guide on the web site that lists clinical internship sites providing training and services relevant to child abuse and neglect for clinical psychology doctoral students (thanks to the efforts of members such as Narina Nuñez), and (d) its participation in "Internships on Parade" at the APA Convention.

Postgraduate Education and Advocacy Training

The Division is also committed to the education of early career professionals and other postgraduate professionals within and outside of its membership. In 2008, it added to its Executive Committee a Member-at-large for Early Career Psychologists. In the late 1990s, the Division sponsored a Continuing Education program for licensed psychologists in collaboration with several state psychological associations and, with APA's Committee on Children, Youth, and Families (CYF), it cosponsored the Task Force on Innovative Training Approaches for Psychologists, chaired by Jane Knitzer and Judith Meyers. This activity led to an APA symposium and resource guide.

A centerpiece of the Division's training activities has been its Advocacy Training Initiative. For years, the Division partnered occasionally with the APA Public Interest Government Relations Office to sponsor free Advocacy Training Workshops in Washington, DC. There, members of Division 37 and other child-relevant divisions would participate in a morning training session, then spend the afternoon on Capitol Hill meeting with Congressional representatives and advocating for child issues. Consistent with the heart of the Division's mission, these sessions taught psychologists to advocate for children's needs with local, state, and national legislators. To expand the reach of these successful sessions substantially, APA Division 37 Task Force on Advocacy (2006) produced the *APA Division 37's Guide to Advocacy* (http://www.apa.org/divisions/div37/division37advocacyguidepart1.pdf). This specific and extensive advocacy training package is disseminated widely via the division's website and on DVD and includes materials that can be used by anyone (students and postgraduate professionals, psychologists and non-psychologists) to teach themselves and others about how to advocate for children's needs—how to approach law and policy makers at all levels, educate them about psychological research, and convince them to support allocations of money to child and family issues. The hope is that these materials will support a "train the trainer" model that will have a snowballing effect across the nation and result in more funding at all levels for children's mental health care, child abuse prevention, juvenile justice concerns, etc. A task force led by Mindy Feinberg Gutow and Carol Falender aimed to disseminate training in advocacy at all levels of education, from high school through professional training, in conjunction with multiple directorates of APA and the Interdivisional Task Force on Child and Adolescent Mental Health.

Awards

Four awards established early in the Division's history recognize outstanding professional accomplishments related to child and youth policy, research, and advocacy. *The Nicholas Hobbs Award*, established in 1984, is presented annually to a psychologist who emulates the efforts of its namesake, a charter member of Division 37 dedicated to child policy and research (Routh & Culbertson, 1996). Past winners have included W. Rodney Hammond, Donald Wertlieb, Lawrence Aber, Dante Cicchetti, Aletha Huston, Barbara Bonner, Joy Osofsky, Gail S. Goodman, John R. Weisz, Robert M. Friedman, and Karen J. Saywitz, Brian Wilcox, and Sheila Eyberg. The *Lifetime Advocacy Award* is a premier honor celebrating individuals who have contributed consistently and sizably to the needs of children, youth, and families. It has been bestowed only twice in the past decade, to Mary Campbell in 2011 (Campbell, 2000) in honor of her 25 years of service as Director of APA's Office of Children, Youth, and Families (CYF) and to Senator Christopher Dodd (in 2005) in honor of his legislative work benefiting children and families. The *Distinguished Contribution to Child Advocacy Award* is given to a non-psychologist who has contributed remarkably to child, youth, and family advocacy. Past recipients include actors, entrepreneurs, executive directors, journalists, lawyers, philanthropists, physicians, and public administrators. In the past decade, winners have been Ellen Bassuk, Olivia Golden, Deborah Prothrow-Stih, T. Berry Brazelton, Beatrice Hamburg, John Myers, Tom Birch, Virginia Weisz, Beth A. Stroul, and Robin Kimbrough-Melton, Laurie Mulvey, and Shay Bilchik.

The *Diane J. Willis Early Career Award* will be bestowed for the first time in 2013. The award honors the significant career of Diane J. Willis, whose child-focused advocacy has informed a range of issues and spanned a variety of disciplines, affecting both national and global public policy arenas. The award will recognize early career psychologists who show promise in advancing public policy concerning the well-being of children and families.

Division 37 and the Section on Child Maltreatment both bestow various awards honoring students and budding psychologists and supporting their early work. These include (a) the Division's and Section's annual *Student Poster Awards* for excellent research presented at the annual APA conference; (b) the Division's annual dissertation award; (c) the Section's Undergraduate Research Award for excellent papers related to child maltreatment; and (d) the Section's $400 dissertation small grant instated in 2001 to encourage excellent dissertation research central to the Section's mission. Gail Goodman led the way for the Section's *Early Career Award for Outstanding Contributions to Research and Practice in the Field of Child Maltreatment,* established in 2001 and given in alternating years to a new outstanding practitioner or researcher. Finally, the Section also provides an important resource that helps researchers and clinical professionals find other monetary awards for their work—*The Alert*, first edited by Lane Geddy, and published in print and as a website. It is a compendium of funding opportunities for research and clinical work in child maltreatment.

Divisional, Interdivisional, and Interdisciplinary Collaborations Promoting Research, Clinical Outreach, and Advocacy

In keeping with its core mission, some of Division 37's most important work is its child- and family-focused advocacy, in the form of direct education of courts and policymakers, clinical outreach, the promotion of relevant research, and so forth.

Collaborations with APA Offices

Of great benefit to the Division and its mission has been the long history of collaboration with the APA Public Interest Government Relations Office (PI-GRO), which performs a range of policy-related functions that dovetail with Division goals, including collaborating with legislators and federal agencies on psychology-relevant issues, engaging in congressional briefings and testimony, partnering to providing advocacy training workshops (as mentioned previously), and maintaining connections with other organizations that have common policy goals. Interactions between the PI-GRO and Division 37 are mutually beneficial. For example, the PI-GRO relies on Division 37 members for knowledge and expertise that inform its undertakings, and the PI-GRO keeps Division members informed of important policy and legislative activities through reports to the executive committee, newsletter articles, and up-to-the-minute email listserv postings. For example, Division 37 members are part of the PI-GRO's Public Policy Action Network listserv, which provides immediate email alerts when there is a legislative issue of relevance to children and families that can be informed by Division 37 members' input. The PI-GRO synthesizes listserv members' feedback, then works directly with congressional offices to ensure that relevant psychological science gets translated into a message that the lawmakers can understand and use to shape better public policy. The PI-GRO also provides Division 37 members with opportunities to influence policy through its public policy column in each *Advocate*, which describes (a) recent and upcoming legislative initiatives and what the issues mean for psychologists, (b) pressing government financial appropriations developments and concerns, and (c) advocacy actions needed from members. Columns have addressed, for example, child maltreatment funding (e.g., Child Abuse Prevention and Treatment Act), education (e.g., Elementary and Secondary Education Act; Individuals with Disabilities Education Act); and mental health prevention and intervention (e.g., Child and Adolescent Mental Health Resiliency Act; Child Health Care Crisis Relief Act; Bullying and Gang Prevention for School Safety and Crime Reduction Act; Safe and Drug-Free Schools and Communities Act). The most powerful aspect of the Public Policy Advocacy Network listserv and the newsletter column is the clear intent to involve readers in practical advocacy efforts. The importance of these methods for providing an avenue for Division 37 to actively engage in policy making cannot be underestimated.

Division 37 and the Section on Child Maltreatment have also enjoyed a strong partnership with APA's Committee on Children, Youth, and Families (CYF), which raises awareness, disseminates information, and develops APA Policy Statements on subjects such as child abuse, sexuality and education, dating violence, school dropout, bullying and violence prevention, and the effects of advertising and media violence on children. The relationship with CYF is strengthened by liaisons who report regularly between the groups and by the fact that Division 37 members are often members of the CYF. Division 37 and CYF members have formed working groups to consider, for example, psychoactive medications for children and innovative treatment and training approaches for the public sector. One collaboration produced a faculty resource guide about training college students to work with youth who have serious emotional disabilities (Vargas, 2000).

Interdivisional Collaborations

Division 37 has formed a variety of successful partnerships with other divisions, especially those with child interests such as 12 (Society of Clinical Psychology), 16 (School Psychology), 43 (Society for Family Psychology), 53 (Society of Clinical Child and Adolescent Psychology), and 54 (Society of Pediatric Psychology). A subset of those (37, 16, 53, 54) plus Division 7 (Developmental Psychology) and 27 (Society for Community Research and Action) collaborated to produce the prior mentioned APA symposium "Psychology and Children: Translating Research into Better Policy and Services," and 37, 16, 7, and 53 produced a special issue of the *Child and Family Policy and Practice Review*.

Perhaps the best example of Division 37's interdivisional efforts is the Interdivisional Task Force on Child and Adolescent Mental Health (2001), which, it is fair to say, is the centerpiece not only of the Division's, but also APA's, advocacy efforts on behalf of children's mental health. To review its history, taking advantage of the national spotlight on children's mental health issues generated in part by the *Report of the Surgeon General's Conference on Children's Mental Health: A National Action Agenda* (U.S. Public Health Service, 2000), APA formed a cross-directorate Working Group on Children's Mental Health. Chaired by future Division president Patrick Tolan, and including then-President Karen Saywitz and future member of the Board of Directors Barry Anton, this working group generated a report that included strategies to assist the APA in promoting the Surgeon General's action agenda. In 2001, to ensure that these recommendations would be implemented, Division 37 joined with Division 7 to establish the Interdivisional Task Force on Child and Adolescent Mental Health, chaired by Karen Saywitz and including Division 37 members Sheila Eyberg, Anne Culp, and Mary Haskett. Later that year, the task force, led by Division 37, was joined by 6 other divisions (12, 16, 27, 43, 53, 54) and its goals were expanded to also promote the goals and recommendations of CYF's *Resolution on Children's Mental Health.* Then, in 2003, the APA Task Force on Psychology's Agenda for Child and Adolescent Mental Health, chaired by Barry Anton and including Karen Saywitz as a member, was formed, and in 2004, it produced a comprehensive report that became the work plan for the Interdivisional Task Force on Child and Adolescent Mental Health. That report, available at http://www. apa.org/pi/cyf/child_adoles_mentalhealth_report.pdf, included directions for using APA policy, research, training, and practice resources to promote the children's mental health issues highlighted by the Surgeon General. It highlighted these priorities: (1) Promoting public awareness of children's mental health issues; (2) Fostering scientifically validated prevention and treatment in children's mental health; (3) Improving assessment and recognition of mental health needs in children; (4) Eliminating racial, ethnic, and socioeconomic disparities in access to care; (5) Improving the infrastructure for children's mental health services; (6) Increasing access to and coordination of quality child mental health care services; (7) Training front line workers to recognize and manage child mental health needs; and (8) Monitoring access to and coordination of quality mental health care services for children.

The Interdivisional Task Force on Child and Adolescent Mental Health has accomplished much in relation to these goals, thereby raising public awareness and supporting more research and better practice related to children's mental health needs. Products include, for example, (a) the article *Crisis in Child Mental Health Care: A Well-Kept Secret,* which has been widely published in the newsletters of numerous APA divisions and state psychological associations; (b) a special issue of *Child and Family Policy and Practice Review* entitled "Prevention for Child Mental Health: Scientific Promise to Practical Benefit" edited by Karen Saywitz and invited by then-President Anne Culp; (c) talking points on the crisis in children's mental health care that were created and disseminated under the direction of Kathy Katz; (d) public service announcements developed with Radio Disney to foster healthy child adjustment and coping; (e) several APA convention symposia; and (f) efforts to train mental health professionals to work with children and adolescents. Task force members have also provided input on numerous congressional legislative issues and expert testimony on various bills.

Finally, the Interdivisional Task Force has arranged for congressional briefings, which are among the division's most important advocacy initiatives. When Congress is about to consider a child or family issue that can be informed by psychological knowledge, organizations may arrange a meeting at the Capital where articulate experts translate psychological research into words that Congress people and their staffers can understand. And often, they listen. In turn, real laws and policies that affect millions of children sometimes get shifted in line with the best available science. In 2007, Karen Saywitz led the Interdivisional Task Force and Division 37 in organizing, "Children's Mental Health: Key Challenges, Strategies, and Effective Solutions," a briefing addressing the reauthorization of SAMHSA, No Child Left Behind, and the Child Health Care Crisis Relief Act. It informed policy makers about the prevalence of children's mental health problems and the failure of the current delivery system. Division 37 was joined in sponsorship by divisions 7, 12, 16, 27, 43, 53, and 54; Senators Pete Domenici (R-NM) and Edward Kennedy (D-MA); Representatives Jim Ramstad (R-MN), Patrick Kennedy (D-RI), Donna Christensen (D-VI), Sheila Jackson Lee (D-TX); and Co-Chairs of the Congressional Mental Health Caucus: Rep. Grace Napolitano (D-CA) and Rep. Tim Murphy (R-PA). Four Congresspersons spoke, in addition to the panelists who included Jane Knitzer, Janice Cooper, Kimberly Hoagwood, Kenneth Martinez, William Pelham, Patrick Tolan, and Mark Weist.

Although the work of the Interdivisional Task Force on Child and Adolescent Mental Health is remarkable, many other important interdivisional collaborations are led by Division 37. For example, in 2000, Divisions 37 and 27 formed the interdivisional task force *Fostering Resilient Children, Youth, and Families,* led by Cynthia Schellenbach and Ken Maton, which organized key symposia at meetings of the APA, the Society for Community Research and Action, and the Society for Prevention Research. It also produced a policy-oriented report and brief advocacy position papers designed for use in advocacy work with legislators as well as a book written by social science and policy experts reviewing the complex contexts of child development, issues in fostering resilience, and implications for policy and advocacy (Maton, Schellenbach, Leadbeater, & Solarz, 2003). Another noteworthy interdivisional collaboration occurred in 2001, when Division President Sheila Eyberg worked with Division 29 (Psychotherapy) to develop "tip sheets" on parenting and behavioral management in the classroom for dissemination to Head Start parents and teachers. Division 37 has also been involved in the APA Interdivisional Coalition for Psychology in Schools and Education. Finally, Divisions 37 and 41 joined in an Interdivisional Task Force on the Prevention of Child Maltreatment, which has, for example, cosponsored national conferences on child maltreatment.

Interdisciplinary Collaboration and Engagement

Division 37 has always embraced collaboration as a goal, not only among psychologists but also with professionals from other fields concerned with child well-being, such as medicine, social work, law, and politics. This is evinced by its election of a non-psychologist to a leadership position (Benjamin Pasamanick, M.D., was President in 1987) and its dedication of an award to non-psychologists. To extend its visibility and influence outside of the APA, Division members have reached out to federal, academic, private, and nonprofit agencies by including reports from outside agencies in its newsletter and sending division members to interdisciplinary meetings.

The Division has had particularly fruitful collaborations with the Consortium on Children, Families, and the Law, which comprises associations and university-based centers across the disciplines of policy, law, psychology, and family studies, and which fosters collaborations to improve child and family policy through research, education, and consultation. For example, Division 37 has contributed both fiscally and substantively to the Consortium's Congressional Briefing Series, on topics ranging from early intervention to the juvenile justice system (Limber, 1998). Examples include O'Donnell and Davidson's 1997 briefing entitled "The seeds of violence: Early childhood abuse, misbehavior and delinquency" and Wilcox and Levine's 1997 briefing entitled "Child maltreatment: issues in reporting, processing and case disposition." In 2002, a briefing entitled "Protecting our nations' children: What we know about child abuse prevention" was organized by the Section on Child Maltreatment and cosponsored by the Division, the APA PI-GRO, the Consortium, and the University of Missouri-Kansas City. Then-APA President Phil Zimbardo introduced the briefing, moderated by Dan Dodgen of the APA Public Policy Office, and Congressional sponsorship was given by Senator Christopher Dodd, D-CT. Division speakers included Jeff Haugaard, who discussed theory and statistics concerning child maltreatment; Sharon Portwood, who presented an overview of child abuse and neglect prevention programs, and Linda Smith, Director of the Golden Strip Family and Child Development Center (Clemson, South Carolina), who described a successful real-life example of a community-based child abuse prevention program. The aim was to encourage appropriations for the Child Abuse Prevention and Treatment Act.

Finally, amicus curiae briefs are also a fine example of Division 37's interdisciplinary advocacy activities. The U.S. Supreme Court, State Supreme Courts, and lower appeals courts tackle many child-relevant cases that could be informed by psychological science, but are not, unless psychologists and attorneys work together to ensure that research makes its way in front of judges deciding the cases. Division 37 members are in unique positions to do this, sometimes individually as expert witnesses. But the division as a whole can also reach the courts through amicus curiae briefs; summaries of psychological research in terms that legal professionals can understand and apply to the issues at hand in a particular case. In turn, the Division has the opportunity to affect case law in important ways. In 2003, under the Presidency of Thomas Lyon, the Section on Child Maltreatment spearheaded an amicus brief reviewing the effects of child sexual abuse and disclosure that was submitted to the U.S. Supreme Court in *California v. Stogner.* The brief was created in collaboration with lawyers from the Washington, DC office of Arnold and Porter and signed by the APA, the National Association of Counsel for Children, and both the American and the California Professional Societies on the Abuse of Children. Such truly interdisciplinary efforts are made easier when the involved division members are interdisciplinary themselves—Lyon holds doctorates in both law and developmental psychology.

Conclusion: The Power of the Group to Effect Change

By relying on collaboration, scientific vision, and advocacy, Division leaders and members have moved it during the past decade into its current state as a dynamic, powerful agent of change. The Division has become a synergistic, interdisciplinary organization that has contributed substantially to improving the lives of children, youth, and families through its effective focus on advocacy, service delivery, and public policies. The hard work of Division 37 members has created an opportunity through which intentions to create a better, safer, more nurturing world for children become reality. Sharing this vision and becoming involved in advocacy makes positive change possible at both local and national levels. Whether advocating for better public policy, conducting and disseminating groundbreaking research, or developing better clinical services, it is evident that Division 37 has and will continue to play an essential role in improving the lives of children, youth, and families.

Acknowledgement For their invaluable contributions to this collective organizational memory, we thank: Mary Campbell, Jan L. Culbertson, Anne McDonald Culp, Carol Falender, Jeffrey Haugaard, Sue Limber, Tom Lyon, Tony Mannarino, Laura Nabors, Cynthia Najdowski, Cindy Perrin, Sharon Portwood, Michael Roberts, Don Routh, Karen Saywitz, Cindy Schellenbach, Carolyn Schroeder, Annie Toro, Luis Vargas, Brian Wilcox, Diane J. Willis, & David Wolfe.

References

APA Division 37's Task Force on Advocacy. (2006). *APA Division 37's guide to advocacy: Legislative support for children, youth and families.* Retrieved from http://www.apa.org/divisions/div37/resources.html.

American Psychological Association. (2013, April 13). *Bylaws of the American Psychological Association.* Retrieved from http://www.apa.org/governance/bylaws/.

American Psychological Association. (2013, April 13). *Society for child and family policy and practice: Division 37 of the American Psychological Association.* Retrieved from http://www.apa.org/divisions/div37/.

APA Working Group on Children's Mental Health. (2001). *Developing psychology's national agenda for children's mental health: APA's response to the Surgeon General's action agenda for children's mental health.* Washington, DC: American Psychological Association.

Bottoms, B. L., & Quas, J. A. (Eds.). (2006). Emerging directions in child maltreatment research: Multidisciplinary perspectives on theory, practice, and policy [Special issue]. *Journal of Social Issues, 62*(4).

Campbell, M. (2000). Committee on children, youth, and families. *The Child, Youth, and Family Services Advocate, 23*(2), 8–9.

Crockett, D. (2003). Critical issues children face in the 2000s. *School Psychology Quarterly, 18*, 446–453.

Goodman, G. S. (2006). A modern history and contemporary commentary on child eyewitness memory research. *Journal of Social Issues, 62*, 653–880.

Grasley, C., Wolfe, D. A., & Wekerle, C. (1999). Empowering youth to end relationship violence. *Children's Services, 2*, 209–223.

Holden, E. W., & Brannan, A. M. (2002). Background for the special issue. *Children's Services, 5*, 1.

Huang, L., Mcbeth, G., Dodge, J., & Jacobstein, D. (2004). Transforming the workforce in children's mental health. *Administration and Policy in Mental Health, 32*, 167–187.

Kutash, K., & Rivera, V. R. (1995). Effectiveness of children's mental health service: A review of the literature. *Education and Treatment of Children, 18*, 443.

Limber, S. P. (1998). Bringing social science to Capitol Hill: The Congressional Briefing Series of the Consortium in Children, Families, and the Law. *The Child, Youth, and Family Services Advocate, 21*(1), 3.

Masi, R., & Cooper, J. (2006). *Children's mental health facts for policymakers.* New York: National Center for Children in Poverty. Retrieved from http://www.nccp.org/publications/pub_687.html

Maton, K. I., Schellenbach, C. J., Leadbeater, B. J., & Solarz, A. L. (2003). *Investing in children, youth, families and communities: Strengths-based research and policy.* Washington, DC: American Psychological Association.

Melton, G. B. (Ed.). (1986). *Adolescent abortion: Psychological and legal issues.* Lincoln: University of Nebraska Press.

Miller-Perrin, C. L. (2000). *An introduction to child maltreatment: A five-unit lesson plan for teachers of psychology in secondary schools.* Retrieved from Education Resources Information Center.

Miller-Perrin, C. L., & Malloy, L. C. (2007, July 3). *Curriculum guide for instruction in child maltreatment. Office of teaching resources in psychology online.* Retrieved from http://www.apadiv2.org/otrp/resources/resources.php?category=Child%20Maltreatment

Morris, P. A., & Gennetian, L. (2006). Welfare and antipoverty policy effects on children's development. In H. E. Fitzgerald, B. M. Lester, & B. Zuckerman (Eds.), *The crisis in youth mental health* (pp. 231–255). Westport, CT: Praeger.

National Institutes of Mental Health. (2001). *Blueprint for change: Research on child and adolescent mental health. Report of the National Advisory Mental Health Council's Workgroup on Child and Adolescent Mental Health Intervention Development and Deployment.* Bethesda, MD: Author.

National Research Council and Institute of Medicine. (2009). *Preventing mental, emotional, and behavioral disorders among young people: Progress and possibilities.* Committee on the Prevention of Mental Disorders and Substance Abuse Among Children, Youth, and Young Adults: Research Advances and Promising Interventions. Mary Ellen O'Connell, Thomas Boat, and Kenneth E. Warner, Editors. Board on Children, Youth, and Families, Division of Behavioral and Social Sciences and Education. Washington, DC: The National Academies Press.

Nightingale, N., & Portwood, S. (1997). Section events at the APA convention. *The Child, Youth, and Family Services Quarterly, 20*(1), 10–11.

Ondersma, S. J., Chaffin, M., Berliner, L., Cordon, I., Goodman, G. S., & Barnett, D. (2001). Sex with children is abuse: Comment on Rind, Tromovitch, & Bauserman (1998). *Psychological Bulletin, 127,* 707–714.

Powell, D., & Dunlap, G. (2005). Mental health services for young children. In R. Steele & M. Roberts (Eds.), *Handbook of mental health services for children, adolescents, and families* (pp. 15–30). New York: Kluwer Academic/Plenum.

President's New Freedom Commission on Mental Health. (2003). *Achieving the promise: Transforming mental health care in America.* Final Report (DHHS Pub. No. SMA-03-3832). Rockville, MD: U.S. Department of Health and Human Services.

Quas, J. A., Bottoms, B. L., & Nuñez, N. (Eds.). (2002). Linking juvenile delinquency and child maltreatment: Causes, correlates, and consequences [Special issue]. *Children's Services: Social Policy, Research, and Practice, 5,* 245–305.

Roberts, M. C., Carlson, C. I., Erickson, M. T., Friedman, R. M., La Greca, A. M., Lemanek, K. L., et al. (1998). A model for training psychologists to provide services for children and adolescents. *Professional Psychology: Research and Practice, 29,* 293–299.

Roberts, M. C., Erickson, M. T., & Tuma, J. M. (1985). Addressing the needs: Guidelines for training psychologists to work with children, youth, and families. *Journal of Clinical Child Psychology, 14,* 70–79.

Roberts, M.C., & Task Force (Eds.). (1996). *Model programs in child and family mental health.* Hillsdale, NJ: Lawrence Erlbaum Associates.

Routh, D. K., & Culbertson, J. L. (1996). A history of Division 37 (Child, Youth, and Family Services). In D. Dewsbury (Ed.), *Unification through division: Histories of the American Psychological Association* (pp. 195–231). Washington, DC: APA.

Tolan, P. H., & Dodge, K. A. (2005). Children's mental health as a primary care and concern. *American Psychologist, 60,* 601–614.

U.S. Public Health Service. (1999). *Mental health: A report of the Surgeon General.* Rockville, MD: U.S. Department of Health and Human Services Administration, Center for Mental

Health Services Administration, Center for Mental Health Services, National Institutes of Health, National Institute of Mental Health.

U.S. Public Health Service. (2000). *Report of the Surgeon General's conference on children's mental health: A national action agenda.* Washington, DC: Department of Health and Human Services.

Vargas, L. A. (2000). Task-force update. *The Child, Youth, and Family Services Advocate, 23*(1), 12.

Weithorn, L. A. (1987). *Psychology and child custody determinations: Knowledge, roles, and expertise.* Lincoln, NE: University of Nebraska Press.

About the Editor

Anne McDonald Culp, **Ph.D.**, is Professor in the Department of Child, Family, and Community Sciences at the University of Central Florida. She has taught at three universities and conducted research as a principal investigator and coinvestigator on several federally funded and state-funded grants, most of which evaluated early intervention effects with young mothers and their infants, and studied children and families of Head Start programs. She is past President of Division 37 of the American Psychological Association, and has been a lifetime advocate for children and families.

A. McDonald Culp (ed.), *Child and Family Advocacy: Bridging the Gaps Between Research, Practice, and Policy*, Issues in Clinical Child Psychology, DOI 10.1007/978-1-4614-7456-2, © Springer Science+Business Media New York 2013

Index

Lightning Source UK Ltd.
Milton Keynes UK
UKHW021114311219
356153UK00005B/393/P